THE ENDOMETRIUM: A CLINICOPATHOLOGIC APPROACH

THE ENDOMETRIUM: A CLINICOPATHOLOGIC APPROACH

Debra S. Heller, M.D.
Assistant Professor of Pathology
College of Physicians and Surgeons
Columbia University
New York, New York

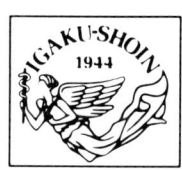

IGAKU-SHOIN   New York • Tokyo

Published and distributed by

IGAKU-SHOIN Medical Publishers, Inc.
One Madison Avenue, New York, New York 10010

IGAKU-SHOIN Ltd.,
5-24-3 Hongo, Bunkyo-ku, Tokyo 113-91.

Copyright © 1994 by IGAKU-SHOIN Medical Publishers, Inc.
All rights reserved. No part of this book may be translated or reproduced in any form by print, photoprint, microfilm, or any other means without written permission from the publisher.

Library of Congress Cataloging-in-Publication Data

Heller, Debra S.
    The endometrium: a clinicopathologic approach / Debra S. Heller.
      p. cm.
    Includes bibliographical references and index.
    1. Endometrium—diseases—diagnosis. 2. Endometrium—histopathology. 3. Endometrium—cytopathology. I. Title.
    [DNLM: 1. Endometrium—pathology. 2. Endometrium—physiopathology. 3. Uterine diseases—diagnosis. WP 400 H477e 1994]
RG316.H45 1994
618.1—dc20
DNLM/DLC
for Library of Congress   93-39684
                                                                     CIP

ISBN: 0-89640-244-4 (New York)
ISBN: 4-260-14244-5 (Tokyo)

Printed and bound in the U.S.A.

10 9 8 7 6 5 4 3 2 1

Preface

Communication between the gynecologist and the pathologist is crucial to optimal patient care. This requires that each physician speak the other's language. Previously, as a practicing gynecologist, I have had the experience of receiving pathology reports that I did not completely understand, or that did not answer all my questions. Now as a practicing gynecologic pathologist, at times I have been frustrated by specimens sent without a clinical history, as the most accurate diagnoses do not always occur in a vacuum. Communication is particularly important in evaluation of the endometrium, where pathologic diagnoses are so often strongly linked to the clinical situation. This book, then, is aimed at both the gynecologist and the pathologist. I hope it will help each side understand what the other is talking about. And to both parties, when in doubt, please pick up the telephone and call the other one!

Debra S. Heller, M.D.

To Allen, Joshua, and Benjamin

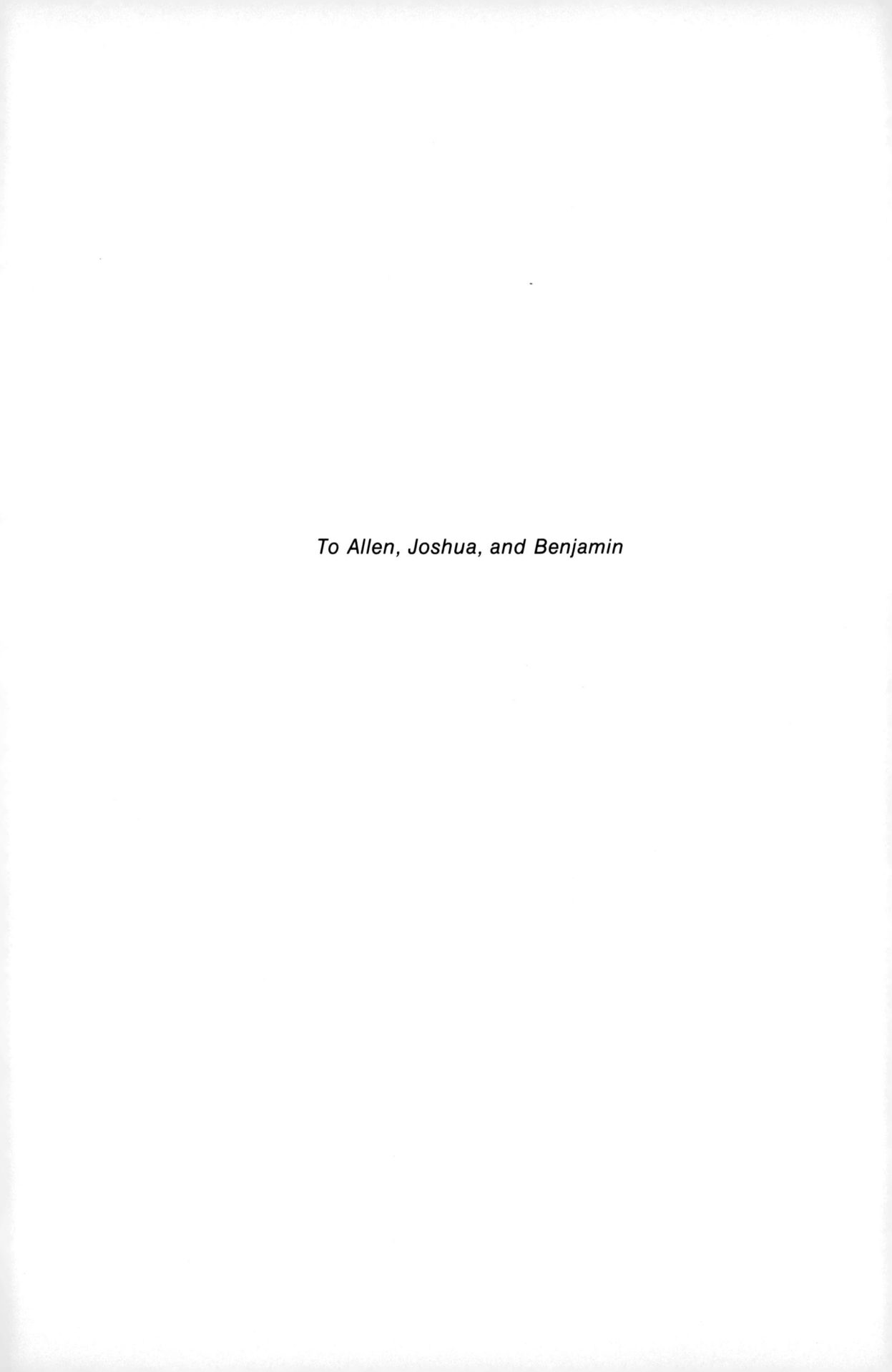

Foreword

Tissue diagnosis is the basis for much of gynecologic therapy, which is why the Council on Residency Education in Obstetrics & Gynecology includes pathology in the residency curriculum and the American Board of Obstetrics & Gynecology includes pathology on the certifying examination.

Unfortunately most practicing gynecologists forego an ongoing interest in pathology and rely on their colleagues in the laboratory for tissue diagnoses that affect their management decisions. At the same time most pathologists are not fully aware of the relevance of their reports to those management decisions. The result is often less then optimal patient care.

We at Columbia are most fortunate. Dr. Heller is a Board-certified pathologist with special training and a primary interest in pathology of the female genital tract. She is also a Board-certified obstetrician–gynecologist with several years of private practice experience in the latter discipline. She is uniquely qualified to comprehend the special bond between the two specialties that affords the best in patient care.

The present volume gives the practicing gynecologist and the general pathologist an opportunity to experience that special bond as it relates to the endometrium. Readers will not only find it educational but may expect it to assist in reaching our universal goal—optimal patient care.

    M. Leon Tancer, M.D.
    Professor of Clinical Obstetrics and Gynecology
    College of Physicians and Surgeons
    Columbia University
    New York, New York

Foreword

The diagnosis that a pathologist issues carries enormous weight in the future therapy and eventual well-being of patients. For this reason, it is critical that the gynecologist have a substantial understanding of pathology. Possibly of even greater pertinence, gynecologists must recognize the limitations and boundaries of diagnostic acumen, such as those related to the marginal or "less than representative" specimen, or when the pathologist's interpretation raises a red flag as to potential processes that might be occurring even if the slide itself is not altogether crystal-clear. In turn, pathologists must thoroughly understand the information the gynecologist wishes to obtain via the operative specimen, if the interest of the patient is to be best served. In this small but comprehensive volume, Dr. Debra Heller presents a well-focused view of endometrial pathology that combines her years of experience as an obstetrician–gynecologist with her work as a practicing gynecologic pathologist in two of the most prestigious universities in New York City. I believe that the general gynecologist and practicing pathologist will find this monograph useful and practical in its spirited presentation.

Stanley Robboy, M.D.
Professor of Pathology, Obstetrics and Gynecology
Duke University Medical Center
Durham, North Carolina

Contributors

Rex Bentley, M.D.
Assistant Professor of Pathology
Duke University Medical Center
Durham, North Carolina

Jody S. Blanco, M.D.
Assistant Professor of Clinical Obstetrics and Gynecology
College of Physicians and Surgeons
Columbia University
New York, New York

Ruth Kreitzer, M.D.
Clinical Instructor
Department of Pathology
Mount Sinai School of Medicine
New York, New York

Jodi P. Lerner, M.D.
Assistant Clinical Professor of Obstetrics and Gynecology
College of Physicians and Surgeons
Columbia University
New York, New York

Robert S. Neuwirth, M.D.
S. Huntington & Dorothy D. Babcock Professor of Obstetrics and Gynecology
College of Physicians and Surgeons
Columbia University
New York, New York

Contents

PART I—Clinical Aspects of Evaluation of the Endometrium

Chapter 1 **Investigating the Endometrium—a Clinical Point of View** 1
Jody S. Blanco, M.D.

Chapter 2 **Ultrasound Evaluation of the Endometrium** 9
Jodi P. Lerner, M.D.

Chapter 3 **Hysteroscopy in Evaluation of the Endometrium** 26
Robert S. Neuwirth, M.D.

PART II—Histology and Pathology of the Endometrium

Chapter 4 **Histopathology of the Endometrium—an Overview** 43
Debra S. Heller, M.D.

Chapter 5 **The Normal Endometrium** 56
Debra S. Heller, M.D.

Chapter 6 **Hormonal Effects on the Endometrium: Dysfunctional Uterine Bleeding, Iatrogenic Hormonal Effects, and Luteal Phase Defects** 76
Debra S. Heller, M.D.

Chapter 7 **Benign Organic Lesions of the Endometrium** 91
Debra S. Heller, M.D.

Chapter 8 **Endometrial Metaplasias** 103
Debra S. Heller, M.D.

Chapter 9 **Endometrial Hyperplasias and Their Distinction from Adenocarcinomas** 114
Rex Bentley, M.D.

Chapter 10	**Endometrial Malignancies** 137 Debra S. Heller, M.D.	
Chapter 11	**Pregnancy and Related Conditions** 166 Debra S. Heller, M.D.	
Chapter 12	**Endometrial Cytology on Cervicovaginal Smears** 185 Ruth Kreitzer, M.D.	
Index		**219**

THE ENDOMETRIUM: A CLINICOPATHOLOGIC APPROACH

PART I

Clinical Aspects of Evaluation of the Endometrium

1
Investigating the Endometrium—a Clinical Point of View

Jody S. Blanco, M.D.

Endometrial sampling, which can be performed in the office, has replaced dilatation and curettage, originally an inpatient procedure, as a diagnostic aid in the evaluation of many of the gynecologic disorders encountered today. The spectrum of indications for endometrial sampling has expanded rapidly as a result of the ease with which the procedure can be performed, and although used primarily as an aid in diagnosis, the procedure is now being investigated as a screening and surveillance tool.

Endometrial sampling is most commonly performed in the evaluation of abnormal vaginal bleeding that is presumed to be uterine in origin. Abnormal uterine bleeding may occur at any time during a woman's life, and the differential diagnosis varies depending on a woman's age (Table 1-1). Menstrual disorders have been reported to account for 21% of gynecologic referrals. Vaginal bleeding may not always arise from an intrauterine source. Abnormal vaginal bleeding can be evaluated using the algorithm shown in Fig. 1-1. It is always important to obtain a complete history and physical exam. Appropriate laboratory and imaging studies should be done to help rule out extrauterine causes of vaginal bleeding. A Papanicolaou smear and a complete pelvic exam will greatly aid in locating the source of the bleeding. Neoplasms of the cervix and vagina may present with vaginal bleeding, which may occur only postcoitus. Diseases of the bladder and urethra, such as neoplasm, stones, and chronic cystitis, may present with vaginal bleeding, in which cases hematuria will be present on a urinalysis obtained following catheterization. Likewise, diseases of the colon and rectum, including neoplasms, colitis, fistulas and hemorrhoids, may present with what appears to be vagi-

TABLE 1-1. Causes of Abnormal Uterine Bleeding

Pubertal
  Endocrine
    Anovulatory bleeding
    Thyroid/Adrenal disorders
  Neoplastic
    Sarcoma
  Congenital
Pre/Perimenopausal
  Endocrine
    Anovulatory bleeding
    Corpus luteal phase defect
    Mid-cycle bleeding
    Thyroid/adrenal disorders
  Anatomic
    Submucous myoma
    Endometrial polyps
  Neoplastic
    Cervical cancer
  Pregnancy-related
    Incomplete/missed/threatened abortion
    Trophoblastic disease
    Ectopic pregnancy
Postmenopausal
  Endocrine
    Hyperplasia
  Anatomic
    Endometrial polyps
    Atrophic endometrium
  Neoplasia
    Endometrial cancer
    Cervical cancer
  Hormone replacement therapy

nal bleeding. In these diseases, frank or occult blood will be found on digital rectal exam.

As mentioned previously, the differential diagnosis of abnormal uterine bleeding changes with age. In adolescent women anovulatory bleeding is the most common cause of abnormal uterine bleeding. This is due to immaturity of the pituitary–ovarian axis. There is a lack of maturation of the ovarian follicles; thus ovulation and progesterone secretion do not occur. Endometrial sampling will confirm lack of progesterone secretion. The usual management is low-dose oral contraceptives, or cyclic progesterone administration (see Fig. 1-1).

In the perimenopausal woman anovulation may also be a cause of abnormal vaginal bleeding. Meldrum in 1993[1] found that in women age 50, only

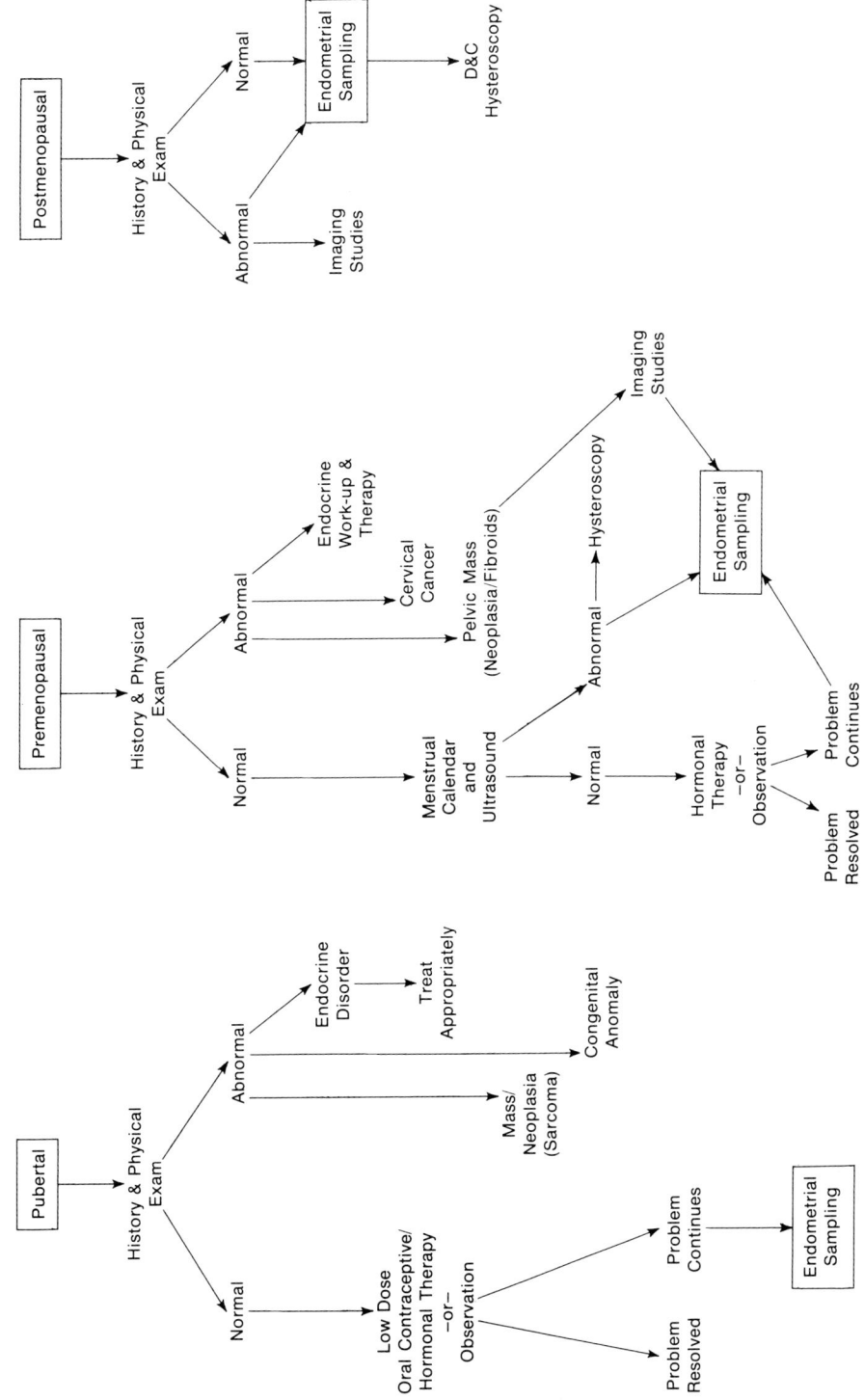

Figure 1-1. Endometrial sampling in the work-up of abnormal uterine bleeding.

10% experienced normal menstrual periods. However, in the perimenopause, there are also pathologic reasons for abnormal bleeding and endometrial sampling is warranted. In the perimenopause abnormal uterine bleeding may be due to a decrease in the sensitivity of the ovaries to follicle-stimulating hormone (FSH) and luteinizing hormone (LH) which causes the ovaries to produce inadequate amounts of estrogen, inhibiting positive feedback of estrogen at the pituitary. The LH surge by the pituitary does not occur, resulting in anovulation. Inadequate amounts of estrogen leads to irregular endometrial development and irregular sloughing of the endometrial lining. In cases where ovulation occurs, progesterone production from the corpus luteum may be insufficient to support the endometrium and bleeding may result. Insufficient corpus luteal function should be considered when dating of an endometrial sample varies from the cycle date by more than 2 days.

Endocrine disorders of the ovary can cause abnormal uterine bleeding. Polycystic ovarian syndrome is associated with anovulation and high blood levels of estrogen and androgen, leading to hyperplasia and abnormal bleeding. The bleeding can be controlled with oral contraceptives or cyclic progestin administration.

Functional ovarian tumors may secrete hormones and cause abnormal uterine bleeding. The most common type are the granulosa–theca cell tumors, which can secrete large amounts of estrogen and cause estrogen breakthrough bleeding; 50% of these tumors occur in postmenopausal women. The endometrial sample will show proliferative to hyperplastic changes and possibly even carcinoma.

In order to maintain the cyclic function of the hypothalamic–pituitary–ovarian axis, thyroid function should be normal. Both hypo- and hyperthyroid states alter the normal pituitary–ovarian axis. Hyperthyroidism can cause anovulation and oligomenorrhea. Hypothyroidism is manifested by anovulatory cycles with menorrhagia or amenorrhea.

Hepatic failure, renal failure, Addison's disease, and Cushing's disease all affect the hypothalamic–pituitary–ovarian axis and are associated with abnormal uterine bleeding. Obesity will lead to excessive estrogen production by adipose conversion of androstenedione to estrone. This can cause a hyperplastic or neoplastic endometrium and abnormal bleeding.

Pregnancy is the most common cause of abnormal bleeding during the reproductive years. Missed, threatened, or incomplete abortion may cause light to heavy bleeding. Hydatiform mole usually presents with irregular bleeding. The incidence of molar pregnancy increases after age 40; 25% of patients with molar pregnancy are between 40 and 50 years old.

Ectopic pregnancy frequently presents with abnormal bleeding. The high progesterone state of pregnancy causes a hypersecretory endometrium with decidual changes. When the ectopic pregnancy starts to "die," the endometrium degenerates and bleeding begins.

The most important role of endometrial sampling in gynecology is in the evaluation of postmenopausal bleeding. The most common cause of abnormal vaginal bleeding in the menopausal period is due to atrophic changes of the lower genital tract. However, since malignancy of the endometrium must be excluded, sampling is always warranted. Studies have shown that office sampling with a Vabra Aspirator (Berkeley Medevices, Inc.), Tis-U-Trap (Milex Products, Inc.), or Pipelle (Unimar, Inc.) endometrial aspirator will contain sufficient tissue for diagnosis in 90% of patients. Hyperplasias of the endometrium and occasionally endometrial polyps can be diagnosed with office sampling.

In-hospital dilatation and curettage with hysteroscopy should be reserved for the following conditions: in patients who were unable to tolerate the office procedure; technical reasons such as cervical stenosis that prevents entrance into the uterine cavity; in patients in whom the biopsy provided insufficient tissue for diagnosis; and in patients who continue to bleed despite therapy after the office procedure. Hysteroscopy will aid in more targeted endometrial sampling by allowing visualization of the lesion in question. It will also increase the accuracy of diagnosing submucous myomas and endometrial polyps. The hysteroscopic exam may confirm the existence of atrophy and reduce the concern of a "missed" carcinoma by allowing direct visualization of the uterine cavity.

The role of sampling in the management of estrogen replacement therapy (ERT) has been controversial. Endometrial hyperplasia and carcinoma are major concerns during ERT. The addition of progestin therapy has reduced the risk of hyperplasia by opposing continuous estrogenic stimulation of the endometrium. In women who have regular withdrawal bleeding after cyclic progestin administration there is no need to perform routine endometrial sampling. Women who take unopposed estrogen therapy or who experience irregular bleeding while on combination or sequential therapy should have an endometrial sample to rule out hyperplasia and/or neoplasia.

In 1989, a report published in The Lancet suggested that women who received tamoxifen as adjuvant therapy after surgery for breast carcinoma experienced an increased risk of endometrial carcinoma.[2] The increased risk appeared to be greatest after 2 years of therapy. This is related to tamoxifen's agonistic estrogenic effect on the endometrial lining, potentially causing hyperplasia or carcinoma. Therefore any woman on tamoxifen who has abnormal vaginal bleeding requires endometrial sampling to rule out hyperplasia and neoplasia. The benefit of routine screening endometrial biopsy during tamoxifen therapy has not been established.

In summary, endometrial sampling is now used as a routine office procedure for the evaluation of abnormal vaginal bleeding. In adolescent women, hormonal therapy is usually instituted without endometrial sampling. However, any abnormal bleeding following the use of hormonal therapy requires an endometrial sample.

In infertility management, the endometrial biopsy with dating is helpful in evaluating corpus luteum function.

In the perimenopausal woman, endometrial sampling aids in the diagnosis of bleeding secondary to an abnormal hormonal milieu and in ruling out bleeding secondary to neoplastic or preneoplastic disease. Hormonal therapy should be initiated when clinically indicated; however, if this therapy is unsuccessful in controlling abnormal bleeding, a dilatation and curettage with hysteroscopy should be done. These procedures aid in the diagnosis of submucous myomata and polyps.

Bleeding in the menopause requires endometrial sampling to rule out hyperplasia and/or malignancy. Women who are on estrogen replacement or other hormonal therapy and have abnormal bleeding also require an endometrial sample to rule out hyperplasia and malignancy.

Office sampling has been shown to be useful and cost-effective in endometrial evaluation. However, one should not hesitate to proceed with a dilatation and curettage with hysteroscopy if the tissue obtained from an endometrial sample is insufficient for diagnosis or if abnormal bleeding continues despite therapy.

REFERENCE

1. Meldrum DR. Perimenopausal menstrual problems. *Clin Obstet Gynecol* 26:762–768, 1983.
2. Fornander T, Cedenar R, Mattsson A, et al. Adjuvant tamoxifen in early breast cancer: occurrence of new primary cancers. *Lancet* 1:117, 1989.

BIBLIOGRAPHY

1. Chambers JT, Chambers SK. Endometrial sampling: when? where? why? and with what? *Clin Obstet Gynecol* 35:28–38, 1992.
2. Coulter A, Bradlow J, Agrass M, et al. Outcomes of referrals to gynecology: outpatient clinics for menstrual disorders. *Br J Obstet Gynecol* 98:789–796, 1991.
3. Garcia CR. Endocrine approach in the management of dysfunctional uterine bleeding. *Clin Obstet Gynecol* 13:460, 1970.
4. Lerner H. Lack of efficiency of a prehysterectomy curettage as a diagnostic procedure. *Am J Obstet Gynecol* 148:1055–1058, 1984.
5. McDonald C, Edman CD, Hensell DL, et al. Effects of obesity on conversion of plasma androstenedione to estrone in postmenopausal women with/without endometrial cancer. *Am J Obstet Gynecol* 130:448, 1970.
6. Nesse R. Abnormal vaginal bleeding in perimenopausal women. *Am Fam Physician* 40:185–188, 1989.
7. Padwick M, Pryse-Davis J, Whitehead M. Single method for determining the optimal dosage of progestin in postmenopausal women. *NEJM* 315:930, 1986.
8. Scommegna A, Dmowski WP. Dysfunctional uterine bleeding. *Clin Obstet Gynecol* 16:221–254, 1979.

2
Ultrasound Evaluation of the Endometrium

Jodi P. Lerner, M.D.

Targeted ultrasound scans utilizing the recently developed high-frequency transvaginal transducers have drastically improved the ability to evaluate the endometrium. This improvement is secondary to the use of higher-frequency probes that yield higher-resolution images. The clinical applications of ultrasound in the visualization of the endometrium include evaluation of (1) the changes in the endometrium during the various phases of the menstrual cycle; (2) the changes secondary to pregnancy, including decidual changes, imaging of early gestations, and evidence of retained products of conception; (3) changes during the postmenopausal years, including use of estrogen replacement therapy; (4) disorders within the endometrial cavity such as leiomyomata and polyps; (5) premalignant and malignant disorders, such as hyperplasia and carcinoma; and (6) the endometrium in the infertility workup, including uterine anomalies, and in ovulation induction and IVF (in vitro fertilization) protocols.

TECHNIQUE

In general, transvaginal sonography (TVS) is utilized in evaluation of the endometrium. In contrast to conventional transabdominal sonography, bladder distension is not required for TVS. The highest-frequency transducer possible should be selected to allow adequate penetration and visualization of the region of interest. Usually, 5.0- and 7.5-MHz transducers are used for TVS of the pelvis, including the endometrium. The transvaginal probe is lubricated with coupling gel and inserted into a condom or surgical glove as a protective sheath. More coupling gel is then applied to the tip of the probe, which is then inserted into the vagina. The probe is directly applied to the vaginal vault, which allows the use of higher frequencies and enhanced picture resolution. A study by Schwimmer et al reports that the commercially available coupling gels have spermicidal properties;[1] therefore, in infertility patients, saline-based solutions are advised for lubrication and coupling. The longitudinal and transverse views are the two most commonly used views in evaluation of the uterus and endometrium. The uterus may then be used as a landmark for depiction of adnexal structures. It is important to remain consistent with measurements of the endometrium, whether measured as a single layer or double layer. This becomes especially important in evaluating postmenopausal women, where upper limits of normal endometrial thickness have been proposed.

NORMAL ENDOMETRIUM AND MENSTRUAL CYCLE CHANGES

The endometrium undergoes normal cyclical changes in reproductive-age women, that is, the time after menarche and prior to menopause. These changes of texture and thickness are related to the relative quantities of estrogen and progesterone at the particular time in the menstrual cycle: menstrual, proliferative, or secretory. In general, the endometrial thickness appears to steadily increase until approximately day 21 of the cycle, when the thickness then remains reasonably constant until menses again.[2]

In the late proliferative phase, the endometrium thickens from its postmenstrual slough, and generally contains three layers, the middle layer representing the lumen of the endometrial cavity[3] (Fig. 2-1). The lumen appears echogenic because the endometrium is mucus-coated, acting as an interface to reflect ultrasound.[3] The endometrial thickness generally ranges from 6 to 12 mm at this time.[4,5] In the periovulatory period, a uniform or trilaminar echo may be visualized. In the subsequent 2–3 days after ovulation, a small amount of fluid can be seen.

During the secretory phase, the endometrium achieves its greatest thickness and echogenicity, measuring between 8 and ≥16 mm (Fig. 2-2). Maximum echogenicity is seen in the midluteal phase when the endometrium is homogenous and universally echogenic. Fluid can often be seen in the endometrial cavity at this time. After the menstrual slough, the endometrium appears as a narrow uniform layer, usually measuring between 1 and 4 mm in anterior–posterior width (Fig. 2-3).

PREGNANCY EVALUATION: DECIDUAL CHANGES, EARLY GESTATION, AND RETAINED PRODUCTS OF CONCEPTION

The recent development of high-quality transvaginal sonography has all but revolutionized the evaluation of the early gestation, especially in the diagno-

Pregnancy Evaluation

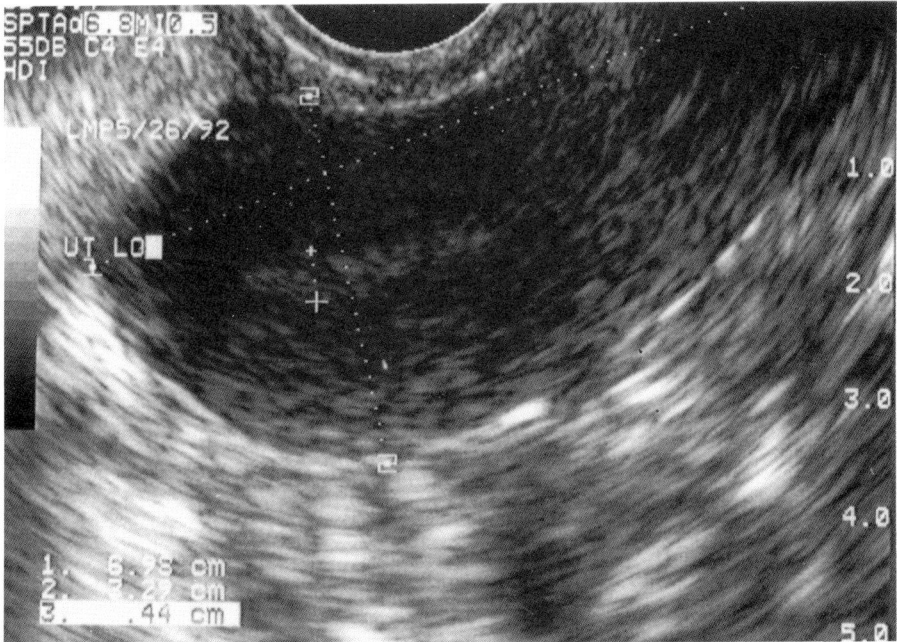

Figure 2-1. Proliferative endometrium, seen between the +.

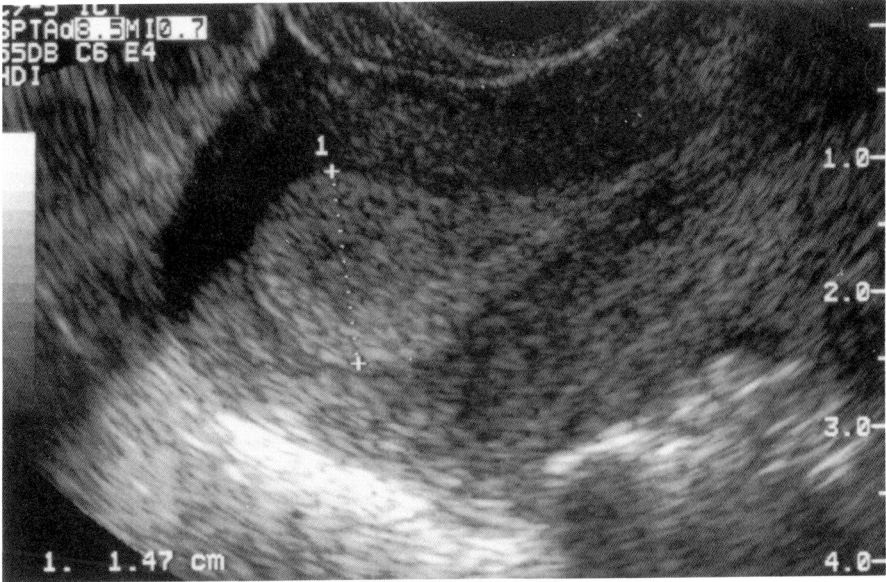

Figure 2-2. Secretory endometrium, appearing thick, homogenous, and echogenic, between the +.

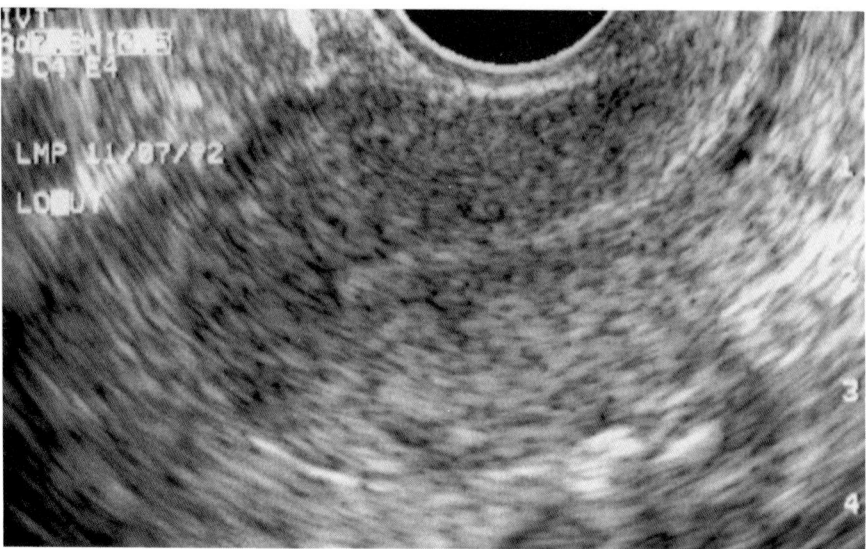

Figure 2-3. Postmenstrual endometrium, uniform and thin.

sis of ectopic pregnancy. An early intrauterine gestation, visualized at 5 postmenstrual weeks, all but excludes ectopic pregnancy, except in the rare case of heterotopic pregnancy. Heterotopic pregnancy, where intrauterine and extrauterine pregnancies coexist, has become more prevalent in recent years, with the increased use of ovulation induction regimens. All embryonic structures, including the gestational sac itself, can be detected at an average of one week earlier than by the traditional transabdominal route.[6] In an intrauterine pregnancy, the chorionic sac can be visualized in the 4th postmenstrual week, appearing as a round or oval hypoechoic structure within an echogenic (chorionic) mass in the endometrial cavity (Fig. 2-4). Occasionally, the two layers of the chorion and decidua may be visualized at this time. By the end of the 5th postmenstrual week, a yolk sac and/or fetal pole will appear within the hypoechoic sac, and an intrauterine pregnancy is confirmed. The pseudogestational sac of an ectopic pregnancy is actually intraluminal fluid within the endometrial cavity, reflecting areas of necrosis and hemorrhage within the decidua.[7] This "sac" is often irregularly shaped and rarely the size expected for a viable intrauterine gestation[8] (Fig. 2-5).

The diagnosis of hydatidiform mole is often made by its characteristic appearance on ultrasound (Fig. 2-6). Multiple small sonolucent areas are visualized that correspond to the "grapelike" vesicles seen on gross pathologic examination. These changes are consistently apparent only after 10 weeks menstrual age,[9] although sonographic recognition has occurred as early as 6 weeks.[10] This can be explained by the understanding that the trophoblastic proliferation and hydropic changes seen grossly are not manifest before this time.[9]

Ultrasound scanning is often utilized in the evaluation of possible retained

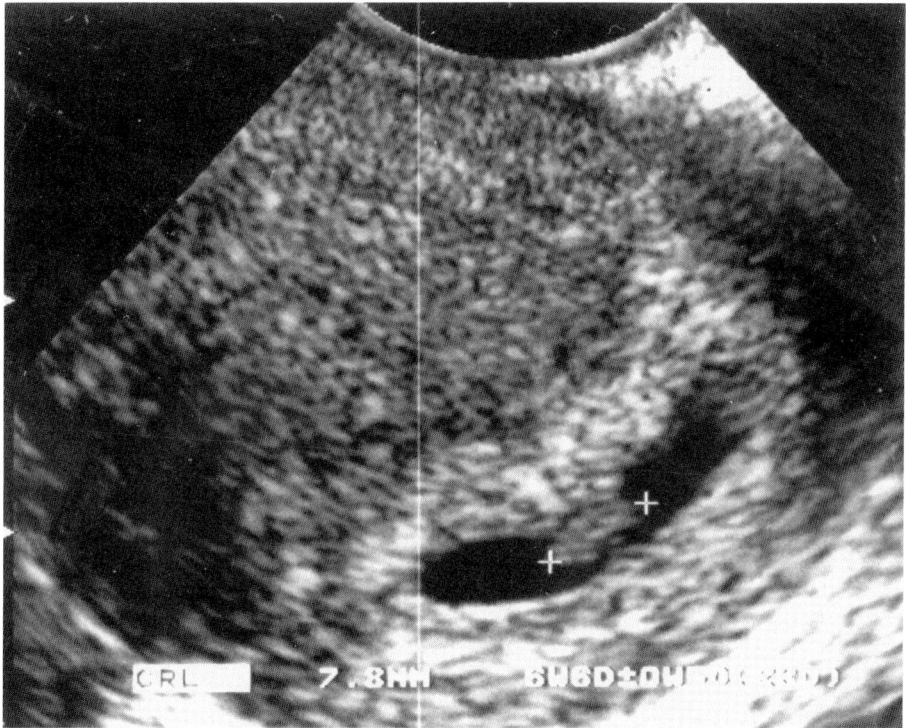

Figure 2-4. Early intrauterine pregnancy, with the gestational sac seen in the cavity.

products of conception in several settings: after a presumed complete miscarriage, in a pregnant patient with bleeding, and in the postpartum patient with hemorrhage. The critical issue is whether ultrasound can differentiate between retained placenta and blood clots or necrotic debris and decidua. The sonographic appearance of retained placenta or products of conception is variable, but visualization of an echogenic mass within the uterine cavity

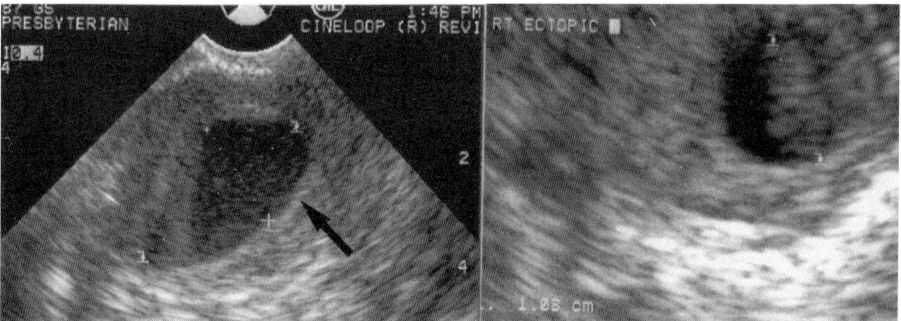

Figure 2-5. Pseudogestational sac, often associated with ectopic pregnancy, can be mistaken for an intrauterine pregnancy (arrow). At right is the live ectopic pregnancy seen in the adnexa.

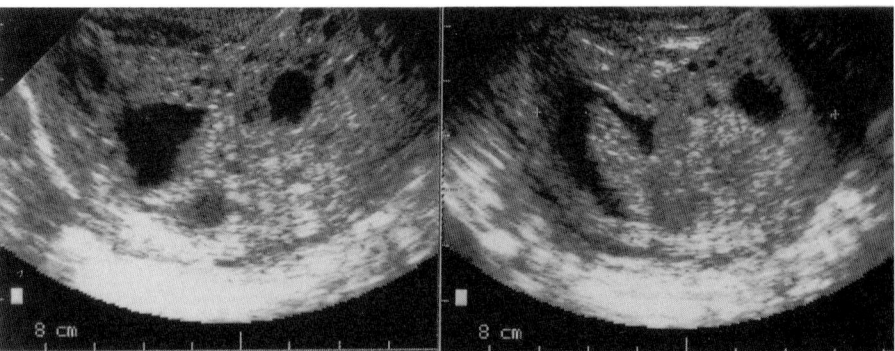

Figure 2-6. Hydatidiform mole. The sonographic appearance is said to resemble a "snowstorm," and contains both cystic and solid-appearing areas.

is highly suggestive[11] (Fig. 2-7). Endometrial thickness, per se, has variable measurements in this setting, and does not appear to be reliable as a sole indicator of retained products. Ultrasound becomes much less accurate as a diagnostic tool in the setting of recent uterine instrumentation, as resulting hyperechoic endometrial foci, representing air within the cavity, are seen even in the absence of concomitant retained products.[11]

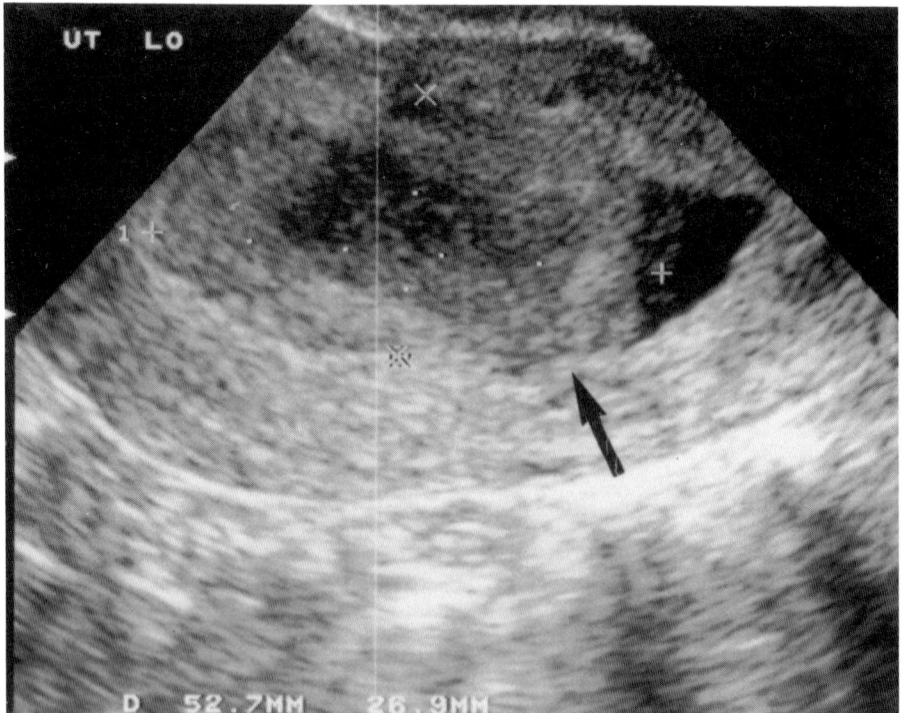

Figure 2-7. Retained products of conception, appears as an irregular echogenic mass in the cavity (arrow).

BENIGN ENDOMETRIAL DISORDERS

Clearly, precise differentiation of benign from malignant endometrial abnormalities cannot be achieved by sonography alone, yet this modality has been used as a noninvasive adjunct in this regard. Leiomyomata can be detected and localized to subserosal, intramural, and submucosal locations within the uterus. They generally appear as well-defined round structures with heterogeneous texture, although calcification (increased echoes) and liquefaction (hypoechoic areas) have also been identified. The visualization of submucosal leiomyomata impinging into the endometrial cavity (Fig. 2-8) has become useful in the evaluation of the patient with abnormal uterine bleeding, as well as in patients with infertility and recurrent pregnancy loss. Benign endometrial polyps as small as 0.5 cm can be visualized[10] as small, well-defined hypo- or hyperechoic defects within the otherwise uniform endometrial echo (Fig. 2-9). Endometritis, while less accurately a sonographic diagnosis, may also appear as a thickened and echogenic endometrium, with or without intraluminal fluid present (Fig. 2-10).

Fusion disorders of the uterus, including uterus didelphys and bicornuate uterus, are able to be identified by ultrasound,[10] although this is not the classic investigative test for this purpose. Typically, these fusion defects are identified by the appearance of two echogenic endometrial cavities imaged in a transverse view of the fundal area (Fig. 2-11). One author has found transvaginal ultrasound of the endometrium a useful adjunct at the time of hysteroscopic evaluation: in almost half the patients with an initially normal sonographic appearance of the endometrium, pathologic conditions including synechiae, myomas, and polyps were seen after filling the cavity with Hyskon (a 32% dextran, high-viscosity liquid).[12]

The intrauterine contraceptive device (IUD), when properly located, is imaged as a highly reflective longitudinal structure within the endometrial cavity (Fig. 2-12). By locating the position of the IUD relative to the cavity, TVS is able to diagnose perforation, malposition, and incomplete removal of the IUD.[13] Partial myometrial implantation may be suspected when a portion of the IUD extends from the endometrial surface into the surrounding myometrium.[13]

PREMALIGNANT AND MALIGNANT ENDOMETRIAL DISORDERS

Endometrial hyperplasia is visualized as a thickened and occasionally irregular shadow sonographically. Carcinoma appears as a highly irregular and thickened endometrium, with occasional pseudostratified or polypoid defects seen within (Fig. 2-13). Malignant polypoid-like masses may be identified as filling the endometrial cavity, and occasionally are seen prolapsing through an open cervical os. The combination of thickened and highly struc-

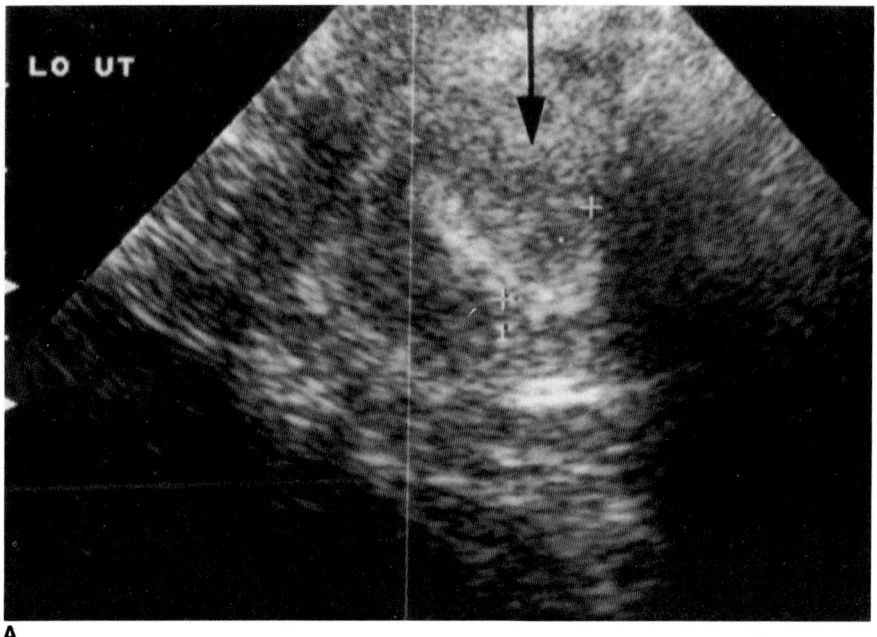

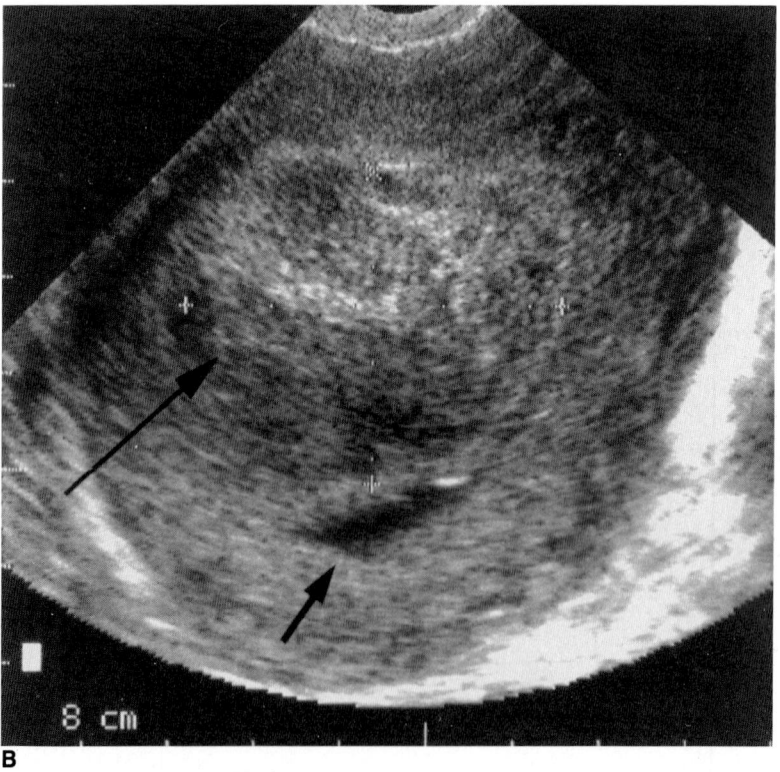

Figure 2-8. Submucosal leiomyomata. (A). A small myoma is seen impinging on the endometrial cavity and distorting the usual linear endometrial echo (arrow). (B). At right is a large submucous myoma (long arrow), also seen distorting the cavity (short arrow).

Premalignant and Malignant Endometrial Disorders

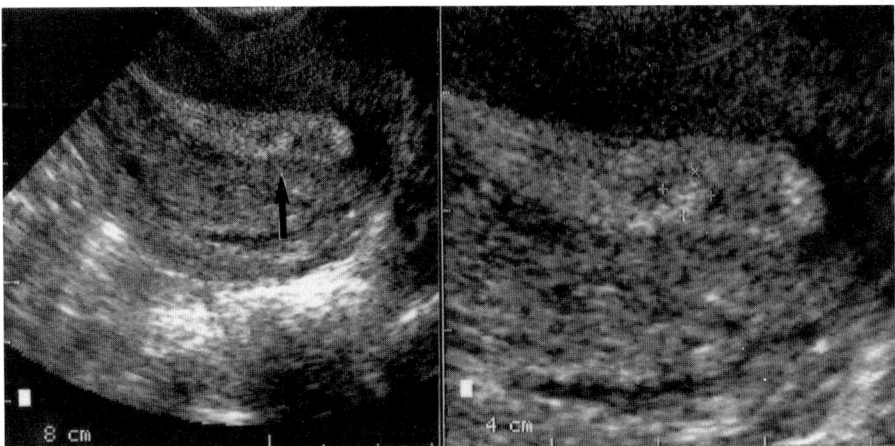

Figure 2-9. Small endometrial polyp, seen as a small echogenic area protruding into the cavity (arrow). At right is a magnified view of the same 0.6 × 0.7-cm polyp.

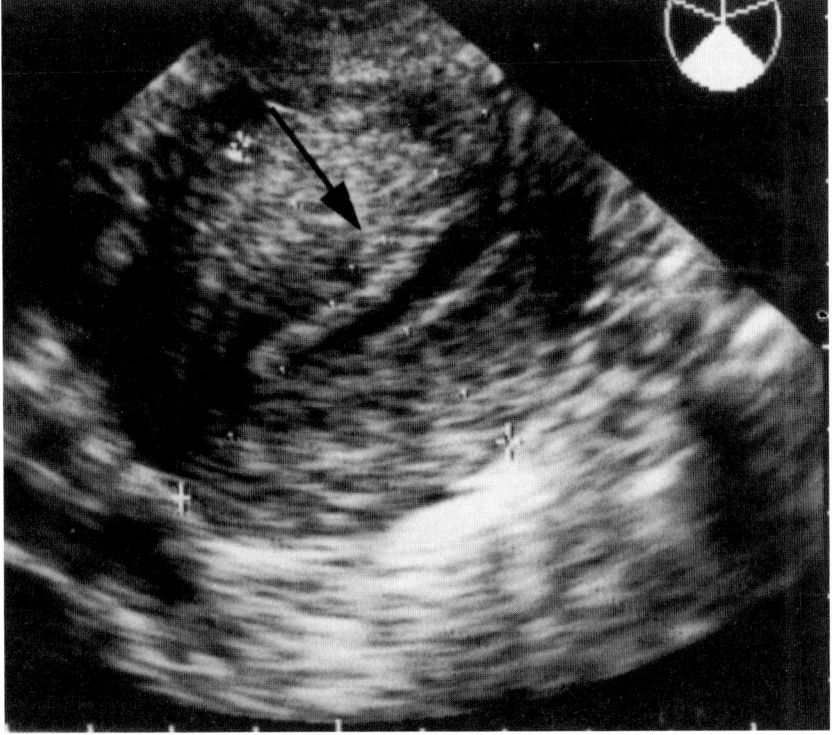

Figure 2-10. Endometritis, often appears as a thickened, irregular, and echogenic endometrium (arrow), often a difficult diagnosis to make sonographically. Here, some fluid in the cavity is present.

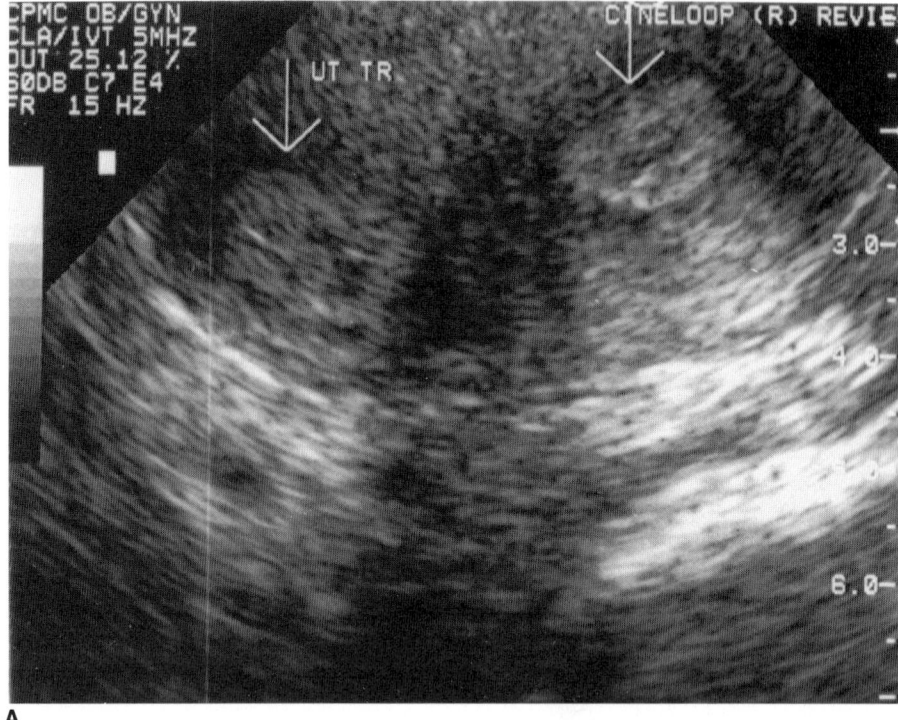

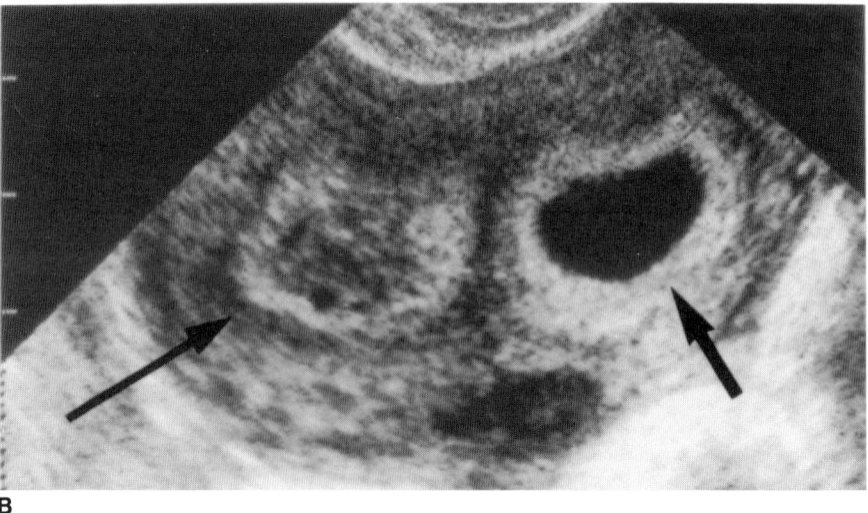

Figure 2-11. Bicornuate uterus or uterus didelphys. (A). Two distinct endometrial cavities can be seen in the transverse view (two white arrows.) (B). At right, a bicornuate uterus with a gestational sac visible in one of the horns (short arrow), and a decidual reaction seen in the other horn (long arrow).

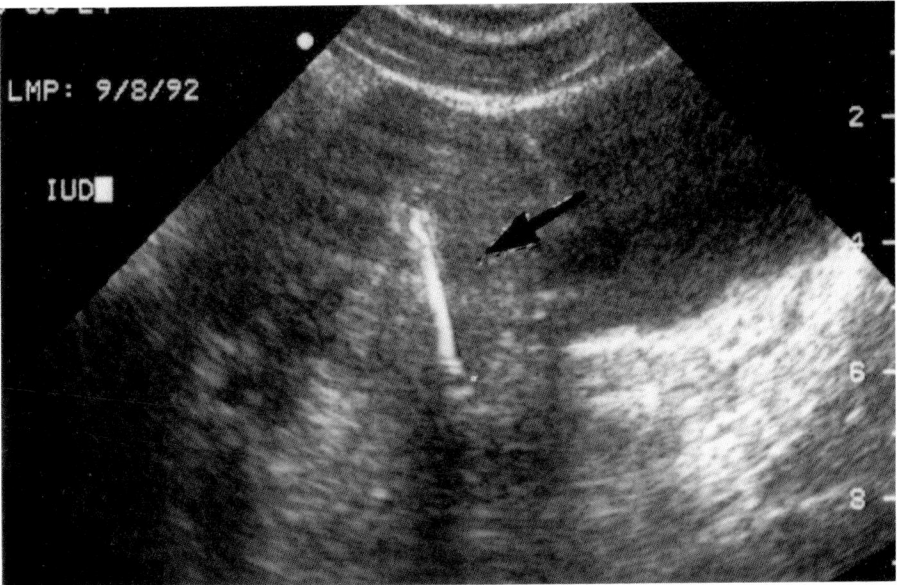

Figure 2-12. IUD within the endometrial cavity appears as a very echogenic linear structure (arrow). This view was from a transabdominal scan.

tured endometrium should raise the suspicion of pathology. Transvaginal sonography appears to be accurate in determining the presence of myometrial invasion,[14,15] although it is often difficult to visually delineate the endometrial–myometrial interface.

POSTMENOPAUSAL ENDOMETRIUM AND HORMONE REPLACEMENT

Although the endometrium in postmenopausal women has been well studied and characterized, there remains no accepted criteria for "normal" endome-

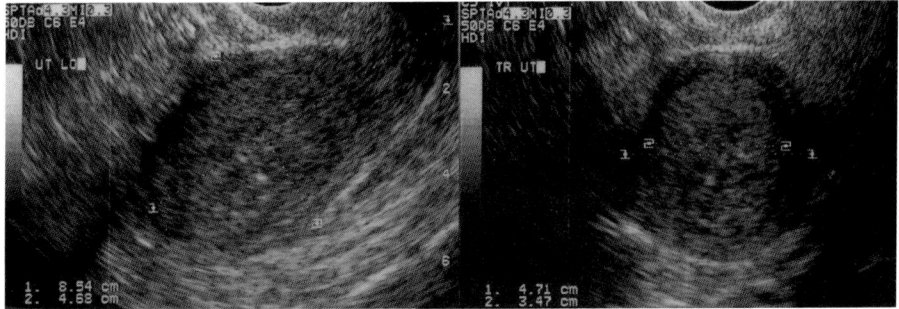

Figure 2-13. Endometrial carcinoma, with irregular and polypoid configuration. The endometrial–myometrial interface is not well defined.

trial thickness, with and without various hormonal replacement regimens. Most authors describe the upper normal limits of postmenopausal endometrial thickness in the 5–10 mm range,[16] but here, some of the authors measure the endometrium as a single layer, and others as a double layer. The double layer is usually used, measured in the anterior–posterior diameter. This sonographic measurement consists of two closely apposed layers of endometrium, and has been shown to be in agreement with pathology specimen measurements.[5] The hypoechoic halo usually surrounding the endometrium histologically correlates with the inner myometrium; therefore, is not included in the measurement (Fig. 2-14).

Certainly, knowledge concerning the presence, absence, and/or schedule of the hormonal replacement regimen of the postmenopausal patient is crucial in the evaluation of the endometrium. Postmenopausal patients not on hormonal replacement require endometrial sampling for episodes of postmenopausal bleeding, although the proportion of these patients with hyperplasia or carcinoma is small. Several authors have attempted to set a cutoff value for endometrial thickness not requiring endometrial sampling in these patients, and generally use 0.5[17] or 0.8 cm.[15,16,18] Endometrial cavity fluid may erroneously increase the sonographic measurement obtained, and must not be included in the calculation. This fluid is seen in the endometrial cavities of many postmenopausal women and is not necessarily associated with endometrial pathology.[19,20]

Patients who are on unopposed estrogen regimens are at increased risk for the subsequent development of endometrial hyperplasia or carcinoma; therefore, it is suggested that any endometrial measurement greater than 0.5 or 0.8 cm should be further evaluated with endometrial biopsy or dilatation and curettage. Patients taking sequential estrogen and progesterone have variations in endometrial thickness depending on the day of the cycle; therefore, sonographic evaluation should take place just after the completion of

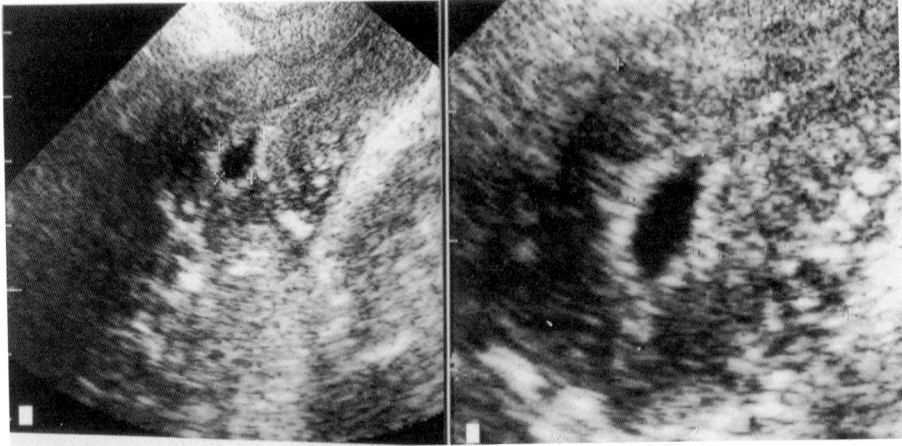

Figure 2-14. Postmenopausal endometrium, thin and homogenous. A small amount of intracavity fluid can be seen. At right is a magnified view.

the progesterone phase, at approximately days 28–30. At this time, the endometrium is expected to be its thinnest.

There is no conclusion to be made in patients on the sequential regimen, especially when the endometrial measurement is between 0.8 and 1.5 cm. It is suggested that patients undergo further evaluation for measurements greater than 1.5 cm and when otherwise clinically indicated, such as in the presence of postmenopausal bleeding.[16] In patients on a continuous regimen, endometrial atrophy is expected, and evidence of endometrial thickening greater than 0.8 cm should be further evaluated as above. The measurement of maximal sonographic thickness alone is not sensitive enough to predict endometrial malignancy, but other parameters, such as homogeneity and echogenicity, must also be included in the evaluation.

IVF AND OVULATION INDUCTION

The most recent development in the use of ultrasound for imaging the endometrium has been in the area of new reproductive technologies, most specifically ovulation induction and IVF. Prior to the development of refined sonographic technique, endometrial thickness was the only parameter available for evaluation. Now, subtle differences in echogenicity of the endometrium at different times of the cycle and utilizing different regimens can be ascertained. It has been concluded that the ultrasound image of the endometrium during the proliferative phase consists of thin echogenic lines and appears similar in stimulated and unstimulated cycles.[21] Endometrial thickness appears to become more important at midcycle, where endometrial thickness measured on the day before oocyte retrieval was significantly greater in the group of patients who went on to achieve pregnancy than in the group who did not.[22] Although there appears to be a trend toward thicker endometria is successfully concepted cycles, there is no universal agreement regarding the minimal endometrial thickness necessary to sustain implantation.

A combination of endometrial thickness and endometrial pattern appears to be a more reliable predictor of successful implantation in stimulated cycles than endometrial thickness alone.[3,22] Several authors have characterized endometrial patterns and correlated these findings with pregnancy implantation rates.[22–24] It appears that a pattern of a multilayered endometrium, consisting of a hyperechoic outer layer and a hypoechoic inner layer (Fig. 2-15), correlated positively with subsequent implantation in ovulation induction protocols, with and without IVF.[25] Some authors have even suggested cancellation of oocyte aspiration or embryo transfer in a patient with a thin, homogenous, hyperechoic endometrium.[23]

Significant differences in endometrial thickness and echogenicity between patients treated with a regimen including clomiphene citrate (CC) or buserelin acetate with human menopausal gonadotropins (hMG) were demonstrable by ultrasound. The women being superovulated with CC/hMG develop a significantly thinner endometrium compared with women receiv-

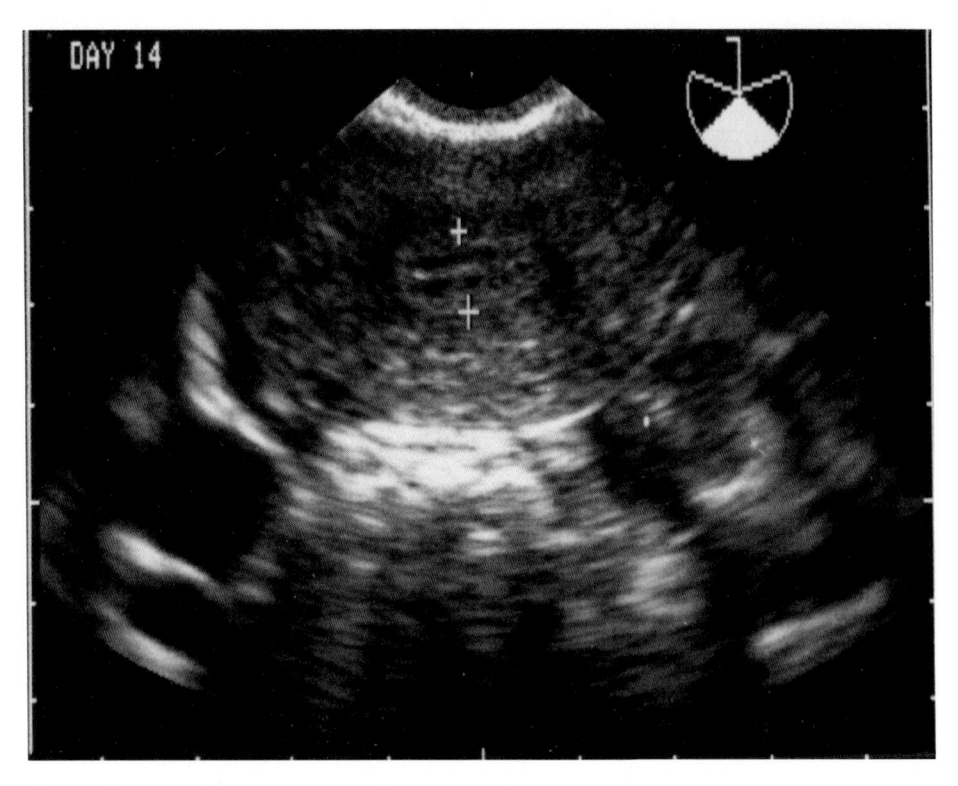

Figure 2-15. Pattern of multilayered midcycle endometrium, seen between the +, in a successful IVF cycle.

ing buserelin acetate/hMG.[26] This has been attributed to the inhibitory action of clomiphene citrate on the endometrium during the proliferative phase.[25,26]

Premature luteal transformation may also be determined sonographically, as Fleischer et al showed that cycles stimulated with gonadotropin-releasing hormone and human menopausal gonadotropins more likely resulted in pregnancy if an echogenic endometrium was not present before oocyte pickup.[25] Each of these observations confirms that when endometrial transformation occurs out of synchrony with embryo readiness, implantation occurs less frequently.[3]

DOPPLER STUDIES AND THE FUTURE

The measurement of blood flow velocity by ultrasound is based on the Doppler effect, which implies that the frequency of a sound wave emitted from a stationary source and reflected from a moving interface changes according to the velocity and direction of the moving interface. If the ultrasound beam is sent toward a blood vessel, the moving erythrocytes act as reflectors and cause a change of the reflected sound frequency. This Doppler effect can be used to measure the mean blood velocity across a vessel, represented as a blood flow velocity waveform and analyzed within the computer of the specialized ultrasound machine. More than 10 indices have been described for velocity waveform analysis, but three—the systolic/diastolic (A/B) ratio, resistance index (RI), and pulsatility index (PI)—are most often used. These measurements are used to identify decreased vascular impedance and increased blood flow, representing neovascularization within the endometrium, and suggesting endometrial cancer. This conclusion is based on Folkman's hypothesis that malignant, rapidly growing tumors contain many newly formed blood vessels, and these vessels contain little smooth muscle within their walls.[27] The resistance to blood flow is therefore decreased. By quantifying this difference, it might be possible to discriminate benign from malignant endometria.

In a recent study by Kurjak et al, the comparison of RI between patients with benign uterine myomas and endometrial carcinoma showed a significantly lower RI in the cases of endometrial carcinoma.[28] In another recently reported series, the PI of the uterine arteries in cases of women with postmenopausal bleeding associated with endometrial cancer was significantly lower than in women with postmenopausal bleeding not associated with carcinoma.[29]

Doppler flow studies of the uterine arteries may be used in the evaluation of early pregnancy failure, and possible in ovulation induction protocols. Doppler flow measurements are proving useful in the assessment of uterine perfusion in patients with failure to conceive during and after IVF protocols. In one study using transabdominal Doppler sonography, the conception rate was increased after oral administration of estrogens and subsequent improvement in uterine perfusion.[30]

Specially designed high-resolution ultrasound transducers placed on the tip of endoluminal catheters are experimentally being placed into the endometrial cavity to evaluate the utility of this approach. Endometrial, uterine, and cervical abnormalities, including myomas, polyps, synechiae, and endometrial and cervical carcinomas, have been visualized and subsequently confirmed by biopsy or surgical removal.[31] This new sonographic technology may become an important diagnostic tool in the near future.

SUMMARY

With the advent of high-frequency transvaginal transducers, the evaluation of the endometrium has become more sophisticated. Essentially the entire gynecologic spectrum is covered: menstrual cycle changes, pregnancy evaluation, the investigation of irregular menstrual bleeding and the identification of leiomyomata, polyps, and hyperplasias, the use of ultrasound in infertility and assisted reproduction, and the evaluation in the postmenopausal woman and identification of carcinoma. The clinical applications for this relatively new technology are continuously expanding, and the most recent developments allude to a promising future.

REFERENCES

1. Schwimmer SR, Rothman CM, Lebovic J, et al: The effect of ultrasound coupling gel on sperm motility in vitro. *Fertil Steril* 42:946, 1984.
2. Santolaya-Forgas J: Physiology of the menstrual cycle by ultrasonography. *J Ultrasound Med* 11:139–142, 1990.
3. Grunfeld L: Physiology of the menstrual cycle. *Infertil Reprod Med Clin N Am* 2:683–687, 1991.
4. Fleischer AC, Kalemanis GC, Entmann SS: Sonographic depiction of the endometrium during normal cycles. *Ultrasound Med Biol* 12:271, 1986.
5. Forrest TS, Elyaderani MK, Muilenburg MI, et al: Cyclic endometrial changes: ultrasound assessment with histologic correlation. *Radiology* 167:233, 1988.
6. Blumenfeld A, Rottem S, Elgali S, et al: Transvaginal sonographic assessment of early embryonic development. In *Transvaginal sonography,* Timor-Tritsch I, Rottem S (eds). Elsevier, New York, 1987, p 87.
7. Fleischer AC, Gordon AN, Entmann SS, et al: Transvaginal scanning of the endometrium. *J Clin Ultrasound* 18:337–349, 1990.
8. Nyberg DA, Filly RA, Laing FC, et al: Ectopic pregnancy: diagnosis by sonography correlated with quantitative hCG levels. *J Ultrasound Med* 6:145–150, 1987.
9. Goldstein S: Early landmarks in the normal and abnormal pregnancy. *Infertil Reprod Med Clin N Am* 2:699, 1991.
10. Lewit N, Thaler I, Rottem S: The uterus: a new look with TVS. *J Clin Ultrasound* 18:331–336, 1990.
11. Hertzberg BS, Bowie JD: Ultrasound of the postpartum uterus: prediction of retained placental tissue. *J Ultrasound Med* 10:451–456, 1991.
12. van Roessel, J, Wamsteker K, Exalto N: Sonographic investigation of the uterus during artificial uterine cavity distension. *J Clin Ultrasound* 15:439–450, 1987.
13. White RG, Lyons M, McDowell M: Transvaginal sonography and the IUD. *Br J Fam Plann* 16:22–24, 1990.
14. Fleischer AC, Dudley BS, Entmann SS, et al: Myometrial invasion: sonographic assessment. *Radiology* 162:297–305, 1987.
15. Schoenfeld A, Levavi H, Hirsch M, et al: Transvaginal sonography in postmenopausal women. *J Clin Ultrasound* 18:350–358, 1990.
16. Lin MC, Gosink BB, Wolf SI, et al: Endometrial thickness after menopause: effect of hormonal replacement. *Radiology* 180:427–432, 1991.
17. Nasri MN, Shepherd JH, Setchell ME, et al: The role of vaginal scan in measurement of endometrial thickness in post menopausal women. *Br J Obstet Gynecol* 98:470–475, 1991.
18. Smith P, Bakos O, Heimer G, et al: Transvaginal ultrasound for identifying endometrial abnormality. *Acta Obstet Gynecol Scand* 70:591–594, 1991.
19. McCarthy KA, Hall DA, Kopans DB, et al: Postmenopausal endometrial fluid collections: always an indicator of malignancy? *J Ultrasound Med* 5:647–649, 1986.
20. Carlson JA, Arger P, Thompson S, et al: Clinical and pathologic correlation of endometrial cavity fluid detected by ultrasound in the postmenopausal patient. *Obstet Gynecol* 77:119–123, 1991.
21. Lenz S, Lindenberg S: Ultrasound evaluation of endometrial growth in women with normal cycles during spontaneous and stimulated cycles. *Hum Reprod* 5:377–381, 1990.
22. Gonen Y, Casper RF: Prediction of implantation by the sonographic appearance of the endometrium during controlled ovarian stimulation for in vitro fertilization. *J in Vitro Fert Embryo Transf* 7:146–152, 1990.
23. Welker BG, Gembruch U, Diedrich K, et al: Transvaginal sonography of the en-

References

dometrium during ovum pickup in stimulated cycles for the vitro fertilization. *J Ultrasound Med* 8:549–553, 1989.
24. Fleischer AC, Herbert CM, Sacks GA, et al: Sonography of the endometrium during conception and nonconception cycles of in vitro fertilization and embryo transfer. *Fertil Steril* 46:442, 1986.
25. Fleischer AC, Herbert CM, Hill GA, et al: Transvaginal sonography of the endometrium during induced cycles. *J Ultrasound Med* 10:93–95, 1991.
26. Rogers PAW, Polson D, Murphy CR, et al: Correlation of endometrial histology, morphometry, and ultrasound appearance after different stimulation protocols for in vitro fertilization. *Fertil Steril* 55:583–587, 1991.
27. Folkman J, Watson K, Ingber D, et al: Induction of angiogenesis during the transition from hyperplasia to neoplasia. *Nature* 339:58–61, 1989.
28. Kurjak A, Zalud I: The characterization of uterine tumors by transvaginal color Doppler. *Ultrasound Obstet Gynecol* 1:50–52, 1991.
29. Bourne T, Campbell S, Whitehead M, et al: Detection of endometrial cancer in postmenopausal women by transvaginal ultrasonography and colour flow imaging. *Br Med J* 301:18–25, 1990.
30. Goswamy RK, Williams G, Steptoe PC: Decreased uterine perfusion: a cause of infertility. *Hum Reprod* 3:955–959, 1988.

3
Hysteroscopy in Evaluation of the Endometrium

Robert S. Neuwirth, M.D.

Hysteroscopy is an extremely useful technique in the evaluation of the endometrium because it offers visual information about the mucosa as well as definitive macroscopic appraisal of the endometrial cavity. No other imaging technique is quite as precise and informative, although sonography, computerized axial tomography, and magnetic resonance imaging can give information about gross lesions in the endometrial cavity as well as some information about the endometrial mucosa. Certainly the endometrial biopsy and curettage are the foundations of endometrial diagnosis but offer little about gross lesions such as polyps or submucous myomas unless they are identified, removed, and examined histologically.

Hysteroscopy consists of introducing a slender, 4–8-mm endoscope into the cervical canal and endometrial cavity for observation. There are rigid (Fig. 3-1) and flexible (Fig. 3-2) panoramic hysteroscopes as well as contact and magnifying hysteroscopes. The panoramic hysteroscopes require a distension system to separate the walls of the endometrial cavity. Carbon dioxide gas (Fig. 3-3) is the most ideal for diagnosis as it has no optical distortions, and is flow-limited to ≤100 ml/min, so that absorbed gas can be handled by the vascular and pulmonary systems. The problems with it are leakage so that adequate uterine pressure (60–80 mmHg) is not achieved, or if blood is present, gas bubbles distort the view. Low-viscosity liquids such as 5% dextrose in water or Ringer's lactate are acceptable but cause some distortion due to the refraction index and in the face of bleeding will disperse the red cells and prevent adequate vision. Hyskon, a 32% dextran product, is a high-viscosity liquid that has a more favorable refractive index

Hysteroscopy in Evaluation of the Endometrium 27

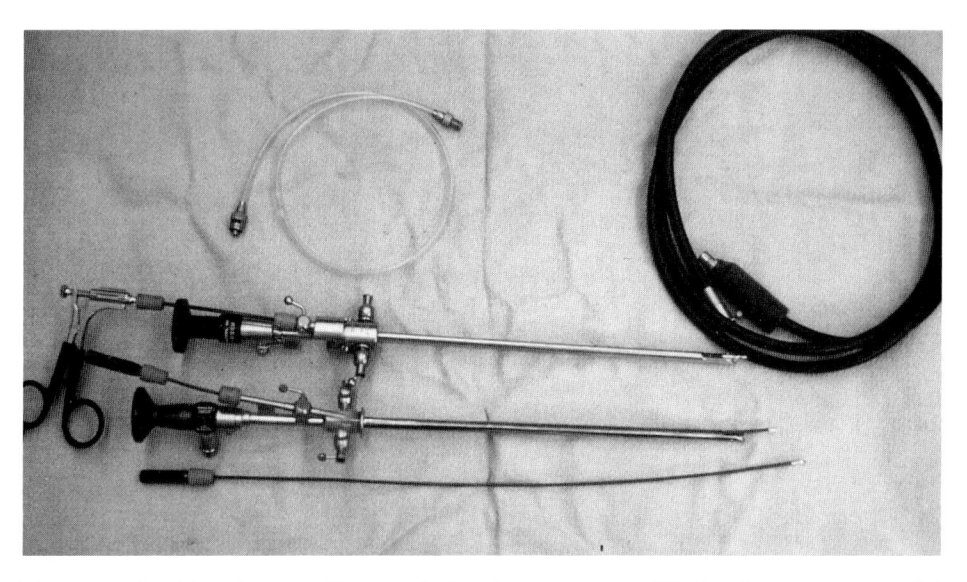

Figure 3-1. Two 5-mm diagnostic hysteroscopes with flexible accessory biopsy forceps and probes plus a catheter for injection of Hyskon to distend the endometrial cavity.

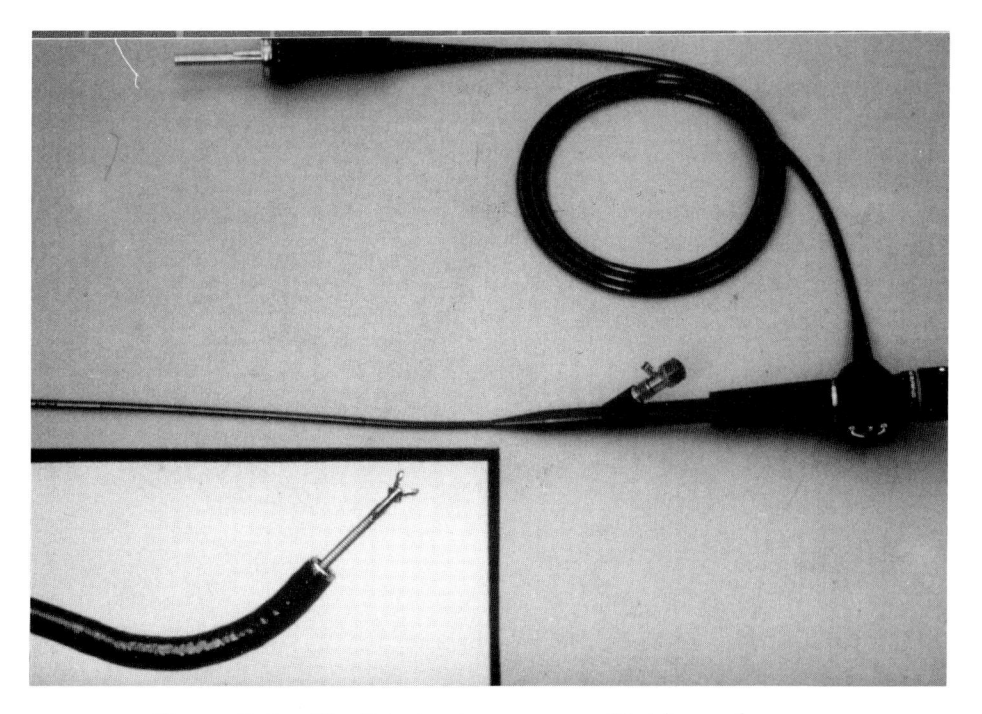

Figure 3-2. Flexible hysteroscope with biopsy forceps.

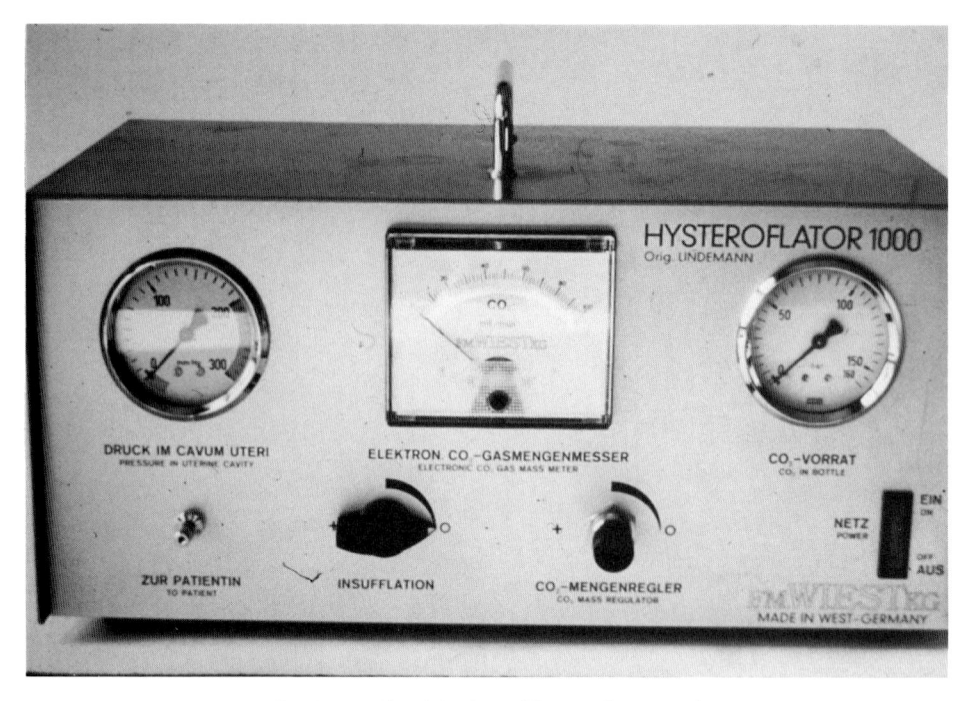

Figure 3-3. Carbon dioxide insufflator for gas hysteroscopy.

and, as a result of high viscosity, promotes rouleaux formation of red cells in the face of bleeding, thereby permitting vision in some circumstances where low-viscosity liquids will not. Absorption of liquids into the vascular system is potentially hazardous as the liquids cannot be flow-limited and absorption of more than 400 ml of Hyskon or 4 liters of low-viscosity liquids can lead to pulmonary edema. Contact hysteroscopes do not require a distension system, but they offer little in terms of the diagnosis of gross lesions such as the submucous myoma. In addition, contact hysteroscopy requires special interpretative ability to understand in vivo microscopic images at varying degrees of magnification.

Hysteroscopy can be done in the office (Figs. 3-4 through 3-6) or the operating room. In the office the procedure can be done under mild analgesia with or without a local cervical anesthetic. A successful procedure requires thorough knowledge of the procedure, equipment, and uterine landmarks (Fig. 3-7) as well as good skills in talking to the patient. Antibiotic prophylaxis is needed only for patients at risk for subacute bacterial endocarditis or general infection. Focal hysteroscopically directed biopsies are possible as well as routine semiblind endometrial biopsies. Biopsies of vascular lesions such as a submucous myoma are not prudent in the office setting. Photographs and television monitoring are possible in the office. The procedure requires about 3–5 min of actual examination time. The patient can be sent home after half an hour of observation.

In the operating room, both diagnostic as well as interventional procedures can be done. The diagnostic procedures may be conducted in the

Hysteroscopy in Evaluation of the Endometrium 29

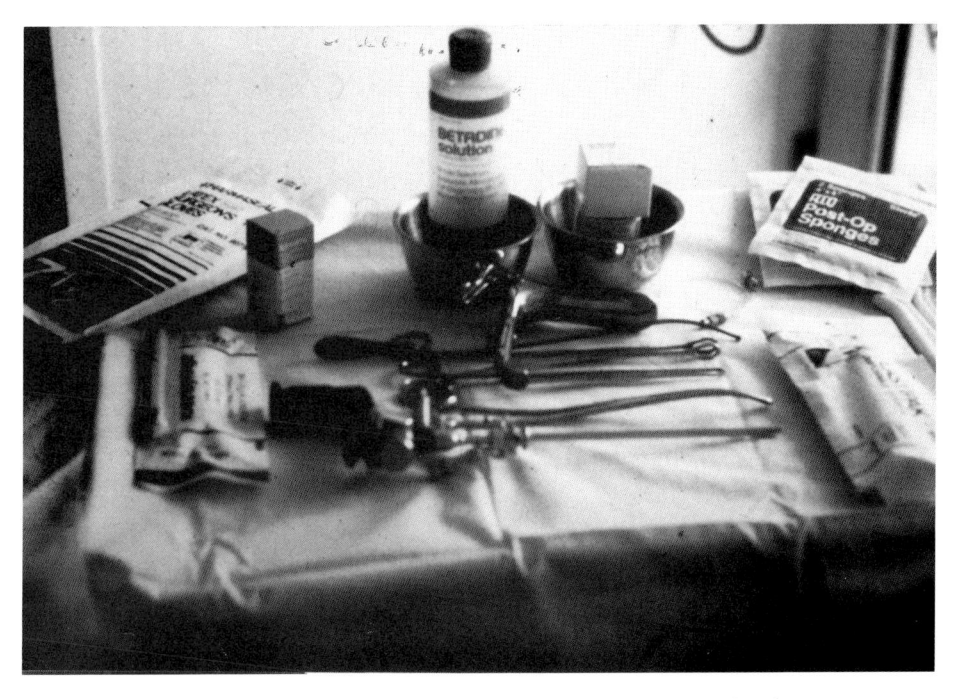

Figure 3-4. Equipment tray for office hysteroscopy including hysteroscope, gloves, prep solution, local anesthesia with spinal needle, one-arm speculum, sound, tenaculum, sponge forceps, dressing forceps and backup catheter, and syringe for Hyskon.

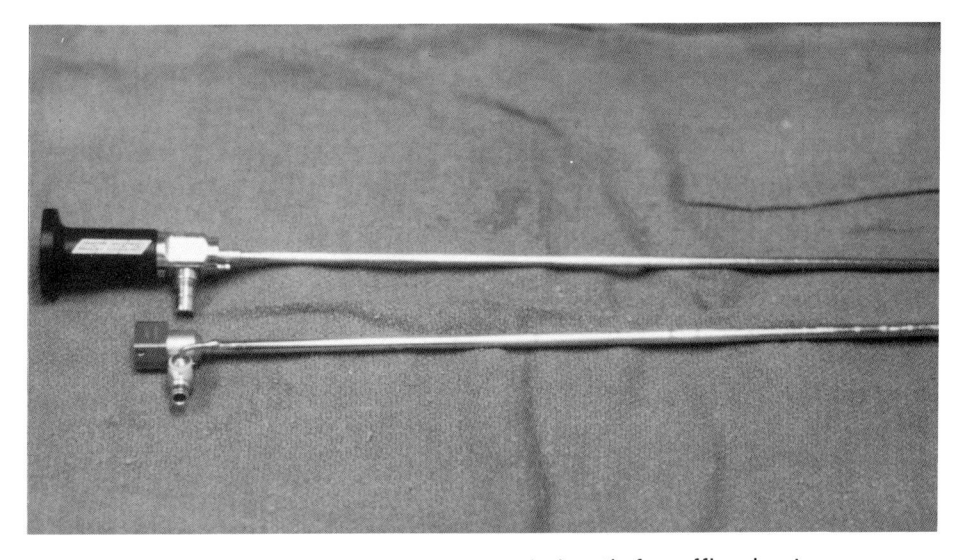

Figure 3-5. A 4-mm hysteroscope and sheath for office hysteroscopy.

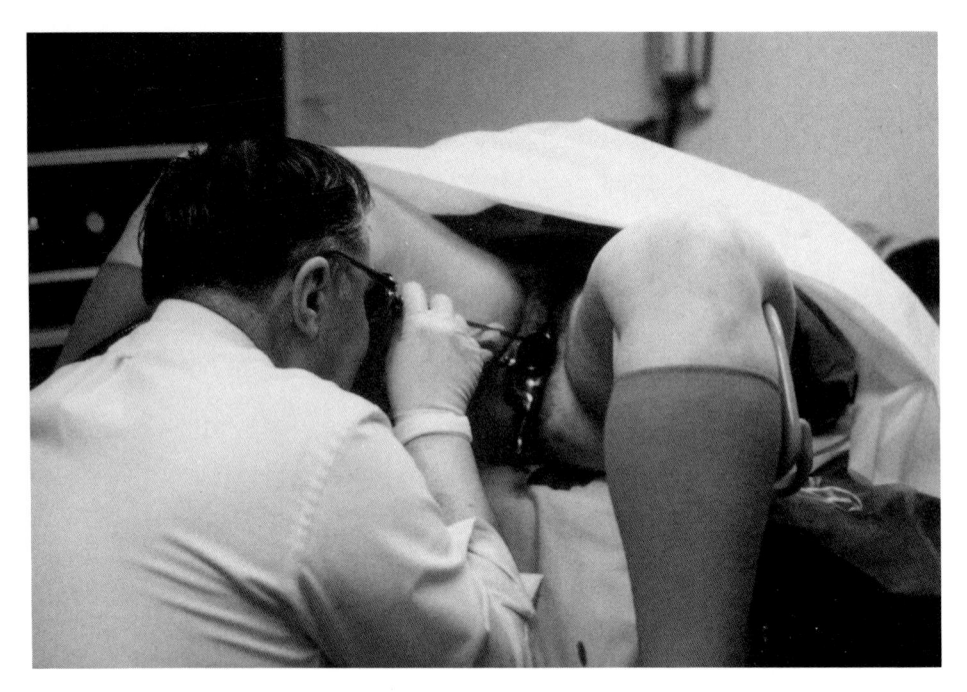

Figure 3-6. Office hysteroscopy.

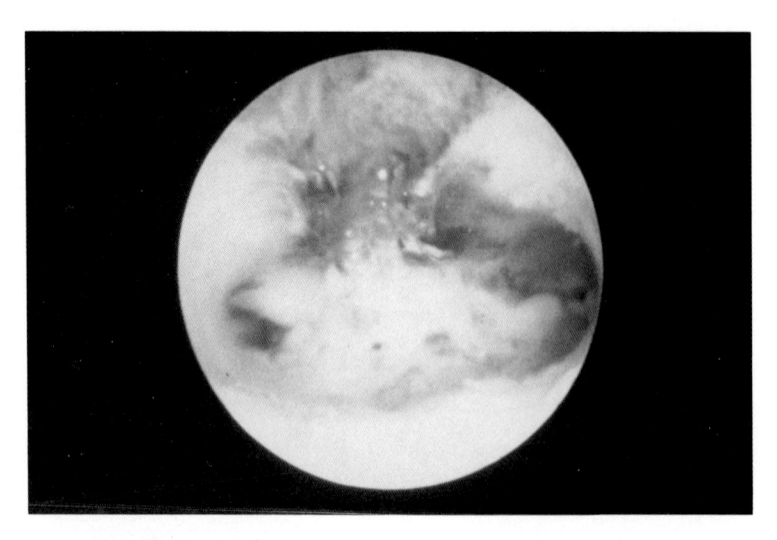

Figure 3-7. Normal endometrial cavity in midproliferative phase; uterine isthmus, fundus and cornual regions are in view.

same way as the office examinations. However, operative procedures are best done under general or regional anesthesia in order to avoid the risk of patient movement during an operative procedure. Liquid distension media are generally used in operative procedures in order to irrigate and wash the endometrial cavity of blood and debris during the procedure. Operative procedures can be performed with mechanical instruments such as scissors, biopsy forceps, and clamps attached to or passed through or around the hysteroscope. Laser and electrosurgical instruments can also be used to cut, coagulate, or take biopsies. The resectoscope has become widely used for this purpose. Postoperative recovery from hysteroscopic diagnosis is usually very brief. Following surgery, the length of observation is dependent on the degree of postoperative cramping, uterine bleeding, and the recovery from anesthesia.

The indications for diagnostic hysteroscopy include vaginal bleeding where endometrial biopsy and hormonal evaluation have not clarified a diagnosis, i.e., to look for polyps (Fig. 3-8), submucous myomata (Figs. 3-9 through 3-11), foreign bodies (Figs. 3-12 through 3-14), or endometrial cancer (Figs. 3-15 through 3-17). Abnormal hysterograms or sonograms may lead to hysteroscopy for confirmation of a diagnosis and further appraisal. Infertility workups should include a hysteroscopy, and an endometrial biopsy in lieu of a diagnostic curettage, possibly at the time of laparoscopy. Specific lesions to be ruled out include uterine septa, polyps, submucous myomas, intrauterine adhesions (Figs. 3-18 through 3-20) or the residua of a prior missed or incomplete abortion. The endocervix can be examined with a magnifying hysteroscope such as the Hamou instrument in cases where there is a cervical neoplastic lesion and extension in the endocervical canal needs appraisal and possible therapy.

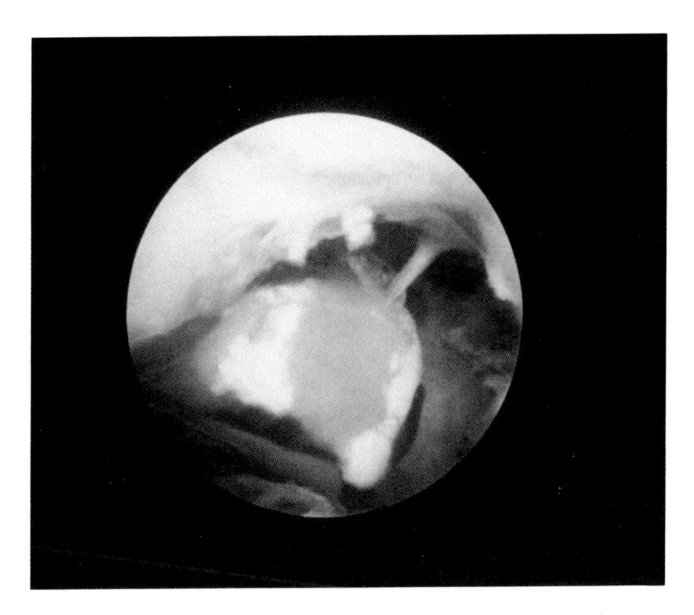

Figure 3-8. Bleeding endometrial polyp missed at prior curettage.

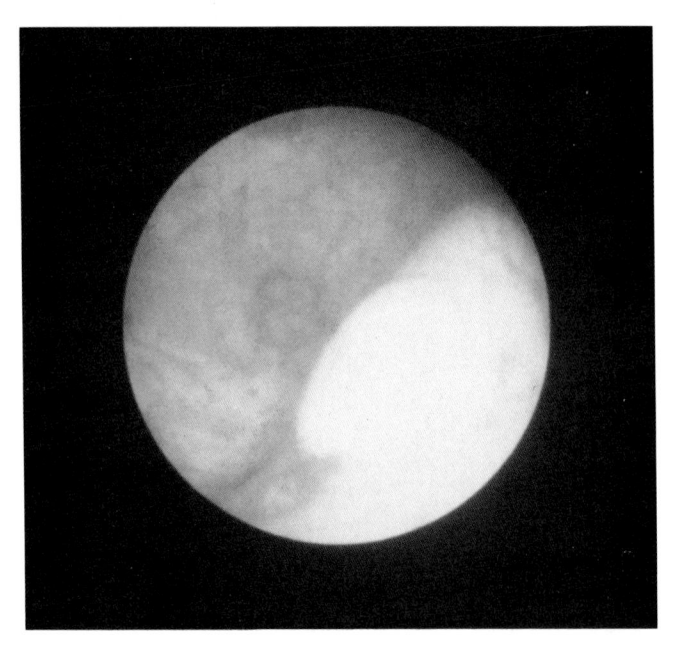

Figure 3-9. Small submucous myoma causing menorrhagia just medial to right tubal orifice.

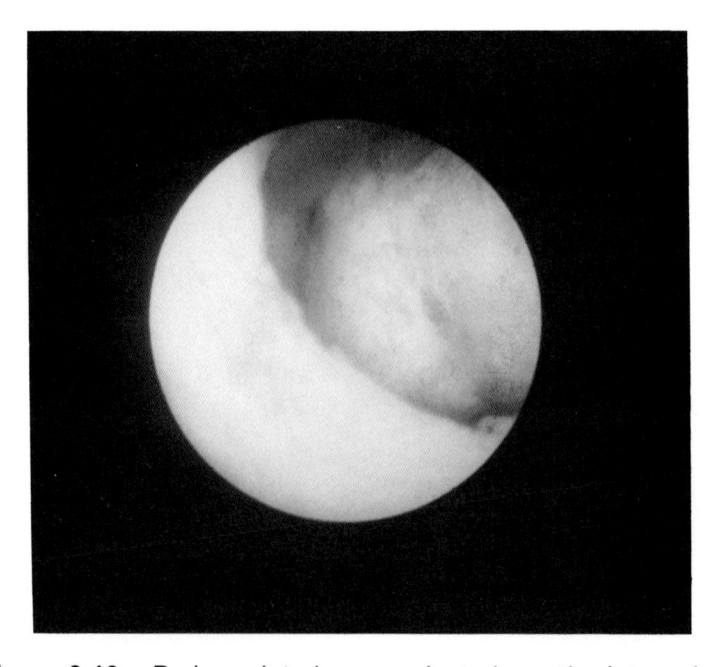

Figure 3-10. Pedunculated myoma just above the internal os.

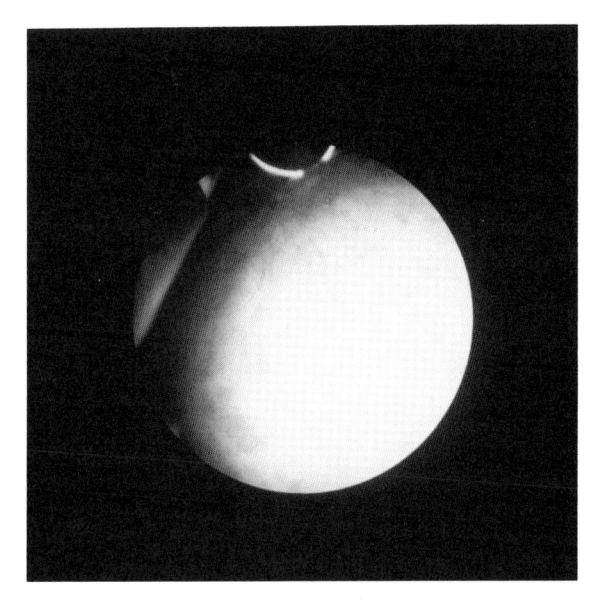

Figure 3-11. Submucous myoma just before resectoscopic morcellation and removal.

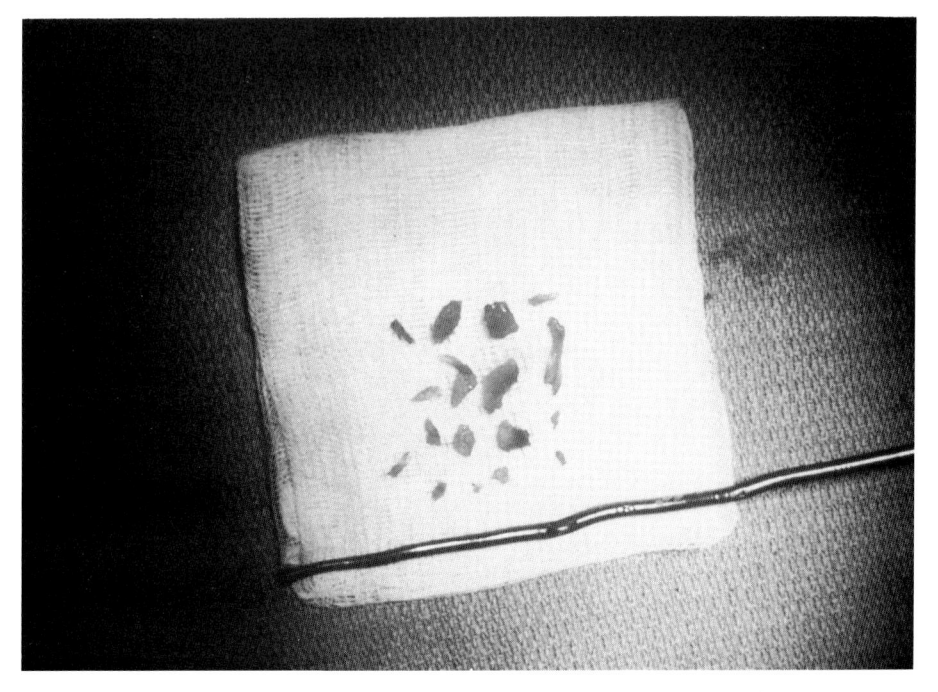

Figure 3-12. Fetal bone fragments removed hysteroscopically 2 years after a curettage for missed abortion.

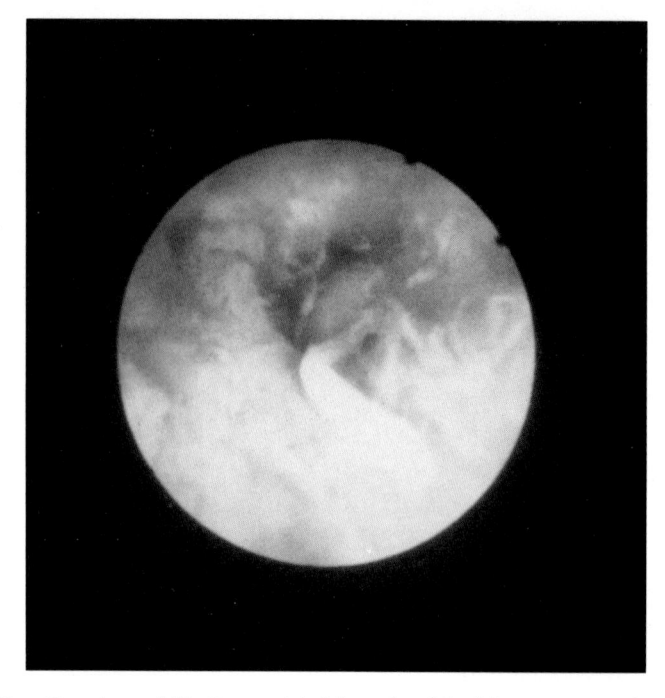

Figure 3-13. Fractured Dalkon shield embedded in myometrium following attempted blind removal.

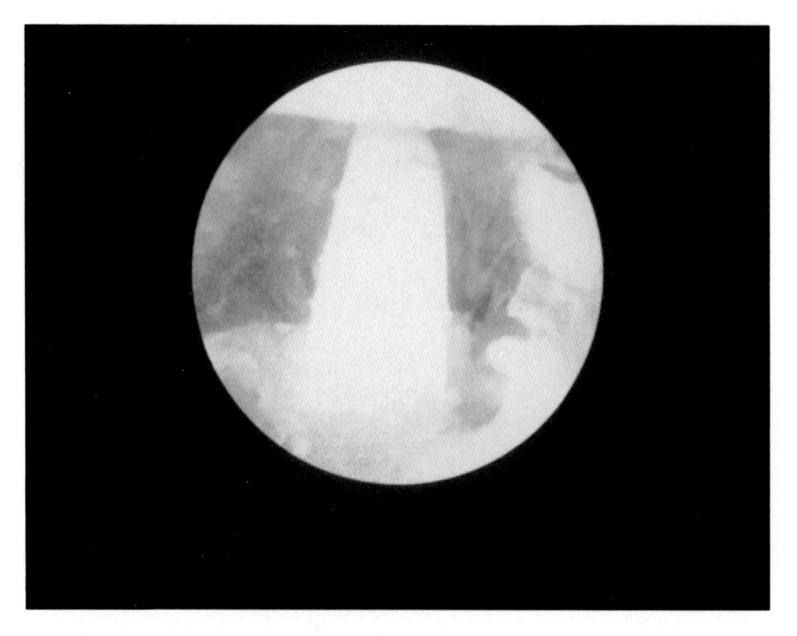

Figure 3-14. Lippes loop embedded in myometrium.

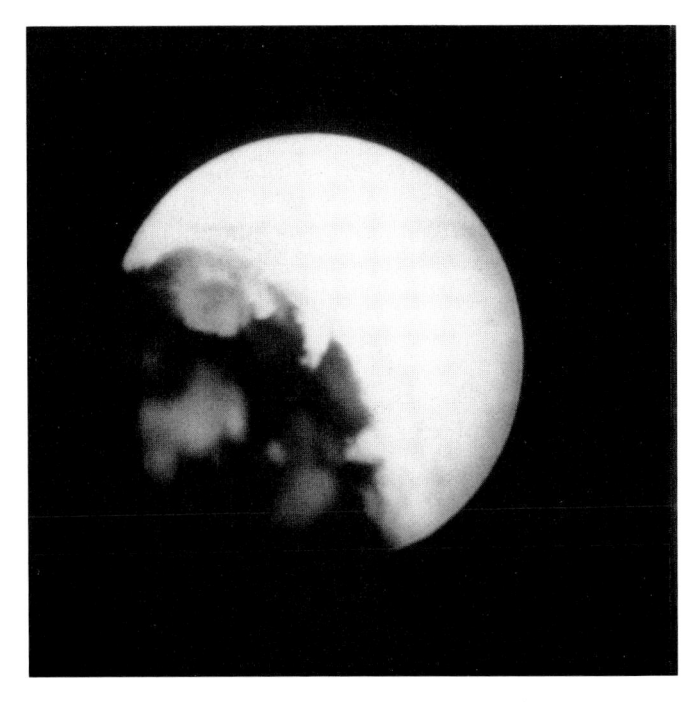

Figure 3-15. Endometrial cancer with involvement of uterine isthmus but not endocervix.

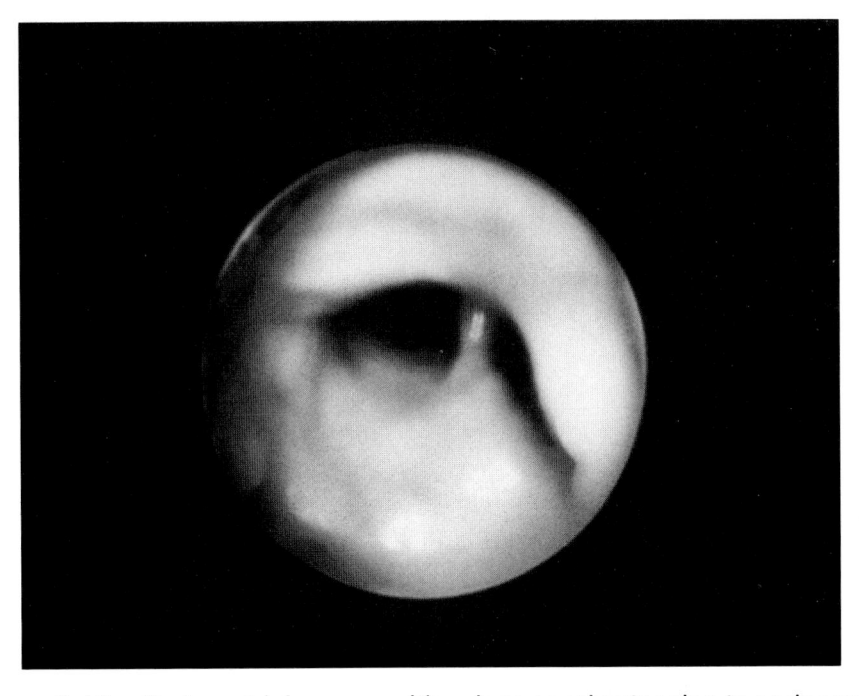

Figure 3-16. Endometrial cancer with submucosal extension to endocervix.

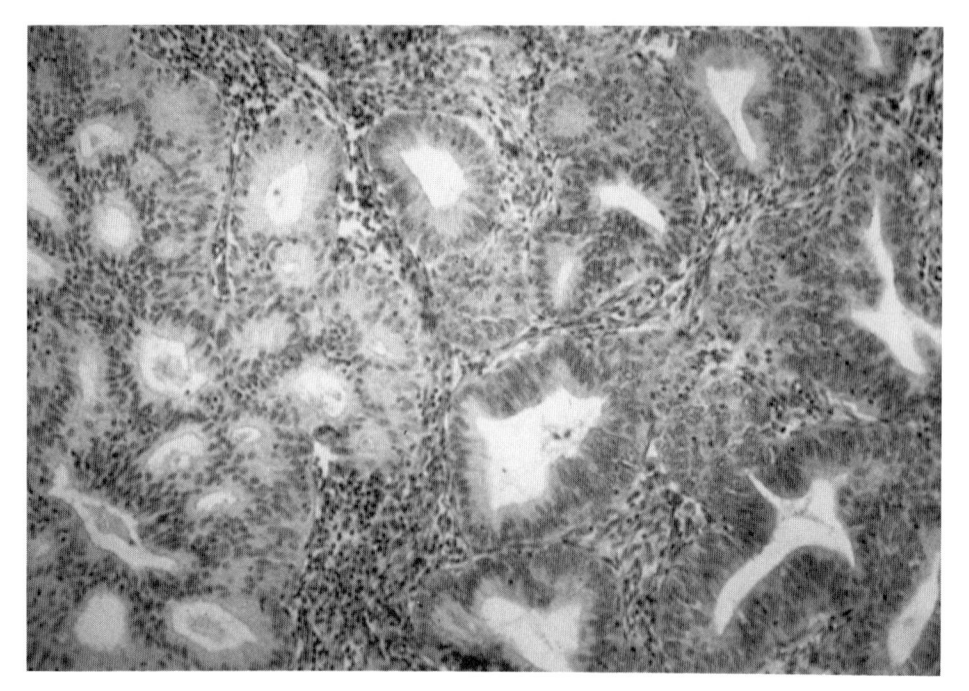

Figure 3-17. Directed biopsy showing endometrial carcinoma and hyperplasia.

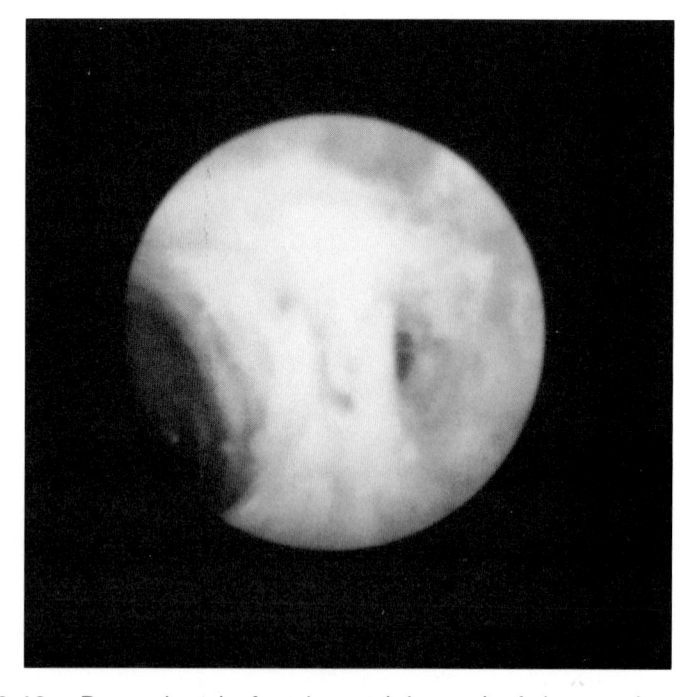

Figure 3-18. Dense band of endometrial scar in Asherman's syndrome.

Hysteroscopy in Evaluation of the Endometrium

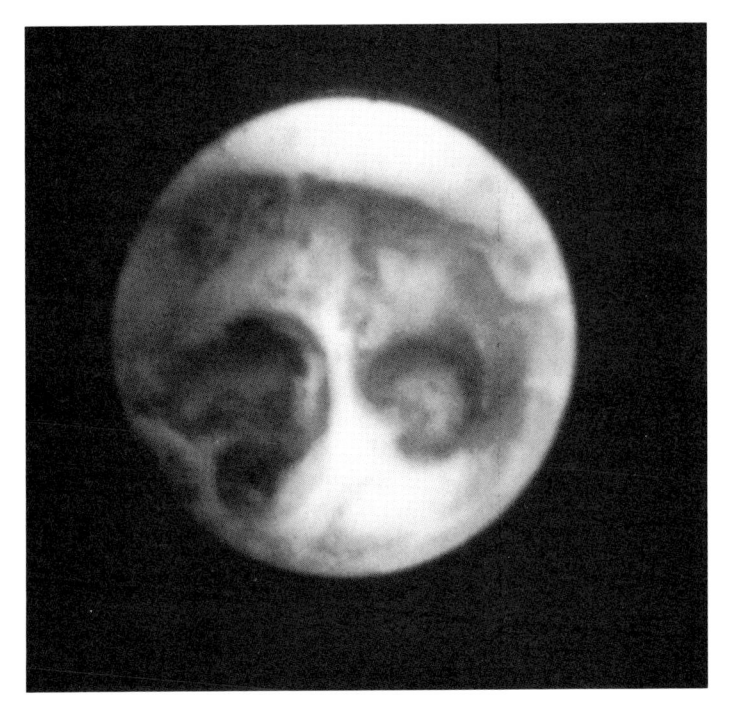

Figure 3-19. Asherman's syndrome with midline scar giving appearance of a septum.

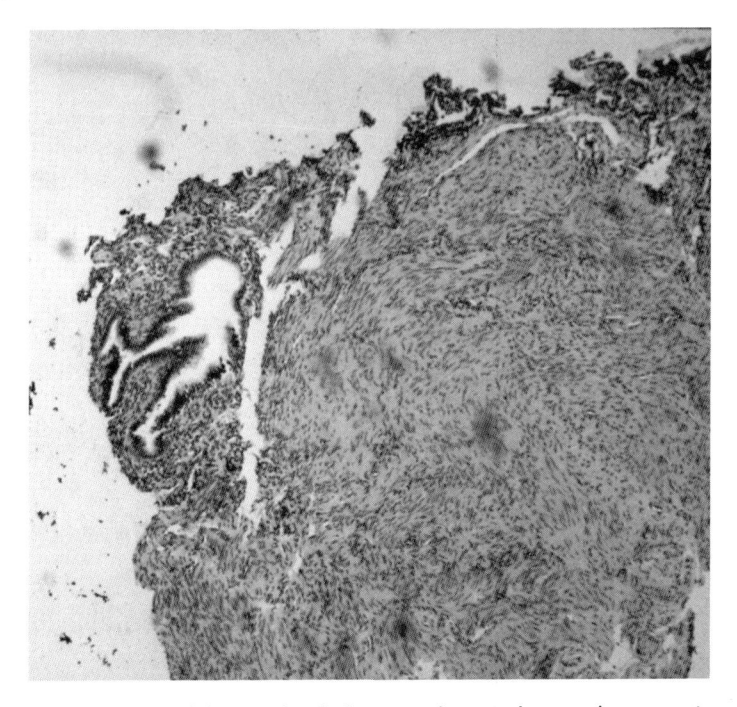

Figure 3-20. Directed biopsy in Asherman's syndrome in secretory phase of cycle showing unresponsive area of mucosa.

Contraindications to hysteroscopy are few and include upper genital tract infection, large uterine perforation, and obvious cervical or endometrial cancer. Heavy bleeding may preclude office hysteroscopy, but it can be done in an operating room with Hyskon or a continuous-flow hysteroscope to raise the intrauterine pressure and wash away the blood.

Hysteroscopic diagnosis is primarily dependent on macroscopic visual appraisal of the mucosa or a lesion distorting the endometrial cavity. Typically these are mass or polypoid protrusions, bands or scars, foreign bodies such as bone or IUD fragments, or diverticular lesions such as an old perforation or necrotic myomas that have eroded into the endometrial cavity. The hysteroscopic diagnosis should always be supported by a histologic diagnosis whenever possible. Although the hysteroscopic appearance can give the gynecologist a strong presumptive diagnosis, a confirmative histologic evaluation will establish an unequivocal diagnosis. It is possible to date the endometrium by hysteroscopic appearance, although it requires substantial experience and is limited to discrimination of early, late proliferative, early and late secretory, and menstrual phases. The typical appearances are demonstrated in Figs. 3-21 through 3-24, which show early growth of vessels, development of tortuous vessels, the evolution of vertical branching to supply the thickening endometrium, the loss of the vessel pattern as the endometrium becomes thick and edematous, and finally scattered endometrial hemorrhage as the shedding begins. Endometrial biopsy to confirm the hysteroscopic impression is useful. The examinations illustrated require a 60× mag-

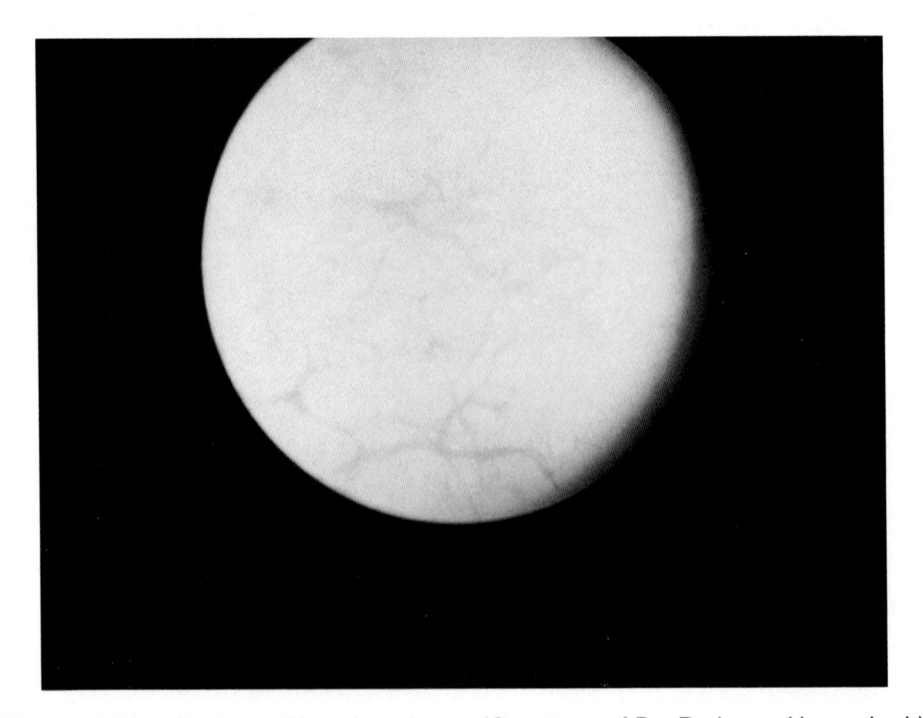

Figure 3-21. Early proliferative phase. (Courtesy of Dr. B. J. van Herendael.)

Hysteroscopy in Evaluation of the Endometrium 39

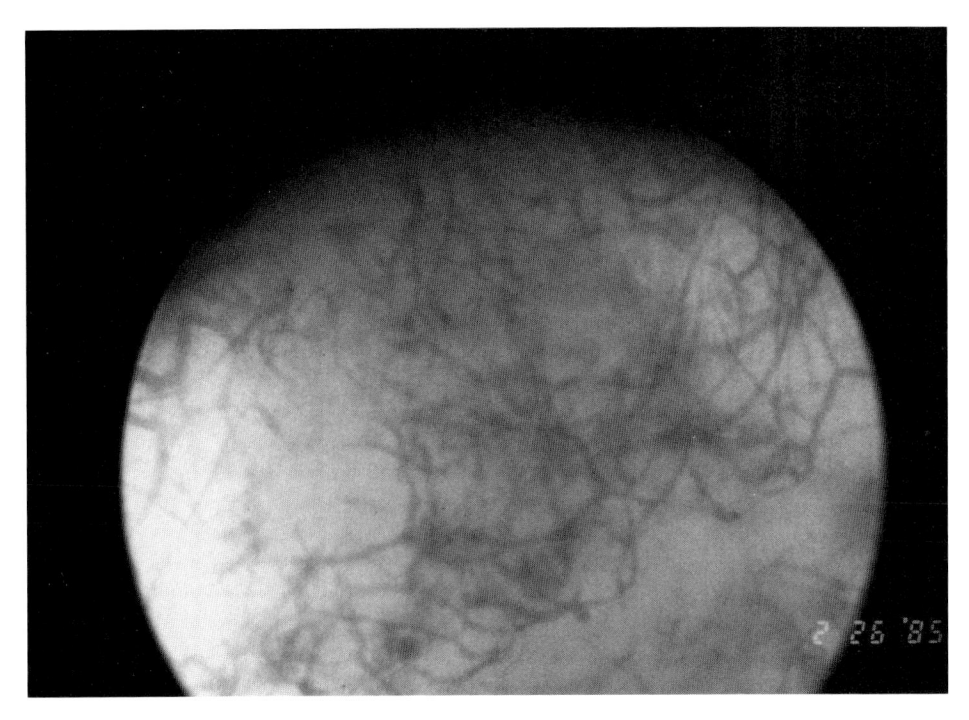

Figure 3-22. Early secretory phase. (Courtesy of Dr. B. J. van Herendael.)

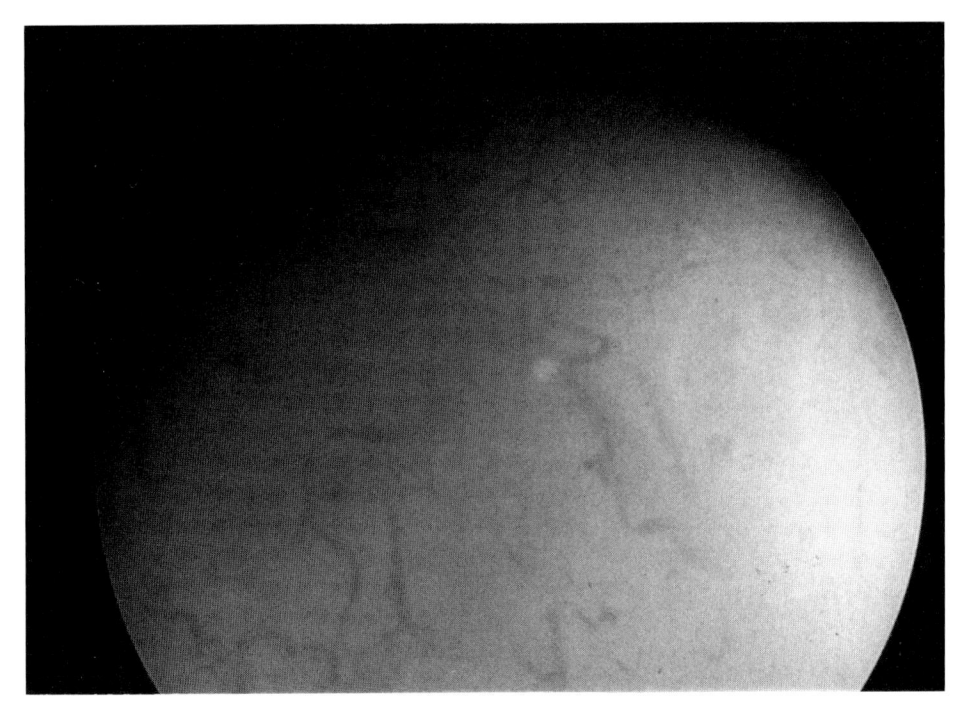

Figure 3-23. Late secretory phase. (Courtesy of Dr. B. J. van Herendael.)

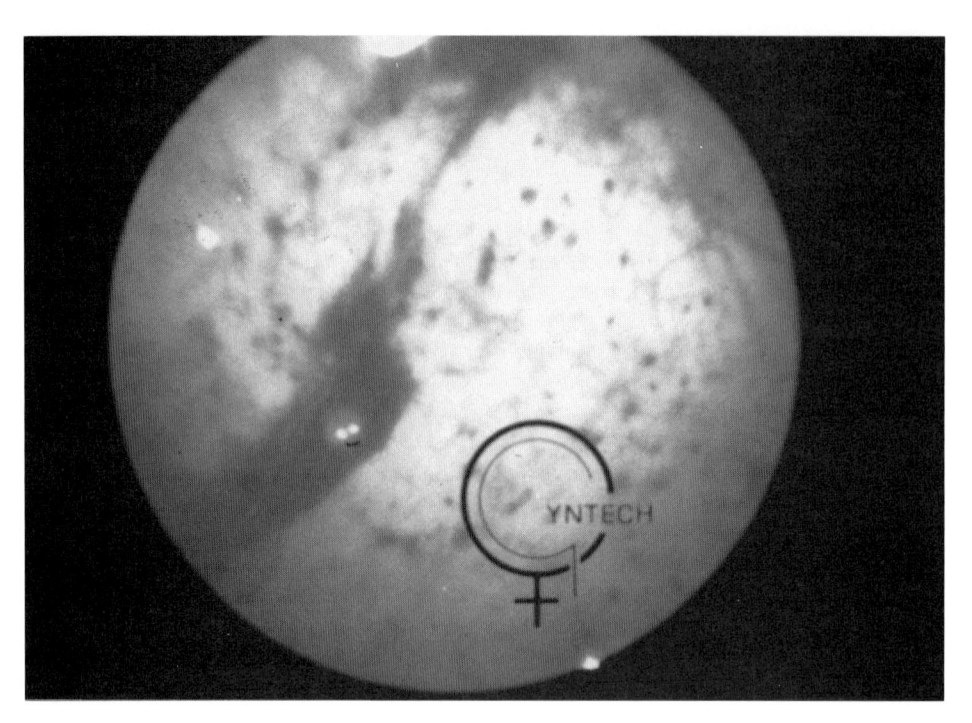

Figure 3-24. Premenstrual/menstrual endometrium. (Courtesy of Dr. B. J. van Herendael.)

nification of the hysteroscopic image and a zoom lens which was used to obtain the photographs, courtesy of Dr. B. J. van Herendael.[1]

In the final analysis, hysteroscopy adds definitive, direct, visual appraisal to the evaluation of the endometrial cavity. It is superior to the curette for anatomic appraisal as well as the other imaging techniques currently available. It provides the opportunity for focal as well as mapping biopsies. It also enables the operative hysteroscopist to perform excisional biopsies of mass lesions such as submucous myomata and polyps, and destroy the endometrium by resectoscopic excision or thermal destruction by laser or electrocoagulation. It is vital in removing some foreign bodies, as well as in correcting the septate anomaly of the uterus, and in selected instances of tubal obstruction at the uterotubal junction. Hysteroscopy has been a major advance in the appraisal of the endometrium and endometrial cavity.

REFERENCE

1. van Herendael BJ, Stevens MJ, Flakiewicz-Kula H, et al: Dating the Endometrium by Microhysteroscopy. *Acta Europaea Fertilitatis* 17:451–452, 1986.

PART II

Histology and Pathology of the Endometrium

4

Histopathology of the Endometrium— an Overview

Debra S. Heller, M.D.

ENDOMETRIAL SAMPLING

While endometrial sampling by cervical dilatation and curettage is regarded by some as the "gold standard," endometrial sampling may be accomplished by other methods. Office sampling devices such as the Pipelle suction curette (Unimar, Wilton CT) have the advantages of cost-effectiveness, safety, and patient acceptability, eliminating the need for anesthesia in most cases. A disadvantage of this technique is that less tissue is obtained than by techniques such as Vabra aspiration (Berkeley Medevices, Berkeley, CA), or by standard dilatation and curettage. While this generally does not cause difficulty in interpreting the sample in most cases, there is the concern that diagnosis may be limited by sampling error. Endometrial polyps and focal neoplasia may be missed, because the entire endometrium is not sampled.[1-3] However, in one study,[3] Pipelle biopsy was found to be accurate in detecting known endometrial carcinomas in the majority of cases. In cases of abnormal bleeding that persists after a normal reading of a Pipelle biopsy, a dilatation and curettage should be performed. The Pipelle biopsy technique is useful for assessing hormonal replacement therapy and for endometrial dating in infertility, since hormonal effects on the endometrium tend to be uniform. It is important for the clinician to realize that a pathology report of scanty tissue from a Pipelle biopsy, particularly in postmenopausal bleeding, may not reflect the amount of tissue present in the uterus. While scanty tissue may truly be present, it is also possible that very little or none of a copious amount of tissue was obtained. This is particularly true if the cervix is stenotic, or if the operator is inexperienced. It is up to the gynecologist to correlate such a report with the clinical situation.

The Vabra aspirator has the advantages of being usable in an office setting, and providing diagnostic accuracy. However, it is less well tolerated by patients.[4] Another office sampling device, in decreasing clinical use, the Novak curette, is also reportedly more painful than the Pipelle.[5]

The type of endometrial sampling device selected, then, is a decision based on a number of factors including cost, convenience, patient preference, and the likelihood of obtaining diagnostic material. In the case of therapeutic curettage, the method chosen must be able to remove a significant amount of tissue. Sampling for diagnostic indications requires less tissue in most cases. Endometrial sampling may be performed, with or without adjunctive hysteroscopy, in either an office or hospital setting.

LIMITATIONS OF ENDOMETRIAL SAMPLING

Satisfactory histologic evaluation of an endometrial sample is dependent on three things: the tissue, the gynecologist, and the pathologist.

Tissue Limitations

An inadequate amount of tissue yields an unsatisfactory or limited diagnosis. This does not mean that all scanty specimens are inadequate for evaluation. It is important to know when to expect scanty or abundant tissue (Table 4-1).

While abundant tissue is not necessary to ensure adequacy of sampling, certain features are necessary in small specimens. As an example, endometrial dating requires the presence of surface epithelium for accuracy, since the surface is where the later secretory changes initially develop. Predecidualization under the surface epithelium occurs on day 25. If no surface is sampled, this change will be missed, and less precise dating is possible. In such cases, the report might state "scanty secretory endometrium. The changes are at least as advanced as day 23." This obviously is less helpful to the clinician. Likewise, if basalis endometrium is obtained without functionalis, normal cyclical changes will not be seen.

Tissue orientation is important, so gentle handling of specimens is advised. Artifacts can be produced by squeezing of the tissue, which may then simulate hyperplasia (Fig. 4-1). Sometimes unavoidable fragmentation of endometrial polyps makes their diagnosis difficult, obscuring the diagnostic criteria.

Prompt fixation of the tissue is crucial, as autolysis develops rapidly (Fig. 4-2). Not only is it important to place the tissue into fixative immediately, but care should be taken that the specimen jar is tightly closed. Unreadable specimens, where the formalin leaked out of the bottle on the way to the laboratory, are sometimes received.

TABLE 4-1. Amount of Expected Endometrial Tissue in a Sample

Scanty
    Some suction biopsy samples, particularly with inexperienced operator or cervical stenosis
    Prolonged bleeding
    Atrophic endometrium
    Asherman's syndrome
    Recent menses
    Some drug effects: prolonged therapy with oral contraceptives, GnRH agonists, danazol (Danocrine), and progestins

Abundant
    Late proliferative endometrium
    Secretory endometrium
    Pregnancy related conditions
    Some drug effects: hormonal therapy with estrogen predominance, some patients on tamoxifen (Nolvadex) therapy
    Endometrial hyperplasia
    Carcinoma or other endometrial malignancy

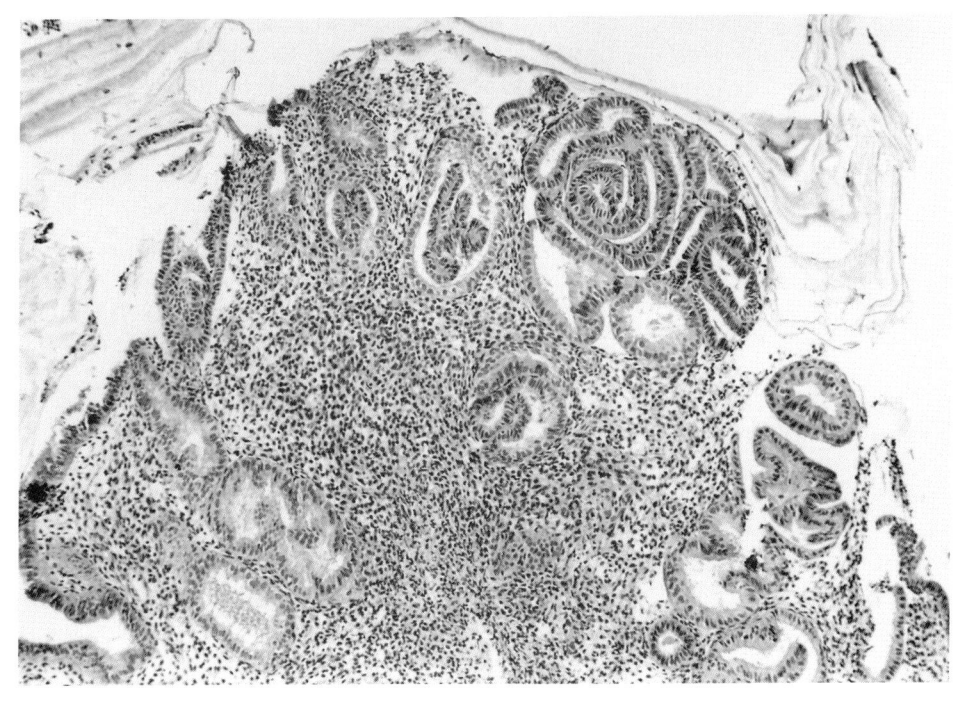

Figure 4-1. Squeezing of endometrial tissue produces glandular crowding, simulating hyperplasia.

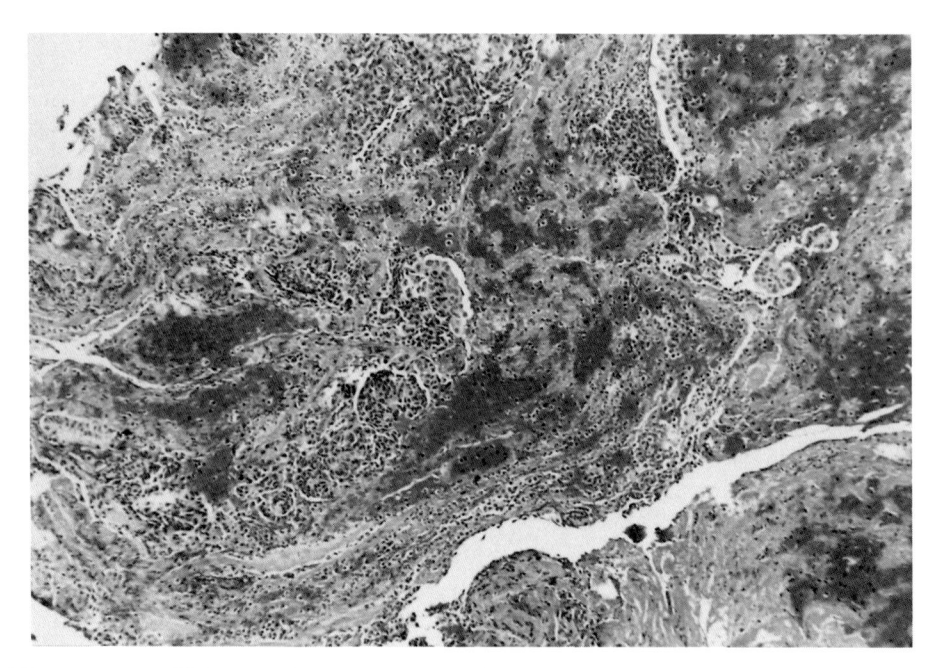

Figure 4-2. This specimen was not fixed properly and underwent severe autolysis. Note the loss of detail.

Timing of endometrial sampling is important in several circumstances. Diagnosis of a luteal phase defect is best made when the biopsy comes from the late secretory period. Irregular shedding due to persistent corpus luteum function is diagnosable after the bleeding has persisted for at least 5 days. When a patient is having heavy bleeding, a precise diagnosis may be difficult, with "menstrual-type endometrium" as the only interpretation possible, with no discernable etiology. However, waiting until the bleeding stops may cause loss of the tissue diagnostic for a hyperplasia,[6] or may be clinically inadvisable. Labeling a specimen "RUSH" sometimes leads to a different processing procedure, with less optimally fixed tissue for evaluation, and should be reserved for circumstances where an earlier report is truly necessary.

The Role of the Gynecologist

It is extremely important for the clinician to provide an adequate history to obtain the most accurate diagnosis. This includes the patient's age, last menstrual period, menstrual pattern if abnormal, any hormonal or IUD usage, pertinent medical history (such as hematologic disorders), and reason for endometrial sampling. An example of lack of history limiting a report is when a pathologist hesitates to report a change consistent with hormonal effect if not given a history of hormonal administration. A clinical correlation made utilizing a pathology report signed out without a history may not be as accurate as one done with a clinical history, and does a disservice to the patient.

The Role of the Pathologist

The pathologist should be liberal in contacting the clinician for more information, particularly if the wording of the report depends on the information. A report of "These changes are consistent with progesterone administration" will be more helpful to the gynecologist than a description of the tissue changes alone.

In difficult cases, direct verbal communication between the gynecologist and the pathologist can expedite diagnoses and ensure greater diagnostic accuracy. Sometimes these conversations lead to additional action that may affect the outcome of the case. For example, if a gynecologist states that curettage yielded copious tissue but the report indicates that the tissue was scant, deeper sections into the block may be made to attempt to identify more tissue, or the clinician can be informed that the abundant specimen consisted primarily of blood clot or mucus.

PITFALLS IN DIAGNOSIS

Given optimally fixed tissue and a relevant clinical history, the pathologist will still encounter pitfalls in evaluation of the endometrium. The quantity of tissue obtained is often related to the clinical situation, and the amount of tissue received should be described grossly prior to processing. Elements seen on the slide may be confusing. These include specimens containing endometrium from the lower uterine segment, basalis endometrium, cervical tissue, smooth muscle, foreign elements, and tissue artifacts.

Lower Uterine Segment

The lower uterine segment responds minimally, if at all, to the cyclic hormonal changes to which it is exposed. The stroma is more fibrous and less cellular than fundal stroma, but more cellular than cervical stroma. The glands may be mixed endometrial and endocervical, or show hybrid features (Fig. 4-3).

Basalis

The basalis is the site of regeneration of the functionalis, and its overzealous removal may lead to Asherman's syndrome, particularly in the gravid uterus. The basalis does not cycle with the functionalis, and is not shed during menses.

Basalis glands are weakly proliferative (Fig. 4-4A), except in pregnancy when secretory changes are seen.[7] The stroma is dense, with thick walled vessels, and may contain lymphoid aggregates (Fig. 4-4B). The lymphoid cells are normal, and should not be construed as inflammatory. If lower

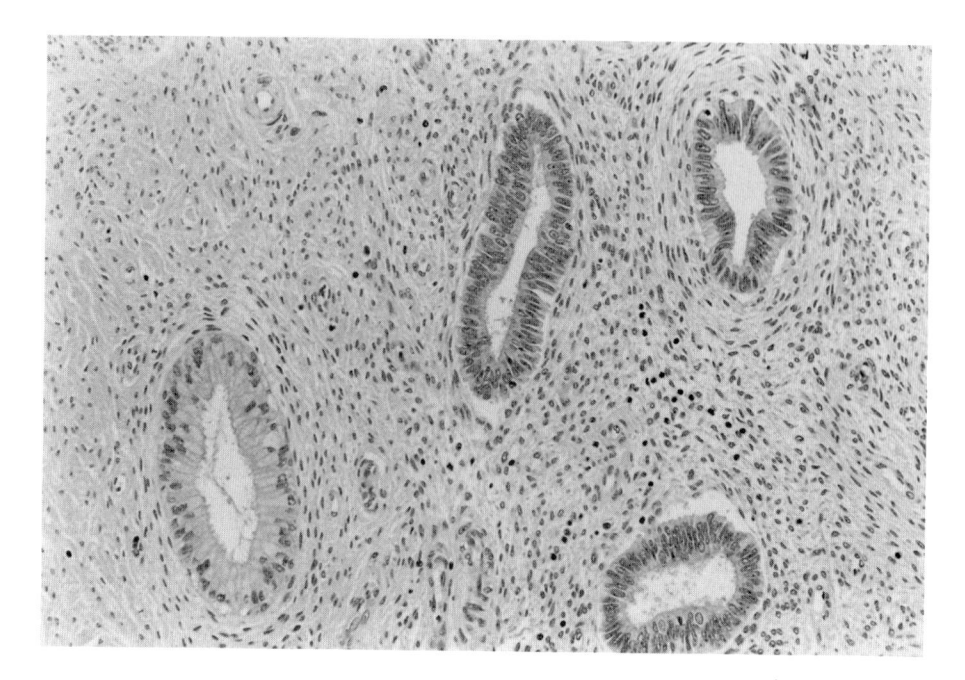

Figure 4-3. In this section of lower uterine segment, there is a mixture of endocervical and endometrial glands in a stroma more cellular than endocervical stroma and more fibrous than endometrial stroma.

uterine segment or basalis endometrium is not recognized, a diagnosis of inactive endometrium may be inadvertently rendered. Basalis meets the myometrium irregularly (Fig. 4-5), and this should not be confused with myometrial invasion by a carcinoma.

Cervical Tissue

Cervical tissue is frequently seen mixed in with an endometrial specimen, and may consist of endocervical tissue, exocervical tissue, metaplastic tissue from the transformation zone, or even neoplastic cervical tissue (Fig. 4-6), which fragments more easily than normal cervical tissue.

Smooth Muscle

Fragments of smooth muscle in a curettage specimen may represent myometrium or a submucous leiomyoma. The distinction is not always possible, but certain features are suggestive of a submucous leiomyoma. A whole microscopic leiomyoma is occasionally obtained (Fig. 4-7). If a fragment of leiomyoma is present, whorled fascicles of smooth muscle, and sometimes compressed overlying endometrium may be seen. Normal myometrium is more likely to demonstrate larger muscle bundles, and overlying endome-

Pitfalls in Diagnosis

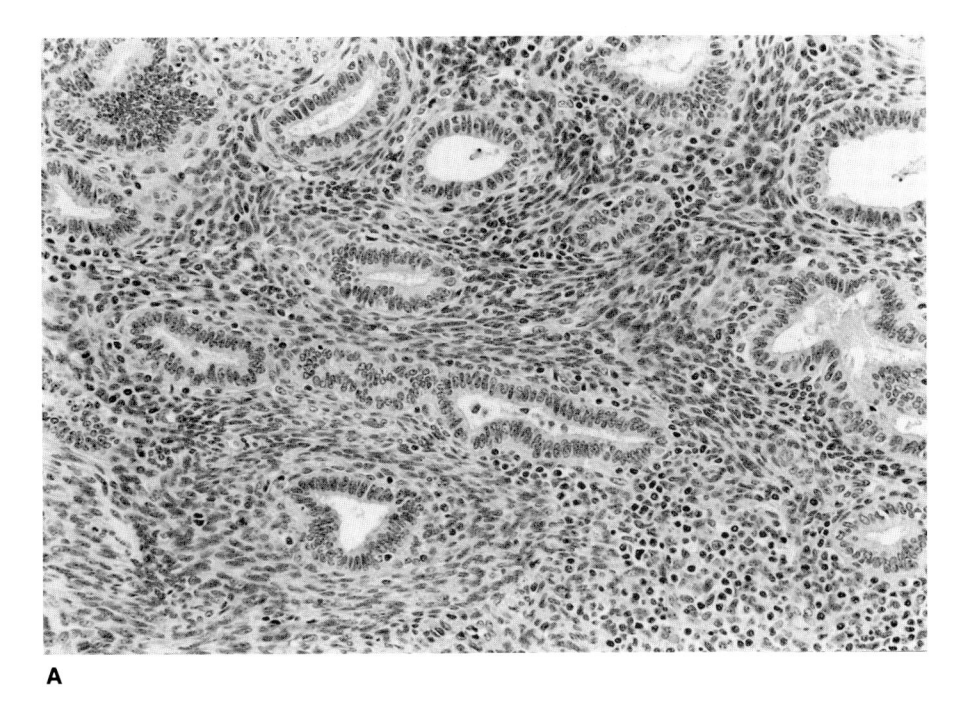

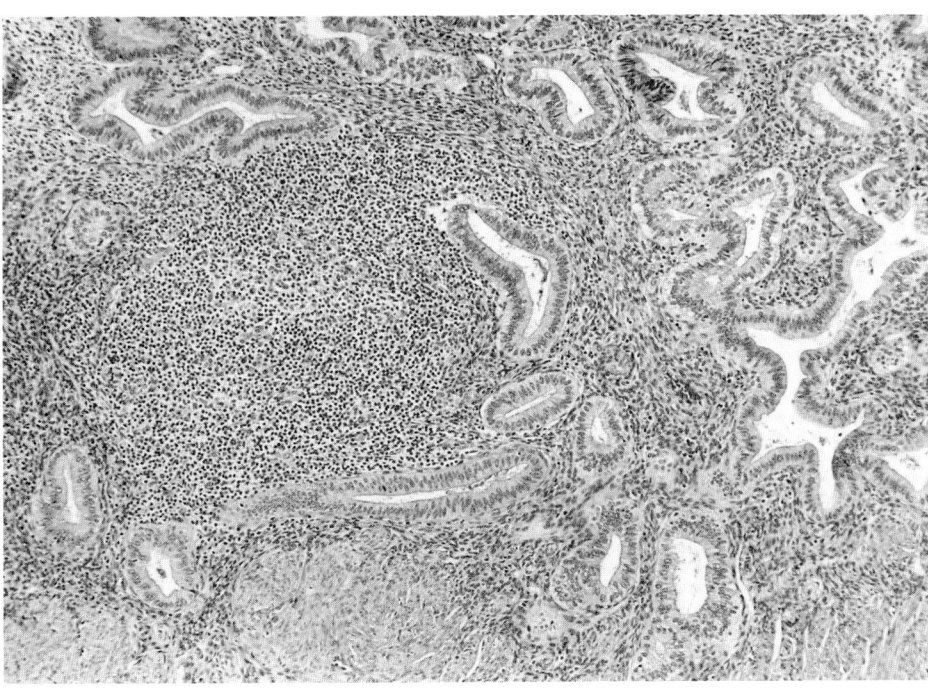

Figure 4-4. (A) The glands of the basalis are weakly proliferative, in a cellular stroma. (B) Lymphoid aggregates are common in the basalis.

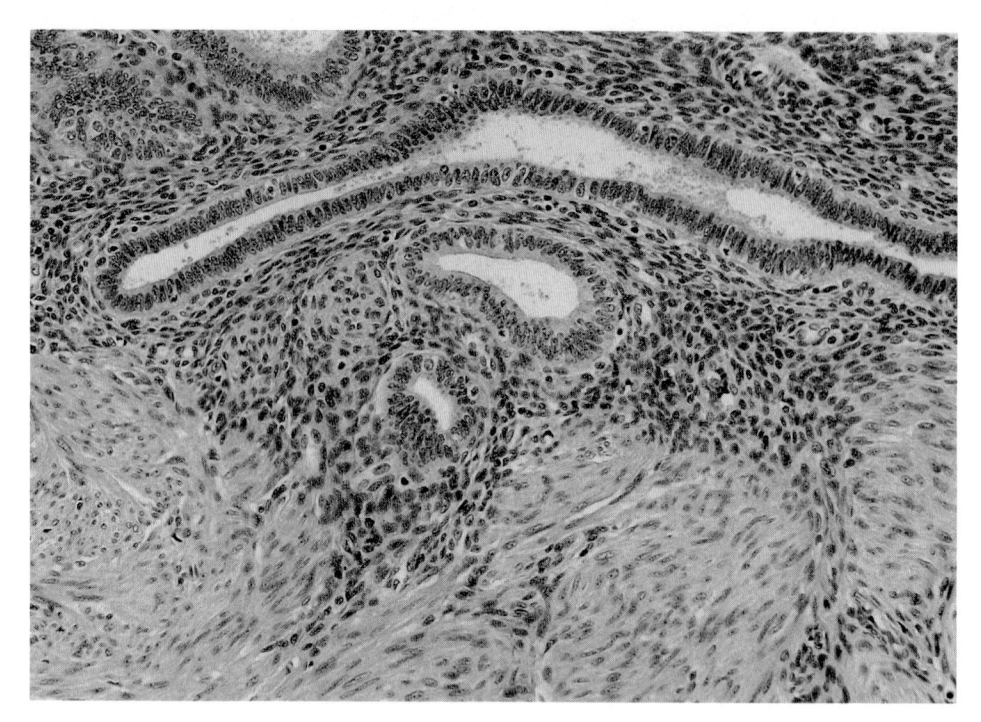

Figure 4-5. The junction between the basalis and the myometrium is irregular, and this should not be confused with myometrial invasion by an endometrial carcinoma.

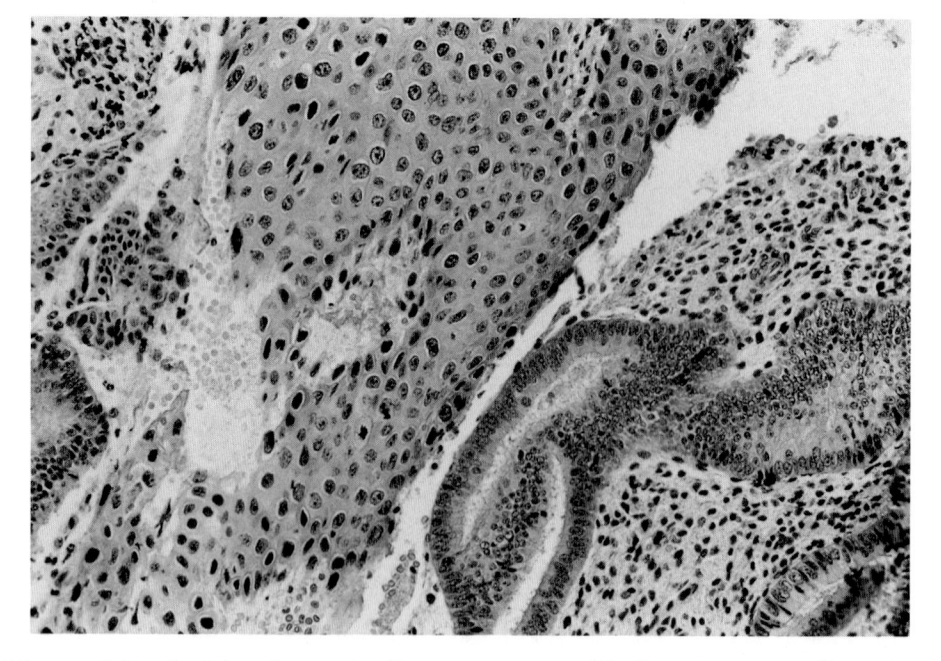

Figure 4-6. A strip of neoplastic squamous epithelium is seen adjacent to proliferative endometrium.

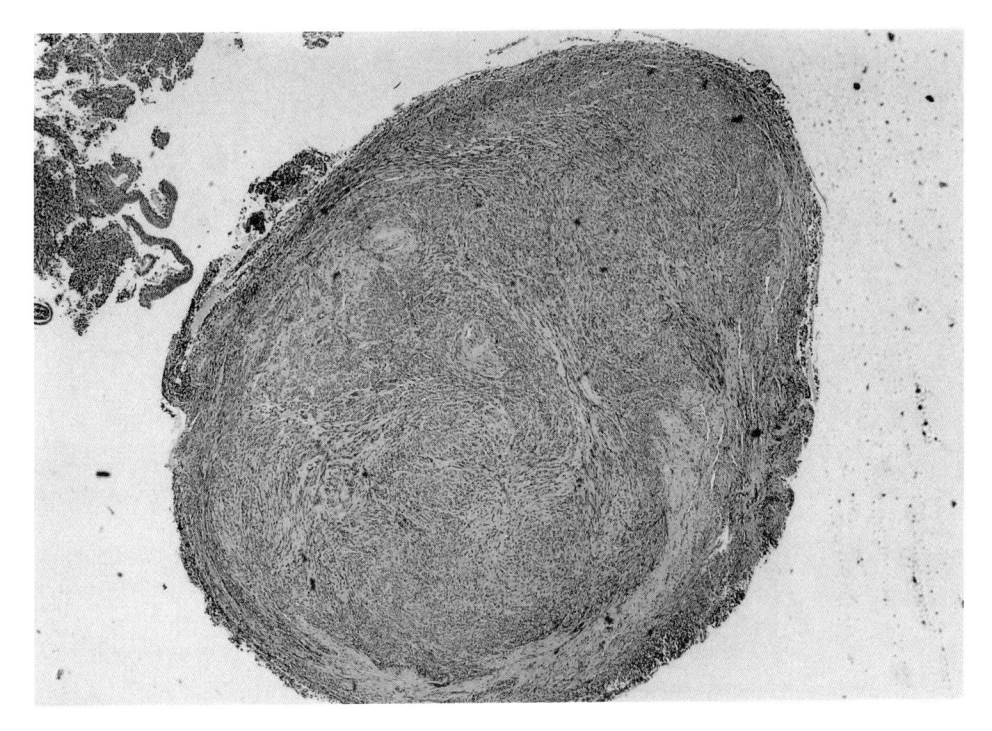

Figure 4-7. An entire small leiomyoma is present in this curettage specimen.

trium tends to be basalis.[6] Sometimes the distinction cannot be made histologically, but the clinician may have felt a submucous leiomyoma with the curette, or seen it with the hysteroscope.

Foreign Elements

When foreign elements are present in an endometrial specimen, there are several possible explanations. These include metastatic disease (Fig. 4-8) contaminants (Fig. 4-9), or evidence of uterine perforation. Adipose tissue on an endometrial slide may be a contaminant, but may be evidence of a uterine perforation,[8] and the clinician should be immediately notified. A contaminant may occur either before or after the tissue block is prepared, with different histologic results.

Tissue is processed by placing it in a tissue cassette where it is embedded in paraffin, forming a tissue block. Slides are prepared by slicing the tissue block at intervals of about 4.5 μm, so that sequential sections can be obtained (Fig. 4-10). A ribbon containing multiple sections of the same piece of tissue is then floated on a water bath, and the slide is prepared by slipping it under the sections. If a contaminant is mixed with the specimen prior to preparing the tissue block, the contaminant will be seen on multiple sections. If it is picked up in the water bath after the ribbon is cut from the block, it

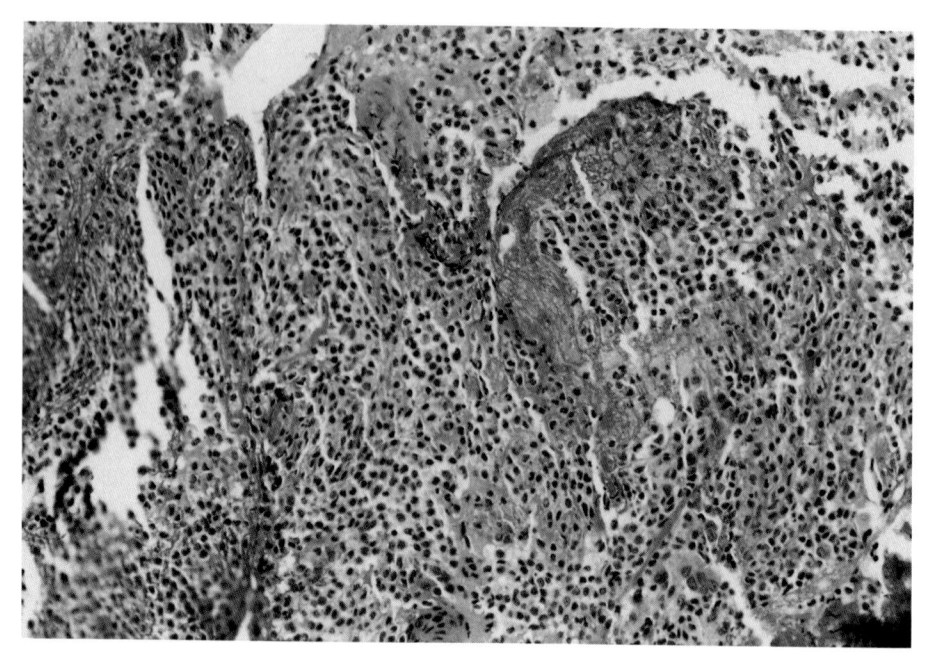

Figure 4-8. Atypical transitional epithelium is present in this curettage specimen from a patient with known transitional cell carcinoma of the bladder.

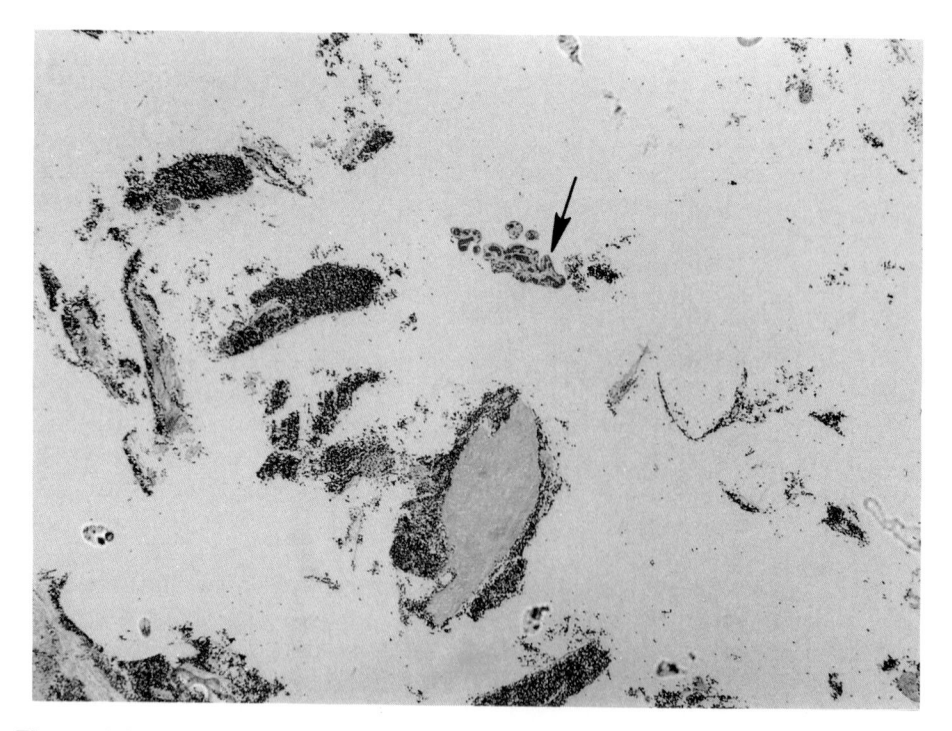

Figure 4-9. A mature chorionic villus (arrow) among fragments of blood clot in this specimen from a postmenopausal woman represents a contaminant. It was present on multiple levels, and was thus present within the tissue block.

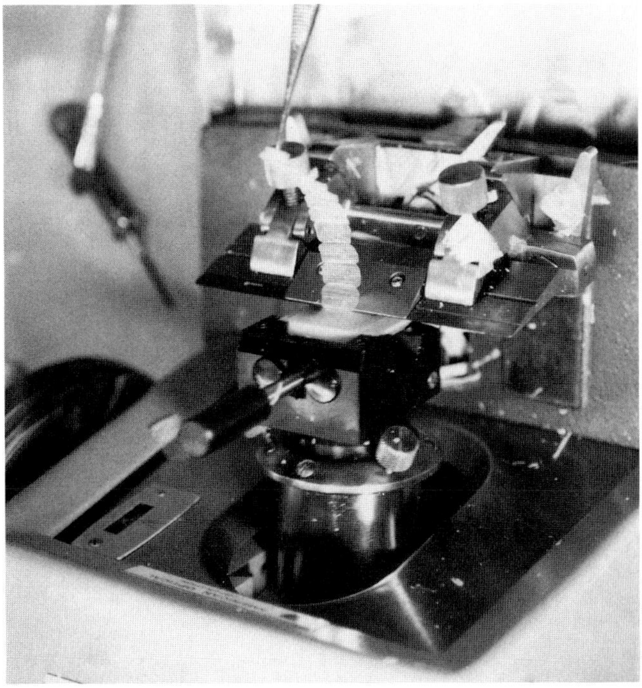

Pitfalls in Diagnosis

Figure 4-10. A ribbon containing multiple tissue sections approximately 4–5 μm apart is cut from the tissue block. This ribbon is floated on a water bath, and picked up on a glass slide.

will be seen in only one section. In this case, cutting additional sections may resolve the problem. In cases where the contaminant is clearly unrelated (e.g., a fragment of prostate in the curettings), there is no diagnostic problem. The difficulty arises when there is one tiny fragment of endometrial carcinoma in an otherwise negative specimen, or one chorionic villus up in the corner of the slide in a case of suspected ectopic pregnancy. Here levels cut from the tissue block may help, as deeper sections may show the carcinoma attached to adjacent endometrium, or additional chorionic villi may be seen. If the problem cannot be resolved, the tissue has to be completely described, with a proviso of "this may represent a floater, clinical correlation is advised." Meticulous laboratory technique minimizes this problem.

Endometrial Artifacts

Intussusception of endometrial glands leads to telescoping, which can be mistaken for hyperplasia (Fig. 4-11). Squeezing of the tissue produces crowding artifacts, which are occasionally mistaken for hyperplasia (Fig. 4-1). A careful evaluation of all the tissue on the slides is helpful in avoiding these pitfalls. Delay in fixation can lead to glands retracting from the stroma (Fig. 4-12), or to simulation of secretory vacuolization of the glands.[7]

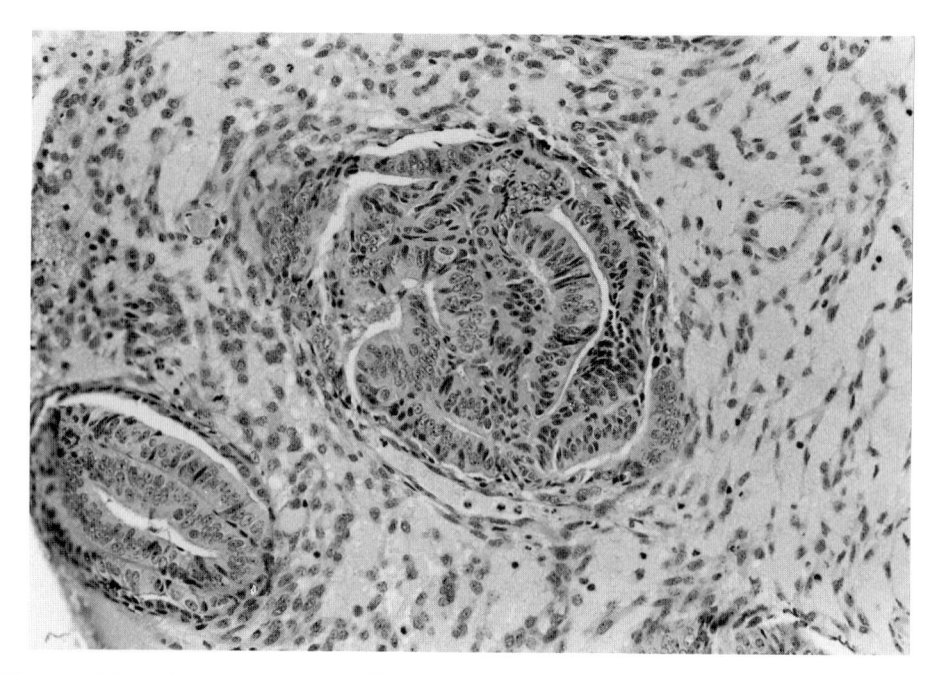

Figure 4-11. Telescoping artifact occurs when there is intussusception of glands. This appearance should not be mistaken for hyperplasia.

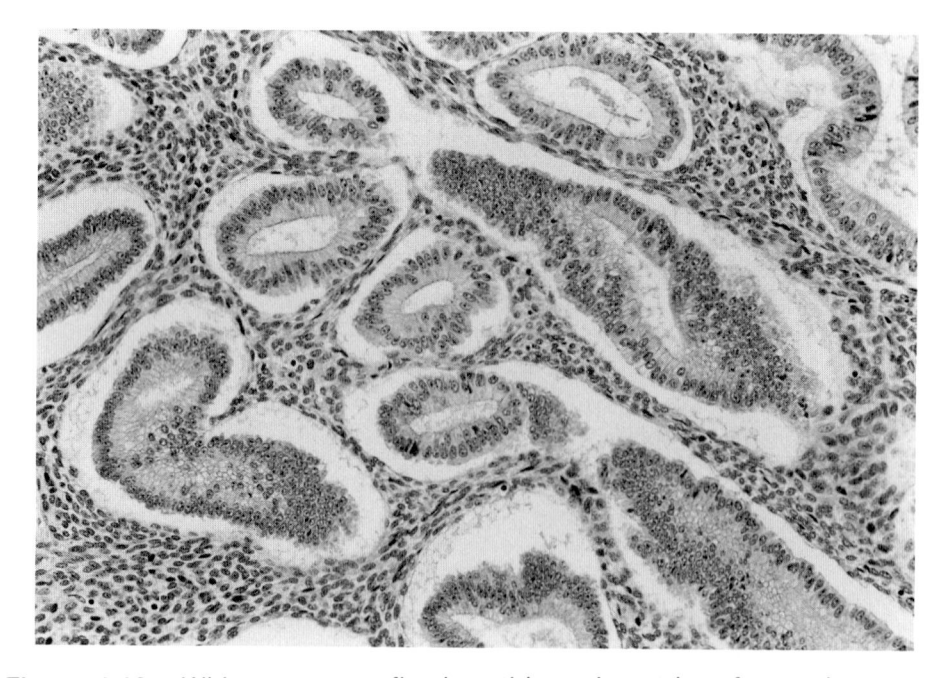

Figure 4-12. Without prompt fixation, this endometrium from a hysterectomy specimen shows retraction artifact, with space between the glands and stroma.

SUMMARY

Optimal evaluation of the endometrium is dependent on clinical information, a sufficient quantity of tissue, adequate fixation, and correct processing. Care taken by all parties involved and good communication between clinician and pathologist will lead to the best possible evaluation of the patient's problem.

REFERENCES

1. Rodriguez G, Yaqub N, King M: A comparison of the Pipelle device and the Vabra aspirator as measured by endometrial denudation in hysterectomy specimens: the Pipelle device samples significantly less of the endometrial surface than the Vabra aspirator. *Am J Obstet Gynecol* 168:55–59, 1993.
2. Friedman F, Brodman ML: Endometrial Sampling Techniques. In Altchek A, Deligdisch L (eds): *The uterus—pathology, diagnosis, and management.* Springer-Verlag, New York, 1991, pp 155–162.
3. Stovall TG, Photopoulos GJ, Poston WM, et al: Pipelle endometrial sampling in patients with known endometrial carcinoma. *Obstet Gynecol* 77:954–956, 1991.
4. Kaunitz AM, Masciello A, Ostrowski M, et al: Comparison of endometrial biopsy with the endometrial Pipelle and the Vabra aspirator. *J Reprod Med* 33:427–429, 1988.
5. Stovall TG, Ling FW, Morgan PL: A prospective, randomized comparison of the Pipelle endometrial sampling device with the Novak curette. *Am J Obstet Gynecol* 165:1287–1290, 1991.
6. Dallenbach-Hellweg G: *Histopathology of the endometrium,* 4th ed. Springer-Verlag, Berlin, 1987, pp 2–3, 18–19.
7. Hendrickson MR, Kempson RL: *Surgical pathology of the uterine corpus.* Saunders, Philadelphia, 1980, pp 40, 811.
8. Blaustein A: *Interpretation of endometrial biopsies,* 2nd ed. Raven Press, New York, 1985, p 20.

5

The Normal Endometrium

Debra S. Heller, M.D.

NORMAL ENDOMETRIUM

The endometrium lining the uterine corpus is composed of the functional layer (functionalis) and the basal layer (basalis). The functional layer is highly responsive to the cyclic changes in estrogen and progesterone that occur during the menstrual cycle, exhibiting predictable morphologic changes. Most of the functionalis is shed during menses, and it is the basalis that gives rise to the next cycle's functionalis. The basalis does not respond to the hormonal changes of the menstrual cycle, and generally remains weakly proliferative throughout the cycle. The following discussion of the endometrial changes seen during the menstrual cycle refers to the functionalis.

ENDOMETRIAL COMPONENTS

The endometrium is composed of epithelial glands contained within a cellular stroma. The glands appear different at different times of the cycle (see Table 5-1), reflecting the nature of the hormonal stimulation. The columnar cells of the glandular epithelium may show proliferative or secretory features. In addition, ciliated cells may also be present, scattered between the columnar cells (Fig. 5-1).

The endometrial stroma is composed predominantly of the stromal cells, whose appearance also changes during the menstrual cycle. The stromal cells are embedded in a reticulin network. Also present may be stromal granulocytes and lymphocytes, including lymphoid aggregates and follicles (Fig.

TABLE 5-1. A Quick Reference for Dating the Endometrium

Point in cycle	Glands	Stroma
Menstrual	Fragmented, nuclear dust	Stromal "balls," fibrin thrombi
Early proliferative	Tubular, +mitoses	Loose
Midproliferative	Coiled, +mitoses	Edematous, +mitoses
Late proliferative	More coiled, ++mitoses; ± occasional subnuclear vacuoles	Compact, ++mitoses
Day 16 (POD 2)	Uniform subnuclear vacuoles ≦ 50% glands	Fewer mitoses
Day 17 (POD 3)	Uniform subnuclear vacuoles throughout, mitoses absent or rare	Rare or no mitoses
Day 18 (POD 4)	Subnuclear and supranuclear vacuoles	
Day 19 (POD 5)	Supranuclear vacuoles	
Day 20 (POD 6)	Peak secretion	
Day 21 (POD 7)	± secretions seen in glands	Beginning edema
Day 22 (POD 8)		Peak edema, naked nuclei
Day 23 (POD 9)	Developing secretory exhaustion	Spiral arterioles prominent, stromal mitoses reappear
Day 24 (POD 10)		Thick predecidual cuffing of spiral arterioles, increased stromal mitoses
Day 25 (POD 11)	Sawtooth glands	Predecidua under surface
Day 26 (POD 12)		Marked predecidual change, +stromal granulocytes
Day 27 (POD 13)		Diffuse predecidual change ++stromal granulocytes
Day 28 (POD 14)	Collapse	Early breakdown and hemorrhage

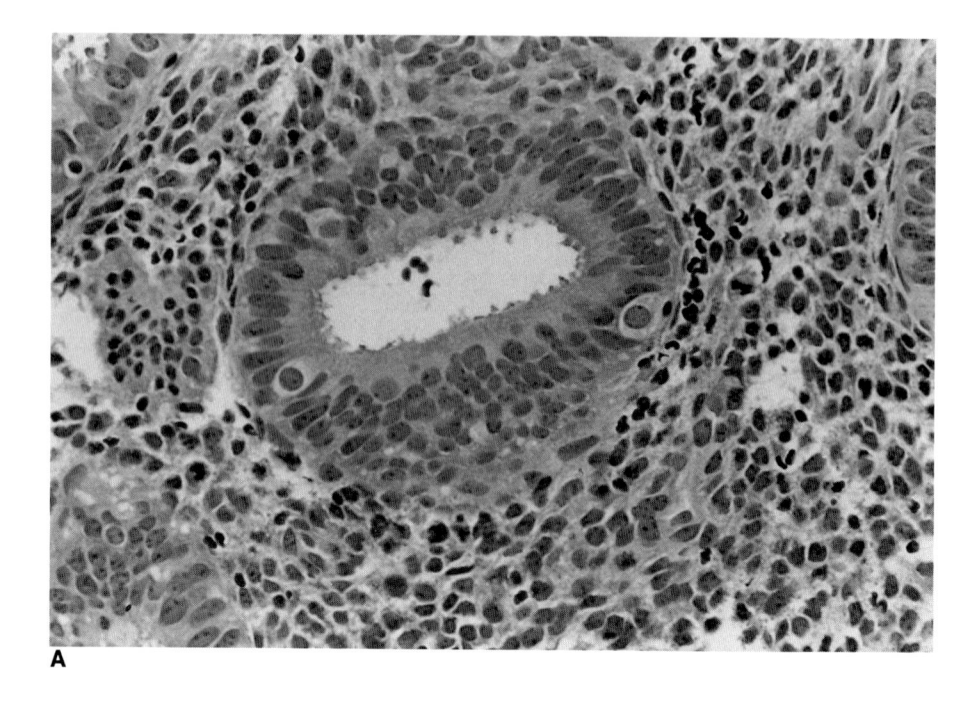

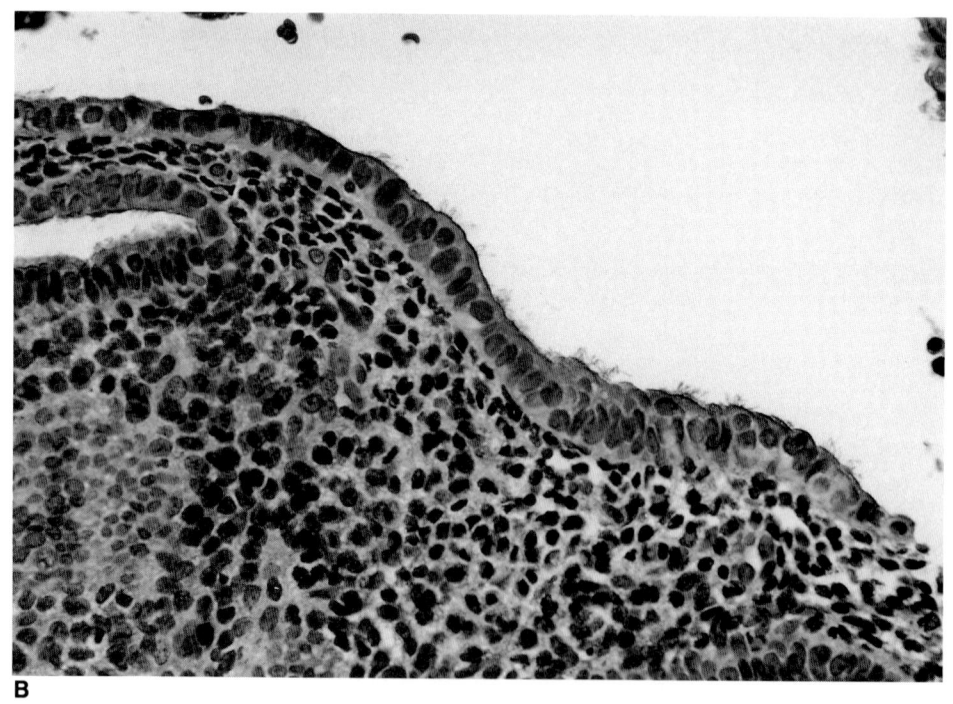

Figure 5-1. (A) Scattered ciliated cells are commonly seen in normal endometrial specimens. Here the characteristic perinuclear halos are seen at the 4 o'clock and 8 o'clock positions. (B) Cilia are seen on some of the surface epithelial cells.

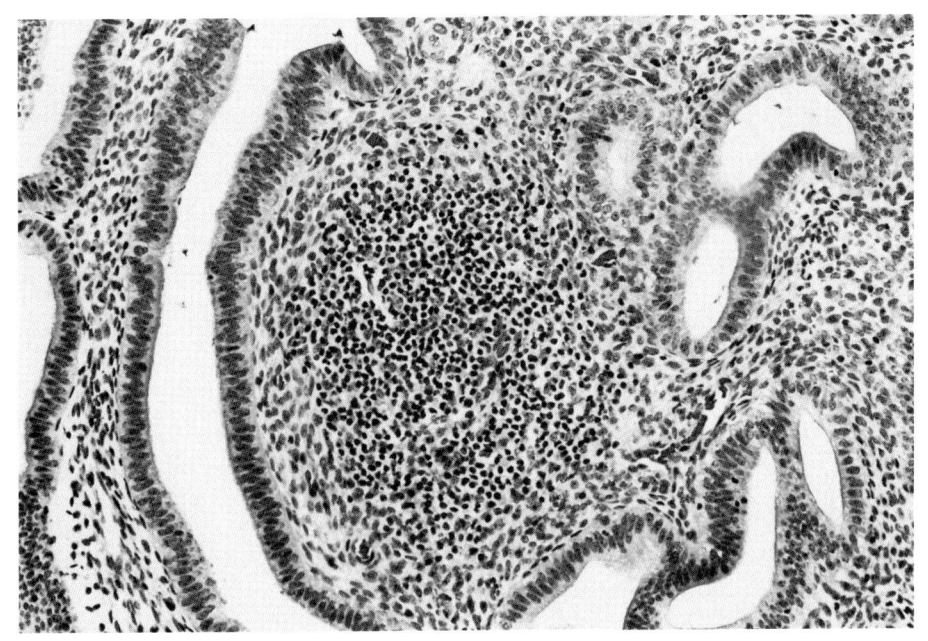

Figure 5-2. Lymphoid aggregates are a normal finding in proliferative endometrium.

5-2). Stromal foam cells may be seen, but these usually occur in hyperplastic and neoplastic processes. Spiral arterioles are also present within the stroma, and their appearance varies with the cycle.

THE MENSTRUAL CYCLE

The criteria established by the classic work of Noyes and colleagues[1] describing in detail the endometrial changes seen during the menstrual cycle are generally used to date the endometrium. Endometrial dating is most commonly employed in the workup of infertility, but it can also be useful in evaluating dysfunctional uterine bleeding. Morphologic endometrial dating is based on the concept of a 28-day cycle, with day 1 being the first day of menses. In this schema, ovulation occurs on cycle day 14, with predictable endometrial changes occurring starting on day 16 [postovulatory day (POD) 2]. While it had been generally accepted that the luteal phase is a constant 14 days, with any cycle variability occurring in the follicular (proliferative) phase, this has been shown to be inaccurate. Fertile women have also been shown to vary in the length of their luteal phase,[2] and predictable endometrial morphology is better related to the LH (luteinizing hormone) surge than the chronologic date.[3] It has been recommended by some that morphologic endometrial dating be correlated with serum hormonal levels;[4] however, many clinicians obtain satisfactory results by timing their biopsies by basal body temperatures, and correlating the results with the subsequent menstrual period.

A few other caveats about endometrial dating are necessary. An endometrial sample may not show the textbook features of a single day, and often demonstrates overlapping features of 2 days. It is perfectly appropriate to report a sample as "Secretory endometrium, day 17–18." It should also be recognized that, as in any subjective endeavor, there will be interobserver variation. (The same pathologist may even assign different dates to the same specimen on different days!)

Proliferative Endometrium

Proliferative endometrium cannot be dated to the day with accuracy, but the early, mid-, and late proliferative endometrial periods may be distinguished.

Early proliferative endometrium (cycle days 4–7) contains straight or minimally coiled tubular glands. Blood vessels are thin-walled and straight. The glandular epithelium is pseudostratified, and mitotic figures are present in the glands (Fig. 5-3). As the proliferative period progresses, glands and vessels become increasingly coiled, creating a more complex histologic picture. There are increased numbers of glandular mitoses, and by the late proliferative phase, scattered subnuclear vacuoles may be seen in some of the glands.

In the early proliferative phase, the stroma is cellular and loosely arranged. Stromal cells have round to spindle-shaped nuclei, and minimal cytoplasm.

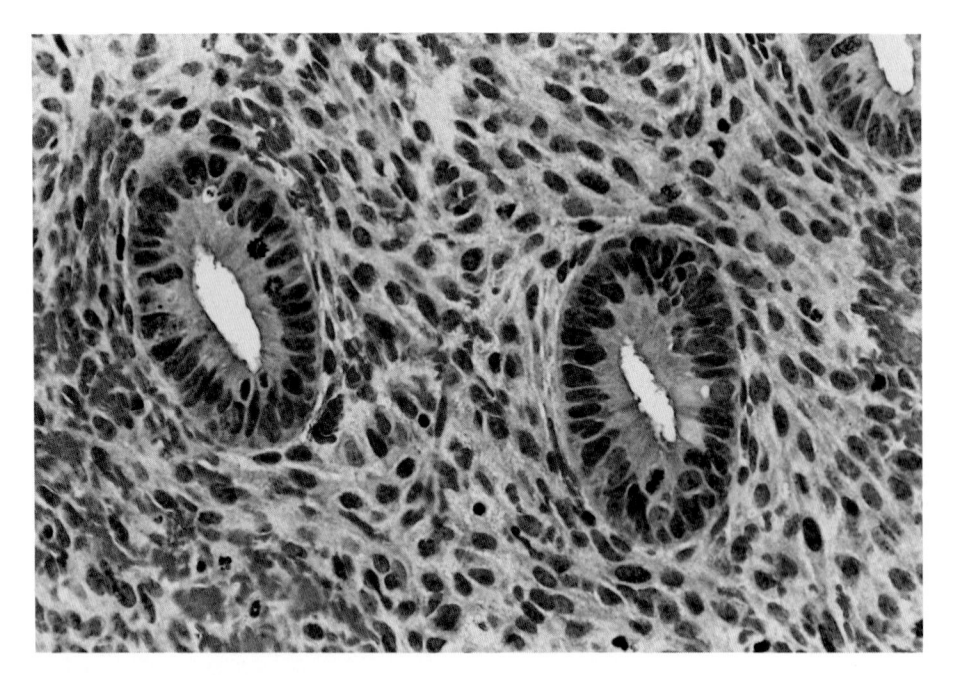

Figure 5-3. Early proliferative endometrium with small tubular glands. The epithelium is pseudostratified, and mitoses are easily seen.

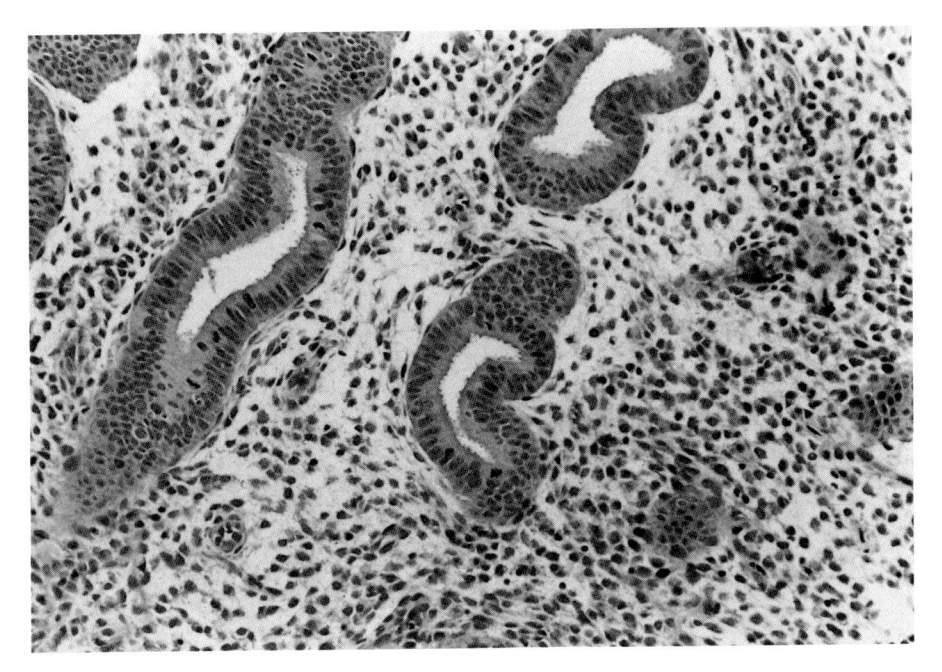

Figure 5-4. Midproliferative endometrium shows stromal edema and increasing complexity of the glands.

Stromal edema is present in the midproliferative period (cycle days 8–10) (Fig. 5-4), but regresses by the late proliferative period (days 11–14) (Fig. 5-5). Stromal mitoses are seen by the midproliferative phase. As with gland mitoses, these increase in the late proliferative period.

Secretory Endometrium

During the late proliferative phase and the first day's postovulation (POD 1 and 2, cycle days 15 and 16), the definite diagnosis of ovulation is not possible by morphologic criteria. The endometrium basically appears late proliferative during this time, and the scattered subnuclear vacuoles in the glands may represent an estrogen effect alone, or may represent ovulation. This period has been called the interval phase.[4] On cycle day 16 (POD 2), there is uniform subnuclear vacuolization in at least 50% of the glands (Fig. 5-6). By cycle day 17 (POD 3), all the glands show uniform subnuclear vacuolization, and mitoses are absent or rare (Fig. 5-7). This is the first definite evidence of ovulation. These secretory vacuoles migrate up around the nuclei, assuming both subnuclear and supranuclear positions on cycle day 18 (POD 4) (Fig. 5-8), and all assume supranuclear positions on cycle day 19 (POD 5) (Fig. 5-9). On cycle day 20 (POD 6), there is peak secretion (Fig. 5-10), with dilated glands filled with secretory material. Secretory "snouts" may be seen on the apical surface of the glandular epithelium. The remaining secretory period is dated by stromal changes. There is progression of glandular secre-

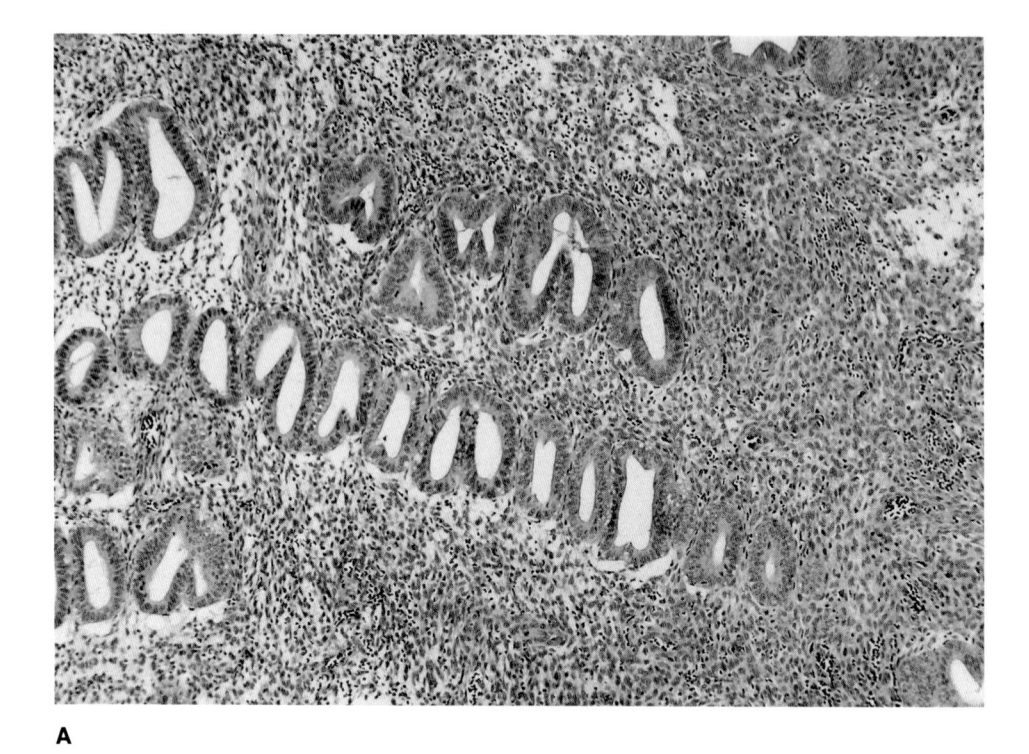

Figure 5-5. (A) In late proliferative endometrium, glands are tortuous. (B) Mitoses are abundant in glands and stroma.

The Menstrual Cycle

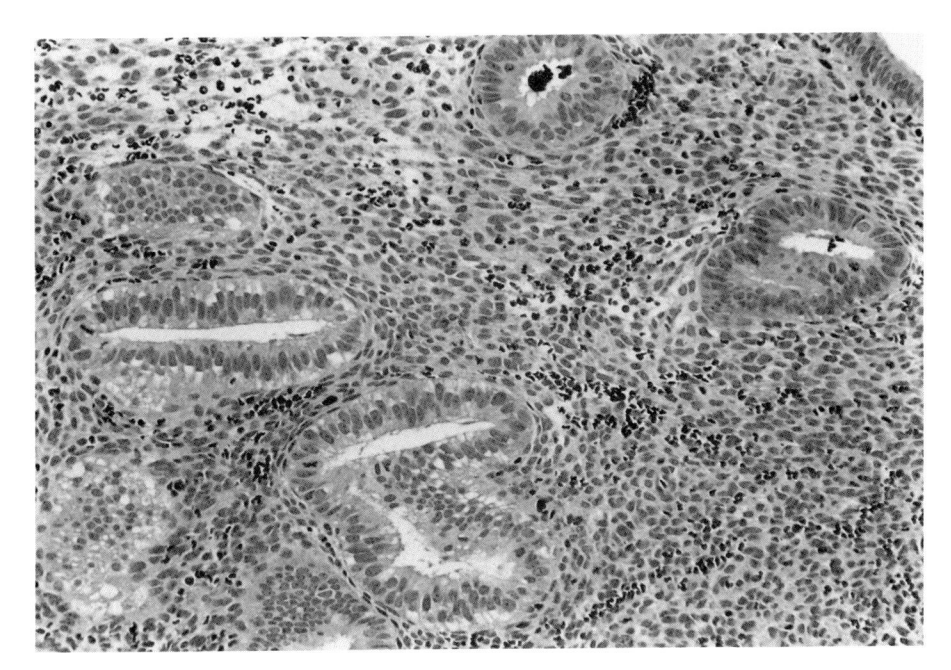

Figure 5-6. On cycle day 16 (POD 2), subnuclear vacuoles are seen in half of the glands, but the rest are still proliferative in appearance.

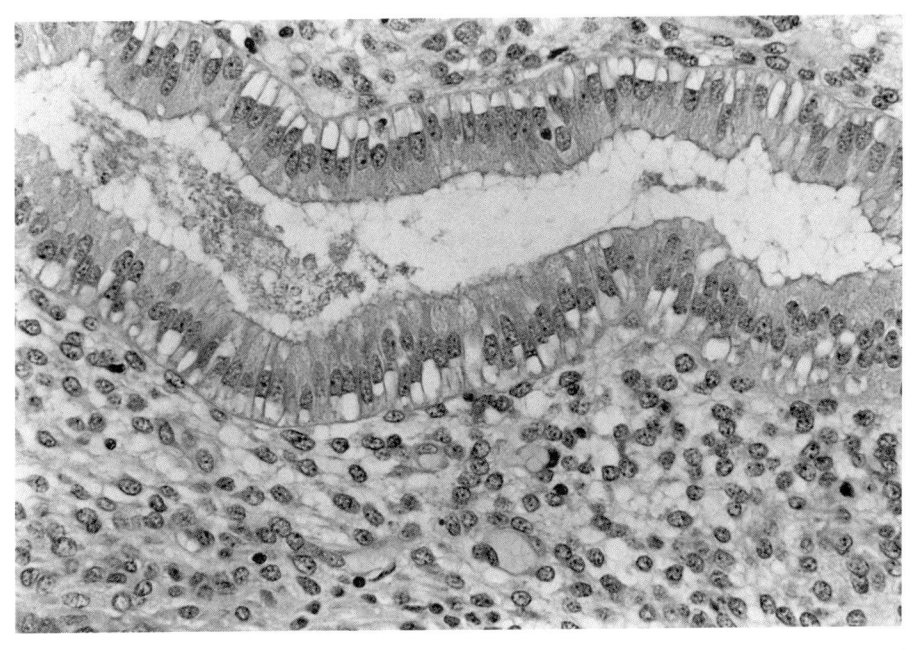

Figure 5-7. On cycle day 17 (POD 3), all of the glands show uniformly aligned subnuclear vacuoles, giving the characteristic "piano keys" appearance. There is no longer pseudostratification of glandular epithelium.

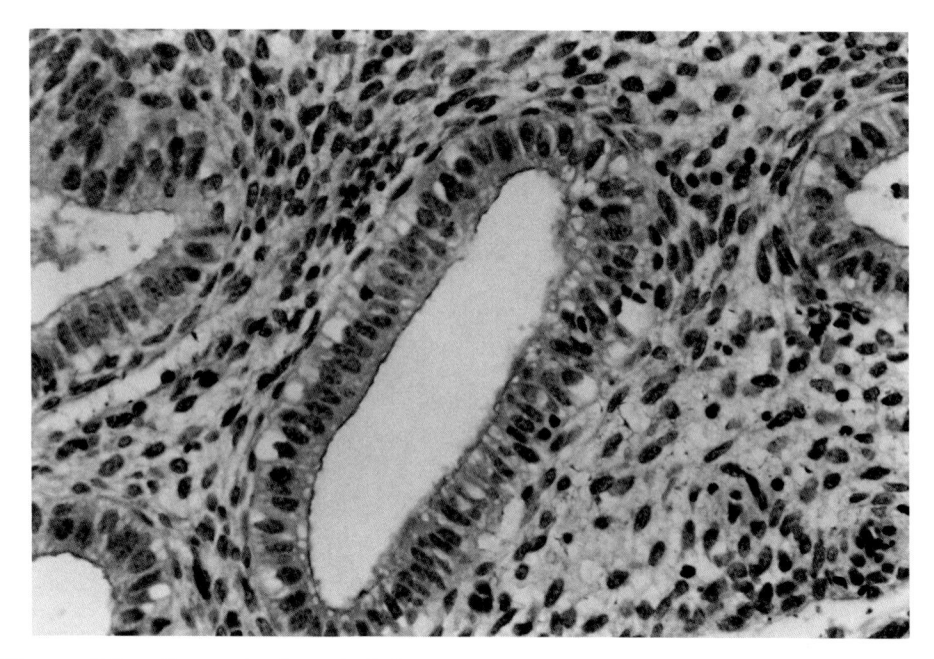

Figure 5-8. On cycle day 18 (POD 4), half of the vacuoles have migrated to the supranuclear position.

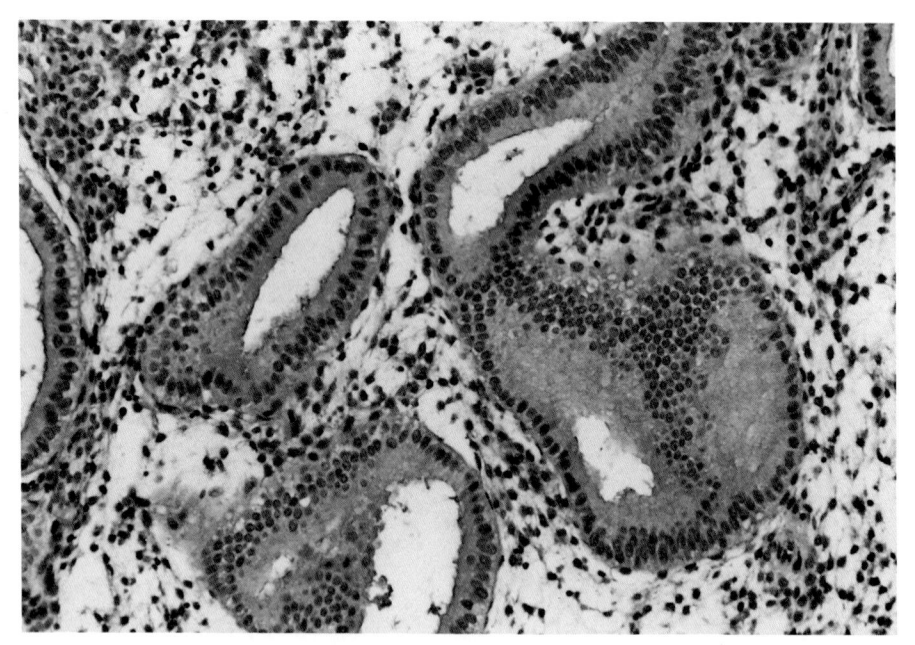

Figure 5-9. On cycle day 19 (POD 5), all vacuoles have migrated apically, giving the cytoplasm a bubbly appearance.

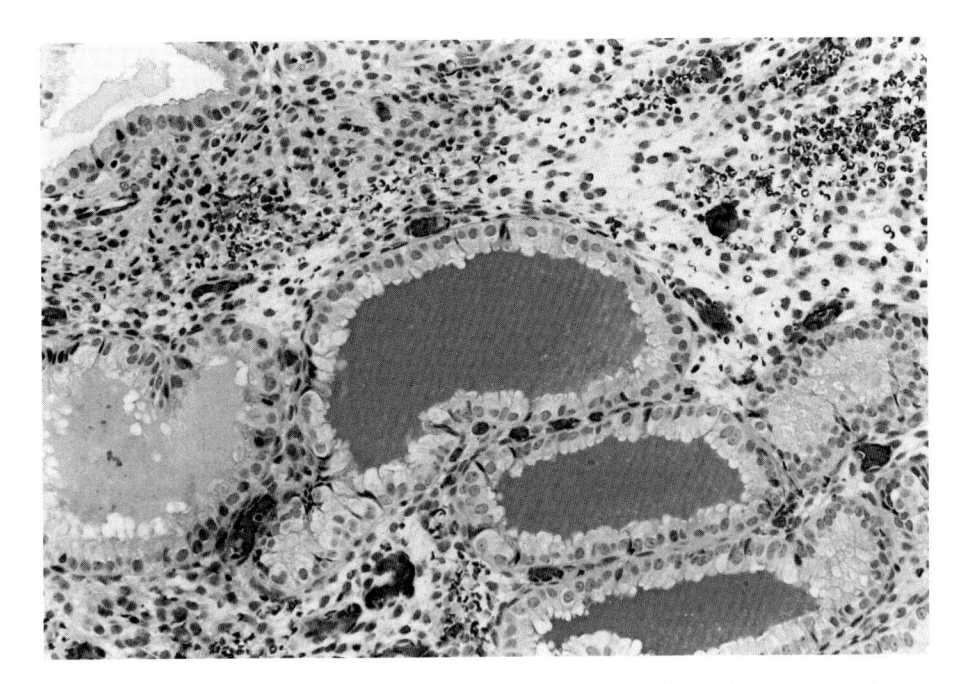

Figure 5-10. Peak secretion occurs on cycle day 20 (POD 6). Glands have become dilated, and secretions can sometimes be seen in gland lumina. This glandular dilatation should not be mistaken for hyperplasia.

tory exhaustion during this time. By cycle day 21 (POD 7), stromal edema begins (Fig. 5-11), peaking at cycle day 22 (POD 8) (Fig. 5-12). On cycle day 23 (POD 9) (Fig. 5-13), there is coiling of the spiral arterioles, which now appear prominent, with a thin predecidual cuff. A few stromal mitoses may be seen, increasing by cycle day 24. On cycle day 24 (POD 10) (Fig. 5-14), the spiral arterioles develop a thicker predecidual cuff. On cycle day 25 (POD 11), predecidualization occurs under the surface epithelium, and the perivascular cuffing further increases (Fig. 5-15). It is for this reason that obtaining surface endometrium is crucial for accurate dating. By cycle day 25 glands usually are sawtooth, exhibiting prominent secretory exhaustion. Cycle day 26 (POD 12) (Fig. 5-16) endometrium shows expanding predecidualization of the stroma, and increased sawtooth appearance of the glands. Stromal granulocytes begin to appear. On cycle day 27 (POD 13) (Fig. 5-17), the entire stroma is predecidualized, and stromal granulocytes are prominent. On cycle day 28 (POD 14), there is early stromal breakdown and hemorrhage and glandular collapse (Fig. 5-18).

Menstrual Endometrium

On the first day of menses, cycle day 1, there is increased stromal hemorrhage and collapse, with vascular fibrin thrombi formation (Fig. 5-19A).

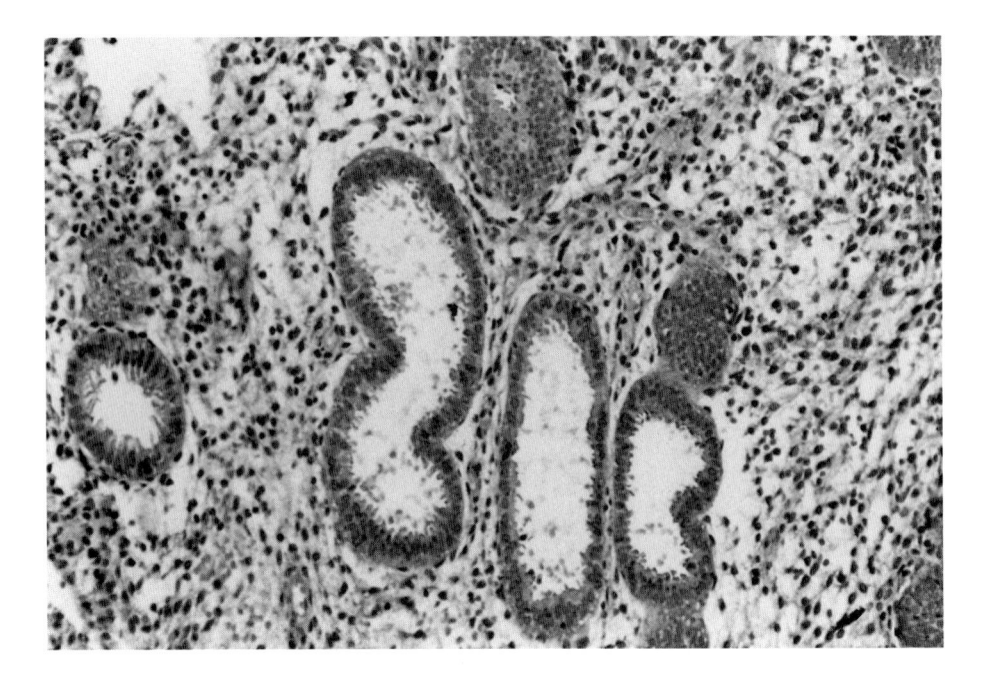

Figure 5-11. On cycle day 21 (POD 7), stromal edema begins. The apical surfaces of the glands are ragged, with "snouts" consistent with secretory activity.

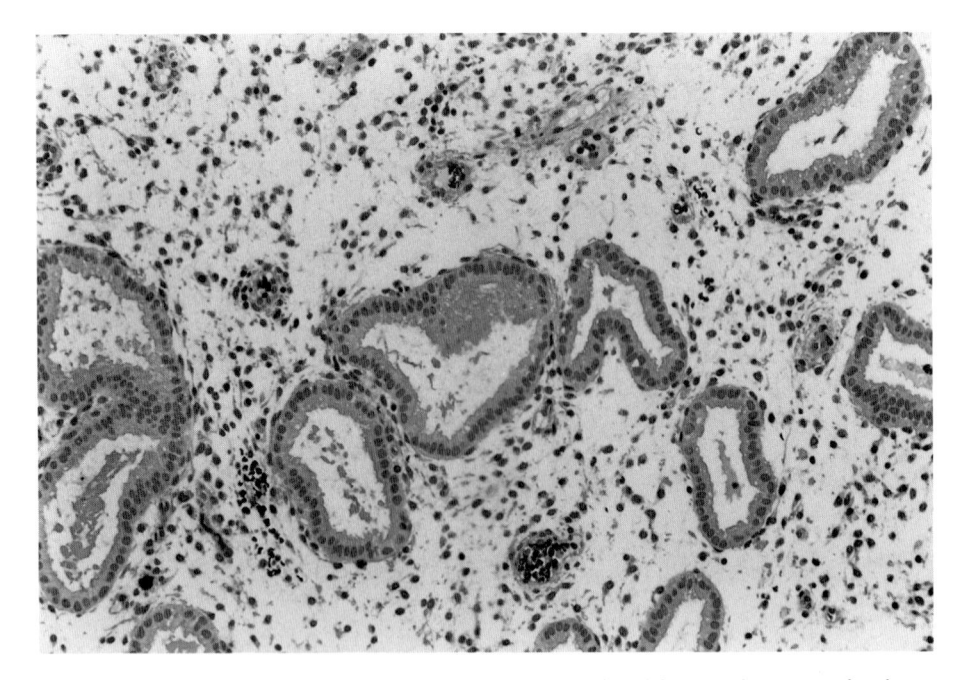

Figure 5-12. Cycle day 22 (POD 8) is characterized by peak stromal edema with "naked nuclei."

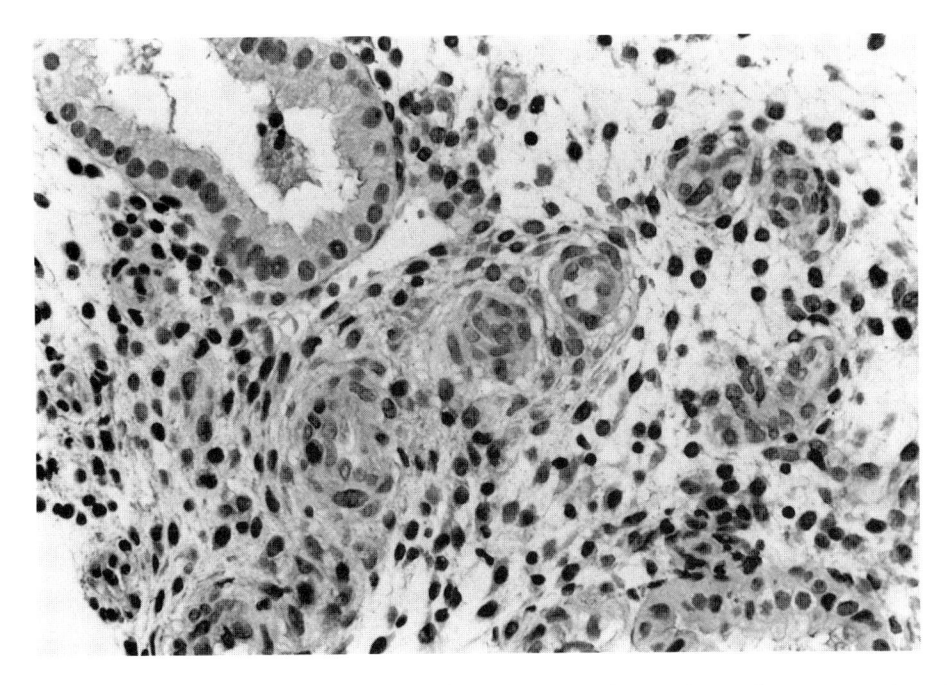

Figure 5-13. On cycle day 23 (POD 9) the endometrium shows prominent spiral arterioles.

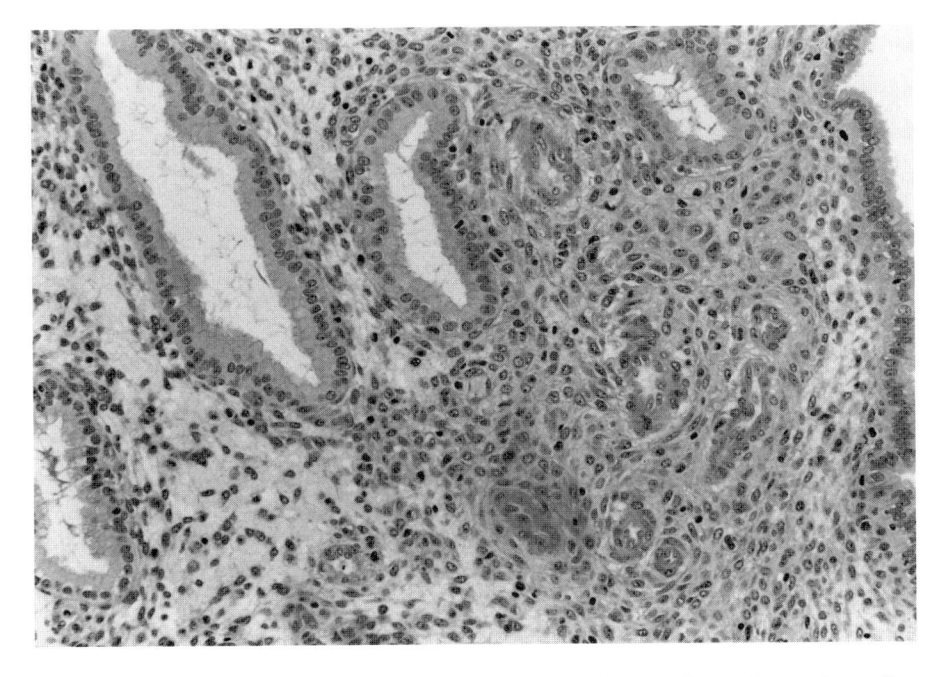

Figure 5-14. On cycle day 24 (POD 10) the endometrium shows broad predecidual cuffing around spiral arterioles.

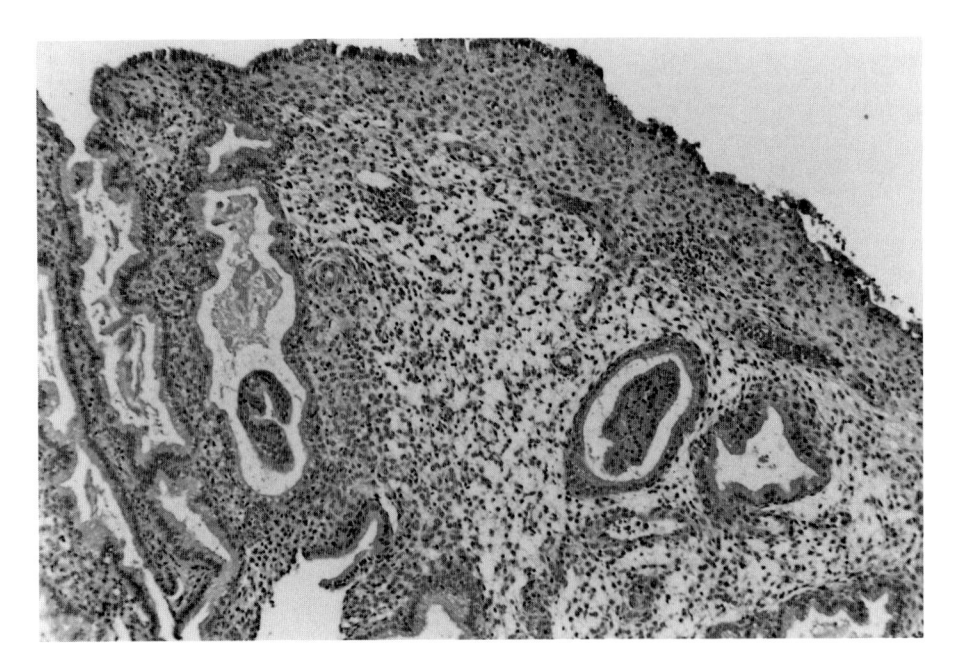

Figure 5-15. On cycle day 25 (POD 11), predecidualization has spread to under the surface epithelium.

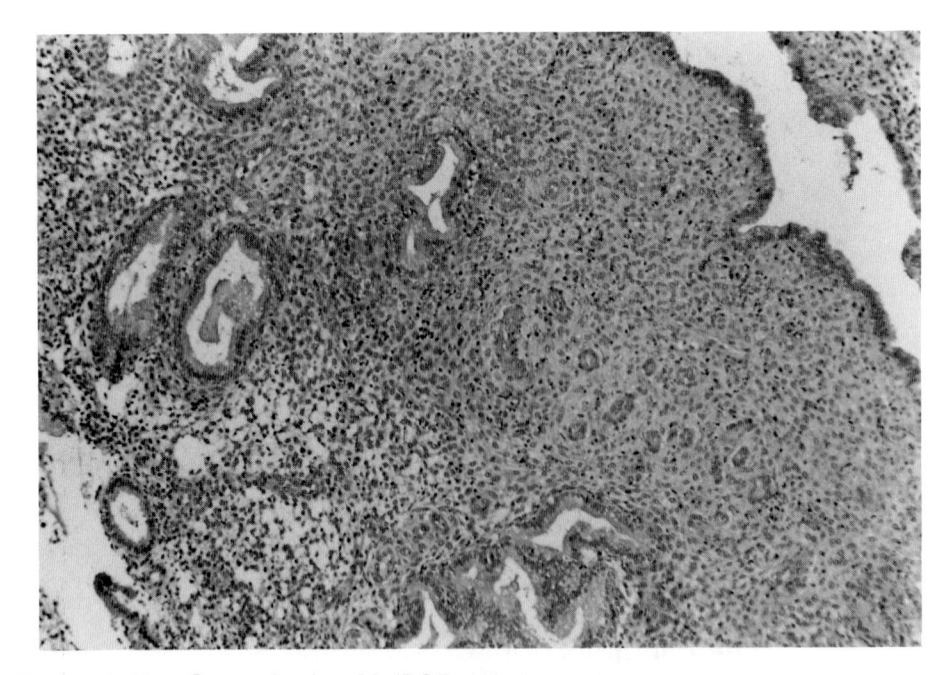

Figure 5-16. On cycle day 26 (POD 12) the endometrium shows continued spread of predecidualization.

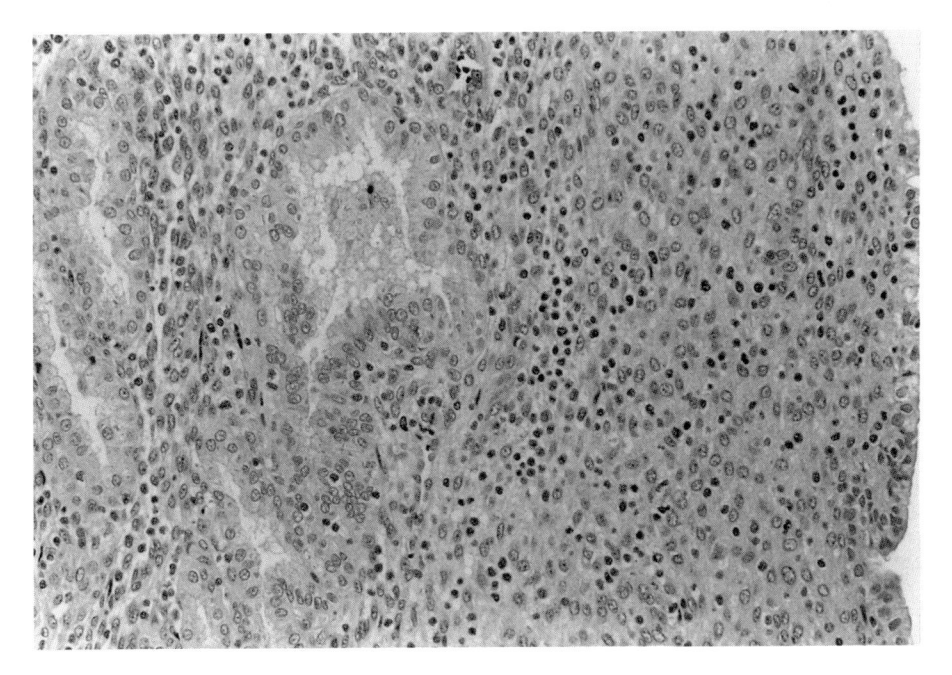

Figure 5-17. Cycle day 27 (POD 13) endometrium shows sheets of predecidua throughout the stroma, and prominent stromal granulocytes.

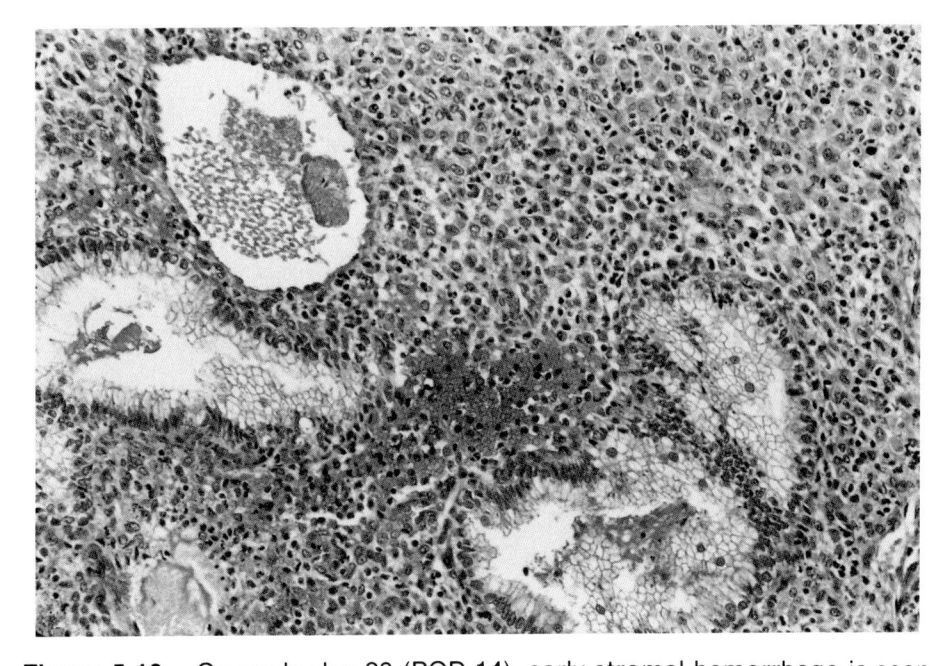

Figure 5-18. On cycle day 28 (POD 14), early stromal hemorrhage is seen.

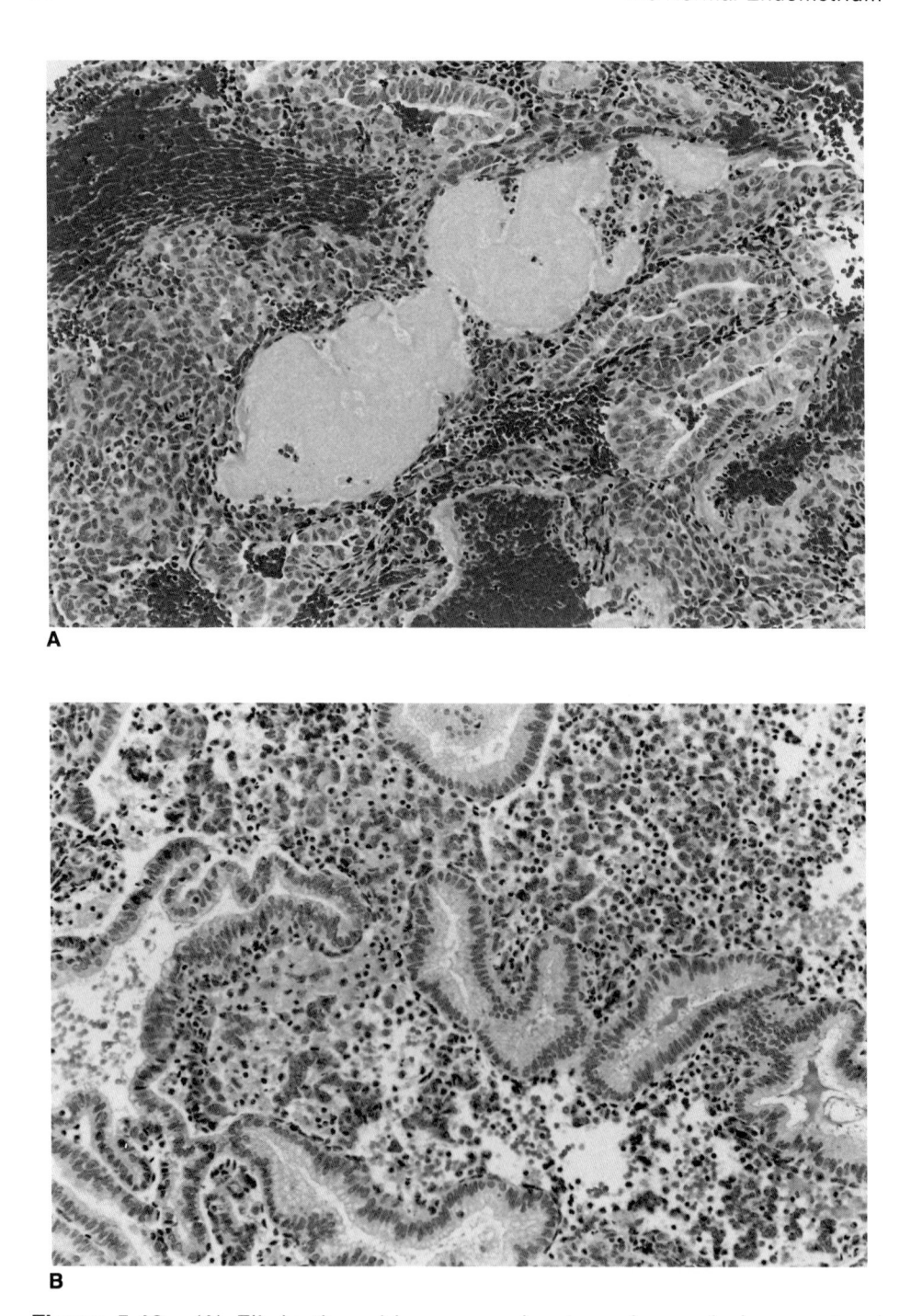

Figure 5-19. (A) Fibrin thrombi are seen in stromal vessels in menstrual endometrium. (B) Early menstrual endometrium shows breakdown, with gland–stroma dissociation, but it can still be determined that this was an ovulatory cycle.

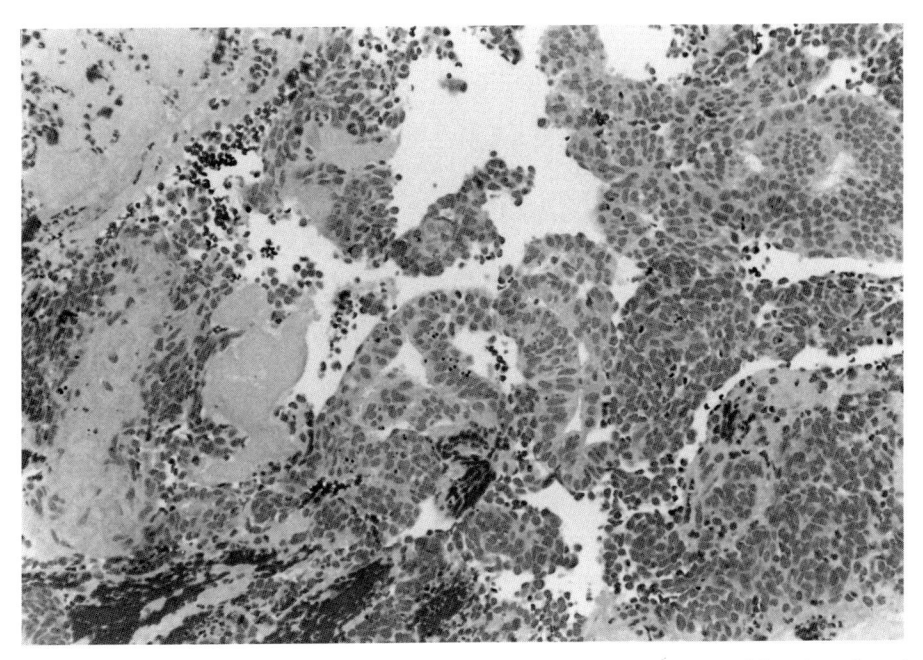

Figure 5-20. Late menstrual endometrium shows total architectural collapse. Round stromal aggregates occur, and nuclear "dust" (fragments) are seen among the glandular fragments. It cannot be reliably determined whether ovulation has occurred at this point.

Glands collapse and nuclear "dust," representing necrosis, is seen. It is still often possible to discern an occasional secretory gland and areas of stromal predecidualization, documenting previous ovulation (Fig. 5-19B). By the late menstrual period, there is complete gland–stroma disassociation, with the formation of stromal "balls," and detached glandular fragments. The etiology of the breakdown is not evident, and may represent ovulatory bleeding, anovulatory bleeding, hormonal withdrawal, or other causes of breakdown (Fig. 5-20). Regenerative changes then begin to occur, usually complete by the 5th day of the cycle.[5] One should not mistake the glandular "crowding" of menstrual endometrium caused by lack of stromal support nor the reparative atypia of the epithelium as a neoplastic process.

Accurate Endometrial Dating

In order to obtain the most accurate reading possible, it is necessary for the endometrial specimen to meet certain criteria. First of all, the specimen must be adequate in amount, and have surface endometrium present. The specimen must consist of functionalis, not basalis or lower uterine segment endo-

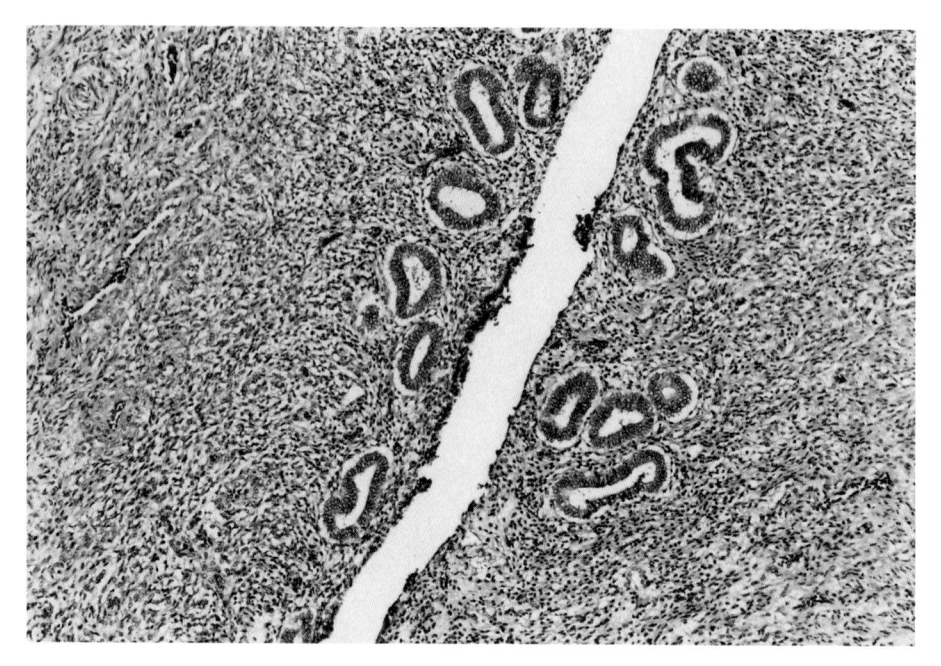

Figure 5-21. Subsequent to the maternal hormones clearing the system of the newborn, the prepubertal endometrium is inactive.

metrium. In the presence of hyperplastic endometria, endometritis, or tissue with nonuniform development, dating cannot be performed.

THE ENDOMETRIUM PRIOR TO MENARCHE

Proliferative changes may be seen in the newborn period due to maternal hormones, but these changes quickly regress. In the absence of abnormal hormonal stimulation, as in a functional ovarian stromal neoplasm, the endometrium of the child is inactive (Fig. 5-21).

THE ENDOMETRIUM DURING MENARCHE

The early menstrual cycles tend to be anovulatory and irregular, and proliferative or disordered proliferative patterns may be seen. As described by Hendrickson and Kempson,[4] disordered proliferation consists of irregular dilated and occasionally budded glands, but with minimal or no increase in the gland/stroma ratio (Fig. 5-22). While some pathologists classify this as a hyperplastic pattern, Hendrickson and Kempson feel that the lack of increased

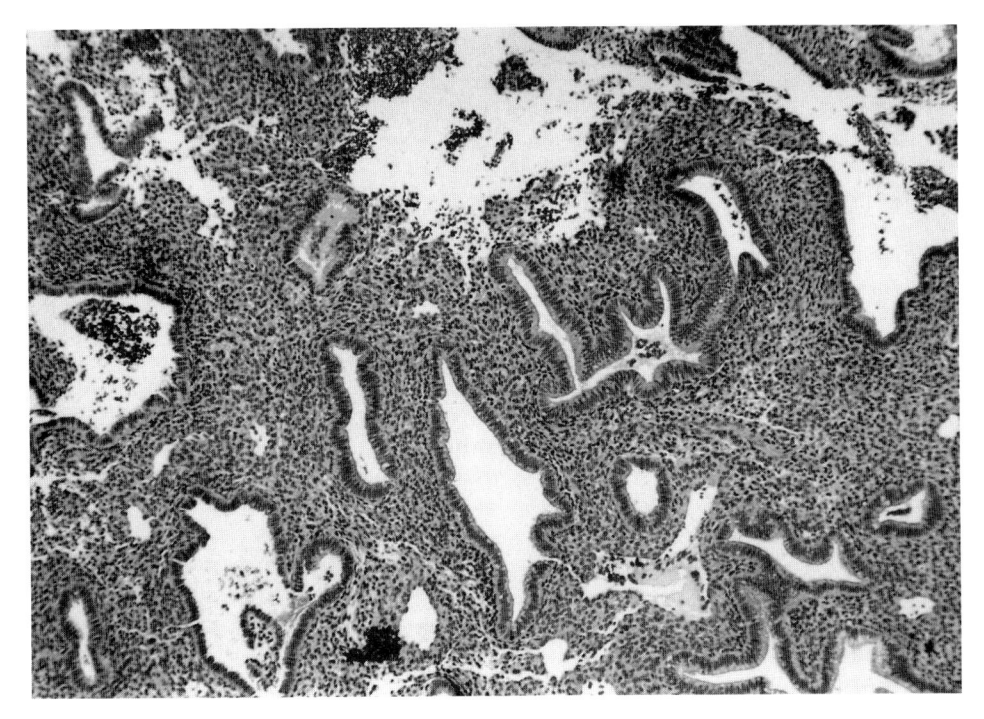

Figure 5-22. One pattern seen at both ends of reproductive life is disordered proliferation, due to mild hyperestrogenism secondary to anovulation. The glands show proliferative features, but additionally there is some dilatation and outpouching, without the increased gland–stroma ratio of a hyperplasia. This is felt to be in the morphologic spectrum of estrogen excess, but insufficient to qualify as a hyperplasia.

carcinoma risk does not justify this terminology. They interpret disordered proliferative endometrium as the earliest manifestation of hyperestrogenic effect on the endometrium, fitting between proliferative endometrium and endometrial hyperplasia in terms of classification.

MENOPAUSAL ENDOMETRIUM

During the perimenopausal period, cycles again tend to become irregular and anovulatory, and disordered proliferation may be seen. As hormonal levels wane, the endometrium becomes weakly proliferative (inactive) (Fig. 5-23), or atrophic (Fig. 5-24). A variant of atrophy is cystic atrophy, which should not be confused with hyperplasia. In cystic atrophy, the glands are cystically dilated, but the proliferative activity of the epithelium seen in hyperplastic glands is absent and the glandular epithelium is flattened (Fig. 5-25).

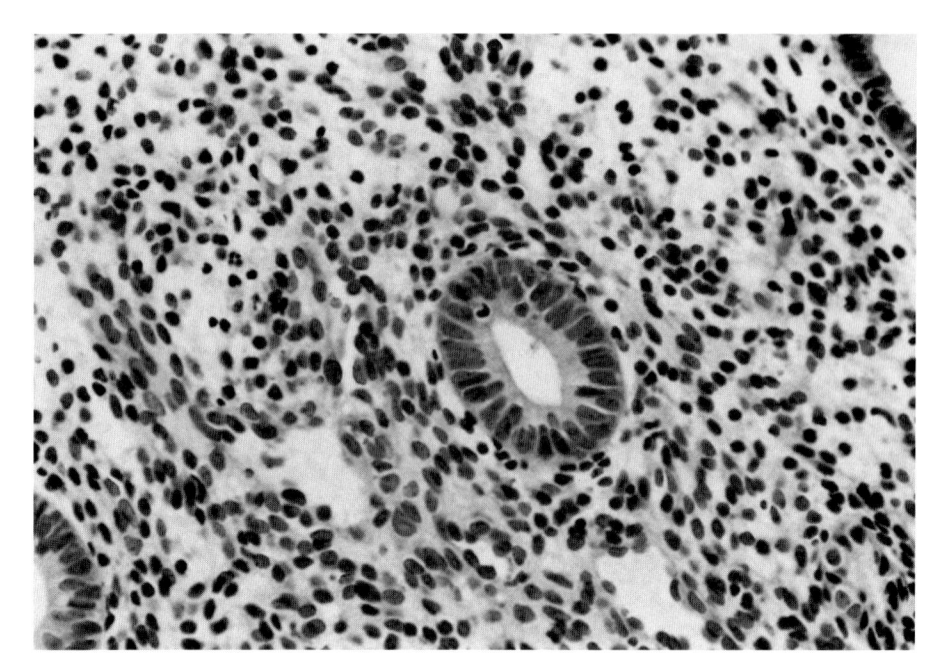

Figure 5-23. In the perimenopausal–early menopausal period, the endometrium can become weakly proliferative (inactive) with the cessation of ovulation, and in the absence of hyperestrogenism or hormonal therapy. The basic pattern is proliferative, but the glandular epithelium is not as tall, and there is loss of pseudostratification and mitotic activity.

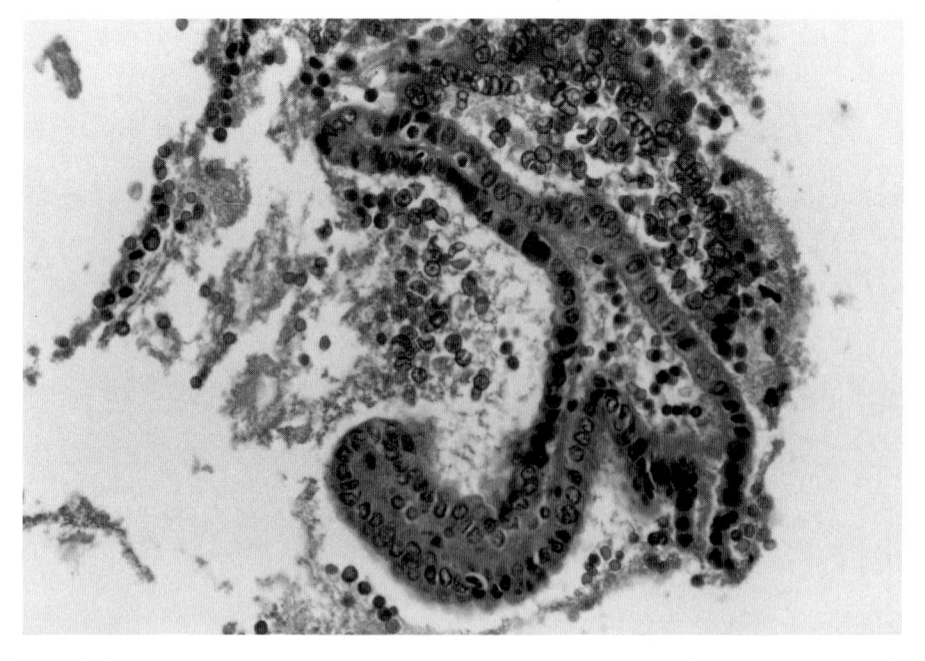

Figure 5-24. In postmenopausal atrophy, scanty strips of inactive glandular epithelium and blood are often all that is seen on sampling the endometrium.

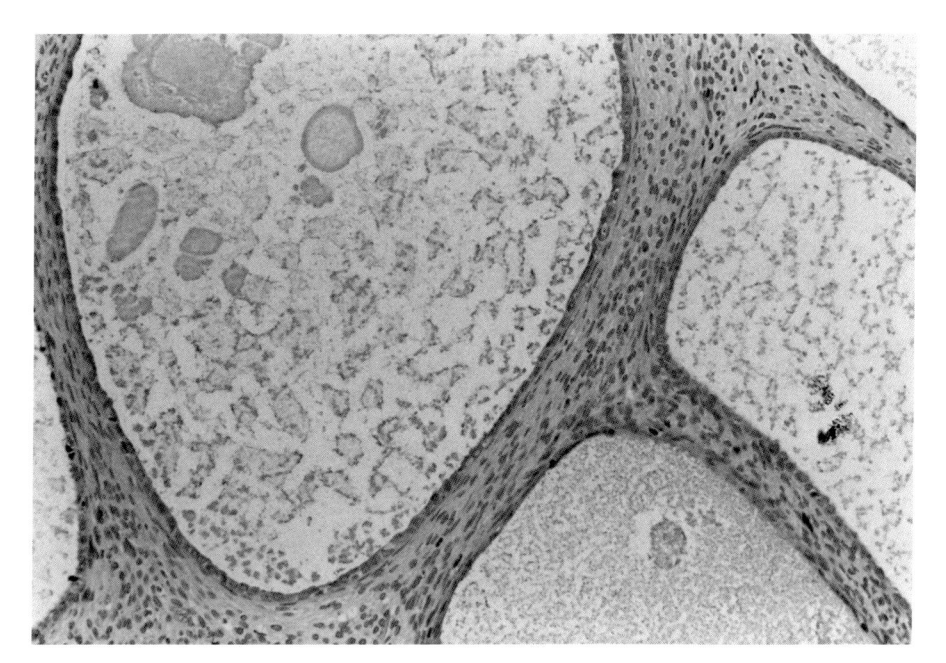

Figure 5-25. Another postmenopausal pattern frequently encountered is cystic atrophy. Glands are dilated, but the epithelium is flat, and not proliferating. This should not be confused with cystic (simple) hyperplasia.

REFERENCES

1. Noyes RW, Hertig AT, Rock J: Dating the endometrial biopsy. *Fertil Steril* 1:3–25, 1950.
2. Langren BM, Unden AL, Diczfalusy E: Hormonal profile of the cycle in 68 normally menstruating women. *Acta Endocrinol* (Copenhagen) 94:89–98, 1980.
3. Johannisson E, Landgren BM, Rohr HP, et al: Endometrial morphology and peripheral hormone levels in women with regular menstrual cycles. *Fertil Steril* 48:401–408, 1987.
4. Hendrickson MR, Kempson RL: Uterus and Fallopian tubes. In Sternberg S (ed): *Histology for pathologists.* Raven Press, New York, 1992, pp 797–834.
5. Dallenbach-Hellweg G: *Histopathology of the endometrium,* 4th ed. Springer-Verlag, Berlin, 1987, p 84.

6

Hormonal Effects on the Endometrium: Dysfunctional Uterine Bleeding, Iatrogenic Hormonal Effects, and Luteal Phase Defects

Debra S. Heller, M.D.

DYSFUNCTIONAL UTERINE BLEEDING

Two diagnoses are frequently scribbled on the pathology requisition slips accompanying endometrial biopsies: menometrorrhagia and dysfunctional uterine bleeding (DUB). These terms are often applied loosely, with minimal history supplied, so that the pathologist has only a vague idea that menstrual cycles are somehow abnormal. Menometrorrhagia implies heavy menses and bleeding between periods, without any reference to causality. Dysfunctional uterine bleeding probably has almost as many definitions in the literature as etiologies.

Dysfunctional uterine bleeding has been defined as abnormal bleeding unassociated with tumor, inflammation, or pregnancy.[1] Others define it as disruption of normal cyclic bleeding unrelated to uterine abnormality or systemic disease.[2] There is dispute as to whether polyps qualify as a cause of dysfunctional uterine bleeding. Some authors[3] feel that polyps are not true neoplasms, but focal hyperplasias, and so qualify as a cause of DUB, but not everyone subscribes to this theory. There has also been dispute as to whether endometrium with secretory changes, such as in luteal phase defects or irregular shedding, should be classified under the heading of DUB, or whether anovulation is a prerequisite for the diagnosis.[4,5]

Abnormal bleeding secondary to hormonal variability may be either endogenous or iatrogenic, and can occur by one of several mechanisms: estrogen withdrawal, progesterone withdrawal, or a relative excess of either hormone. Bleeding after estrogen withdrawal can occur after oophorectomy, or more commonly after withdrawal of exogenous therapy. Likewise, progesterone withdrawal bleeds commonly occur after therapy. Progesterone breakthrough bleeding is seen with some oral contraceptive agents. In general, most cases of DUB are due to unopposed estrogen excess, secondary to anovulation (Fig. 6-1). In addition, a relative paucity of estrogen, as in postmenopausal atrophy, can lead to abnormal uterine bleeding.

Histopathologic correlation with the abnormal bleeding process can only be achieved with an adequate history, which includes the patient's age, last menstrual period (LMP), any hormonal therapy, and the basic abnormal bleeding pattern. Endometrial samples in cases of DUB may be abnormal, but may be normal but out-of-phase; this cannot be determined without clinical information.

In this chapter, abnormal bleeding secondary to hormonal variations, ovu-

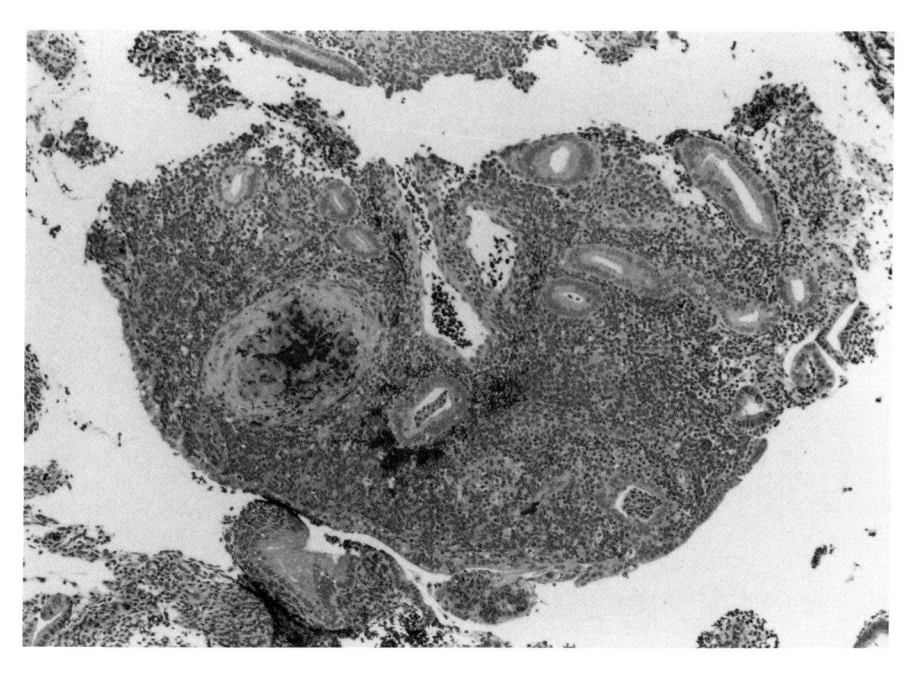

Figure 6-1. Anovulatory menstrual endometrium. Stromal breakdown, as evidenced by hemorrhage and vascular thrombosis, is present in this nonsecretory endometrium.

TABLE 6-1. Endometrial Patterns Seen in DUB

Nonsecretory patterns
  Atrophic endometrium
  Weakly proliferative endometrium
  Proliferative endometrium
  Disordered proliferative endometrium
  Endometrial hyperplasia

Secretory patterns
  Underdeveloped secretory endometrium
  Out-of-phase secretory endometrium
  Dyssynchronously developed secretory endometrium
  Irregular shedding
  Irregular ripening

latory and anovulatory, will be considered. Endometrial polyps are discussed in Chapter 4. For the purposes of this discussion, DUB will be defined as abnormal uterine bleeding, whether ovulatory or anovulatory, in the absence of intrinsic uterine disease, pregnancy, or contributory systemic disease. The effects of exogenous hormonal therapy will be considered separately, as will the hormonal variations related to the endometrium in infertility.

A rational classification of endometrial patterns has been advanced by Hendrickson and Kempson,[6] who divide the endometrium into secretory and nonsecretory patterns (see also Table 6-1). Nonsecretory patterns include atrophic endometrium, weakly proliferative endometrium, proliferative endometrium, disordered proliferative endometrium, and the endometrial hyperplasias. The farther end of the spectrum of hyperestrogenic stimulation of the endometrium—the hyperplasias, metaplasias, and carcinomas—are discussed elsewhere. Secretory patterns may be either normal or abnormal. Abnormal secretory patterns may be underdeveloped, dyssynchronous, or show irregular ripening, as in some cases of luteal phase defect. They may also be superimposed on a nonsecretory endometrium, as in irregular shedding.

Nonsecretory Patterns Seen in DUB: Atrophic Endometrium, Weakly Proliferative Endometrium, Proliferative Endometrium, Disordered Proliferative Endometrium

Although all episodes of postmenopausal bleeding should be investigated by endometrial sampling, not all cases are due to hyperplasia or neoplasia. In many cases, postmenopausal bleeding is due to atrophy. Biopsy in these cases yields scanty tissue, and often merely strips of inactive endometrial glands are seen [see Fig. 5-24 (in Chapter 5)]. In these cases, it is up to the clinician to decide whether the specimen was scanty due to little tissue inside the uterus, or scanty as a result of incomplete sampling, as when the cervix is stenotic. In hysterectomy specimens, atrophic endometrium shows thinning, with small inactive glands devoid of mitotic activity in a compact stroma. A common variant of atrophic endometrium is cystic atrophy, which must be distinguished from cystic (simple) hyperplasia. In cystic atrophy, the glands, although dilated, show a flattened epithelium without mitotic activity (see Fig. 5-25).

With the decreasing levels of estrogen accompanying the perimenopausal period, weakly proliferative endometrium is sometimes seen (see Fig. 5-23). The histologic appearance is similar to proliferative endometrium; however, there is less pseudostratification of glandular cells, and essentially no mitotic activity.

Often biopsies for dysfunctional uterine bleeding show normal proliferative endometrium, and may reflect an ongoing pattern of anovulatory cycles. If the unopposed estrogenic stimulation persists, a pattern referred to as *disordered proliferative endometrium* may be seen.[6] This is a nonneoplastic pattern with disordered proliferative glands, some cystically dilated, but with overall preservation of the gland/stroma ratio (see Fig. 5-22). Eventually, with unopposed estrogen, hyperplasias or carcinoma may develop.

Secretory Patterns Seen in Dysfunctional Uterine Bleeding: Weakly Secretory Endometrium, Out-of-Phase Secretory Endometrium, Dyssynchronous Secretory Endometrium, Irregular Shedding, Irregular Ripening

Weakly or poorly developed secretory patterns may be due to poor corpus luteum function, or possibly poor endometrial response to progesterone. Similar patterns are sometimes seen with hormonal replacement therapy with estrogen or progestins (Fig. 6-2). The out-of-phase secretory endometrium is morphologically normal but lags behind the clinical dates, and must be correlated with the clinical history. Dyssynchronous patterns, where the glands and stroma meet different dating criteria, are most commonly seen in ovulation induction. (See the section on the endometrial biopsy in infertility.) Irregular shedding is felt to be secondary to persistent corpus luteum function into the next follicular phase. As such, the diagnosis cannot be made unless the biopsy is taken at least 5 days after the onset of bleeding. The usual picture is one of shrunken stellate glands in a dense stroma. Adjacent proliferative changes may also be seen (Fig. 6-3).

A combination of proliferative and secretory glands may also be seen in irregular ripening, which is a form of luteal phase defect. Again the findings may represent either poor ovarian function or regional variations in endometrial receptiveness to normal hormonal levels. Here normal or underdeveloped secretory glands may be seen in proximity to proliferative glands (Fig. 6-4). The situation is temporally different from irregular shedding, in that it occurs during the secretory phase of the cycle.

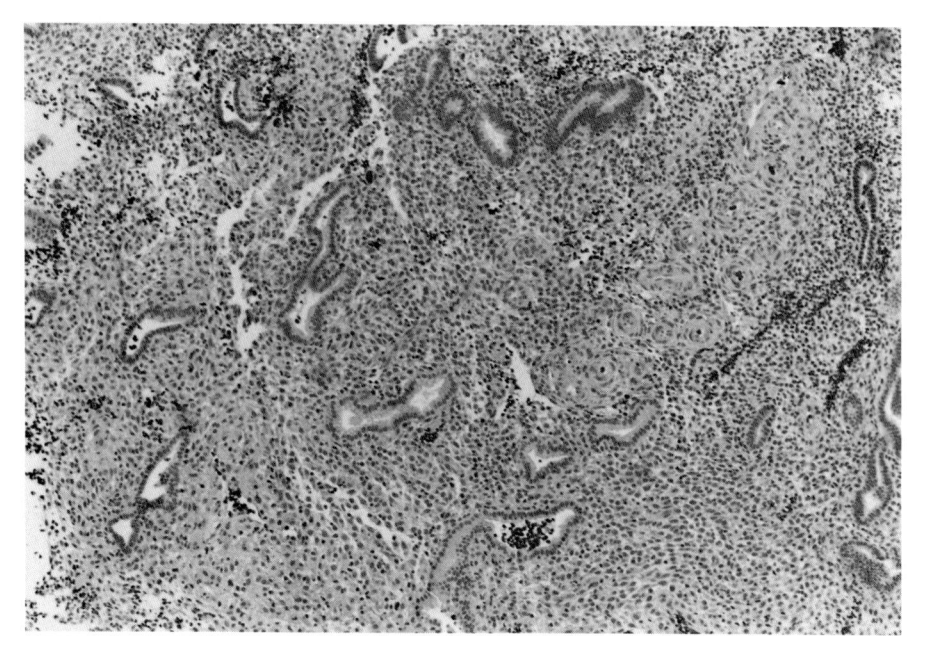

Figure 6-2. Underdeveloped secretory endometrium, showing diffuse stromal predecidualization, but poorly developed glands, in a patient on hormonal replacement therapy.

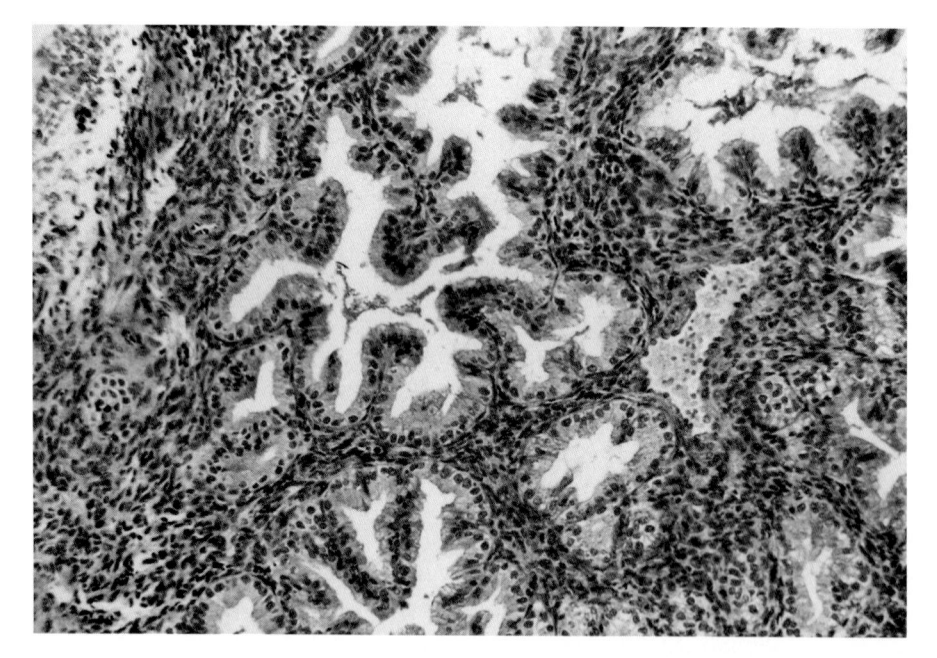

Figure 6-3. Irregular shedding. Persistent corpus luteum function into the next follicular period produces a picture of stellate, shrunken secretory glands in a dense stroma. Adjacent proliferative changes are sometimes present.

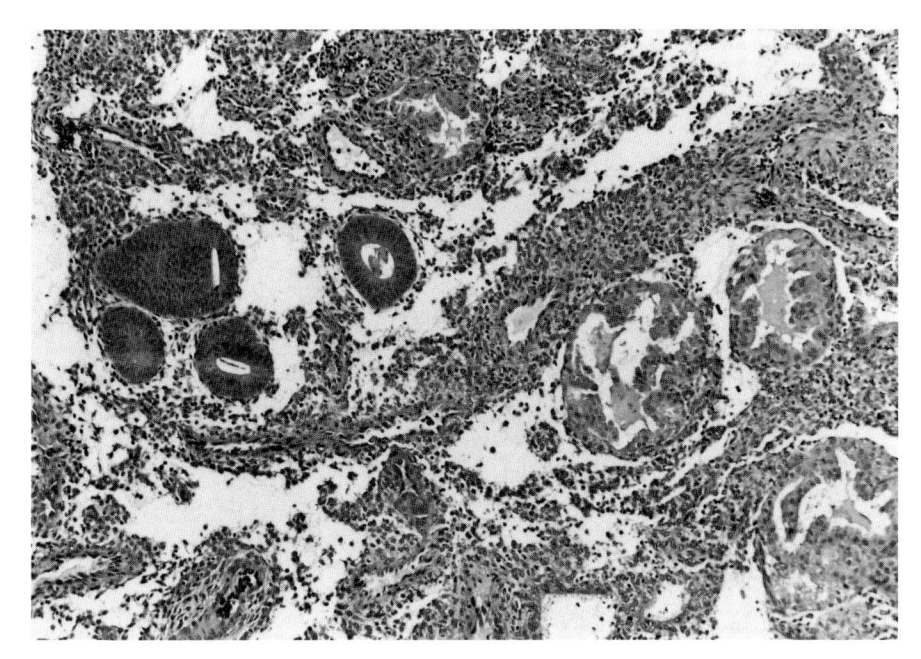

Figure 6-4. Irregular ripening—a focus of proliferative glands (left) is seen in this secretory endometrium.

EFFECTS OF ENDOGENOUS HORMONAL THERAPY

The morphology of endometrium that has been exposed to exogenous hormonal stimulation is extremely variable, depending on which hormones have been administered, in what combination, for how long, and on the background of the patient's own underlying hormonal milieu. In addition, responses between individuals vary as well, and this may relate to the hormone receptor status in the endometrium.

Oral Contraceptive Therapy

With prolonged oral contraceptive use (combined estrogen–progesterone), the progestational effect predominates, and small inactive glands are seen in a pseudodecidualized or hyperplastic stroma (Fig. 6-5).

Hormonal Replacement Therapy

Estrogen administered to a postmenopausal woman with an atrophic endometrium may initially induce weakly proliferative changes. Prolonged unopposed estrogen may produce any of the known sequelae of hyperestrogen-

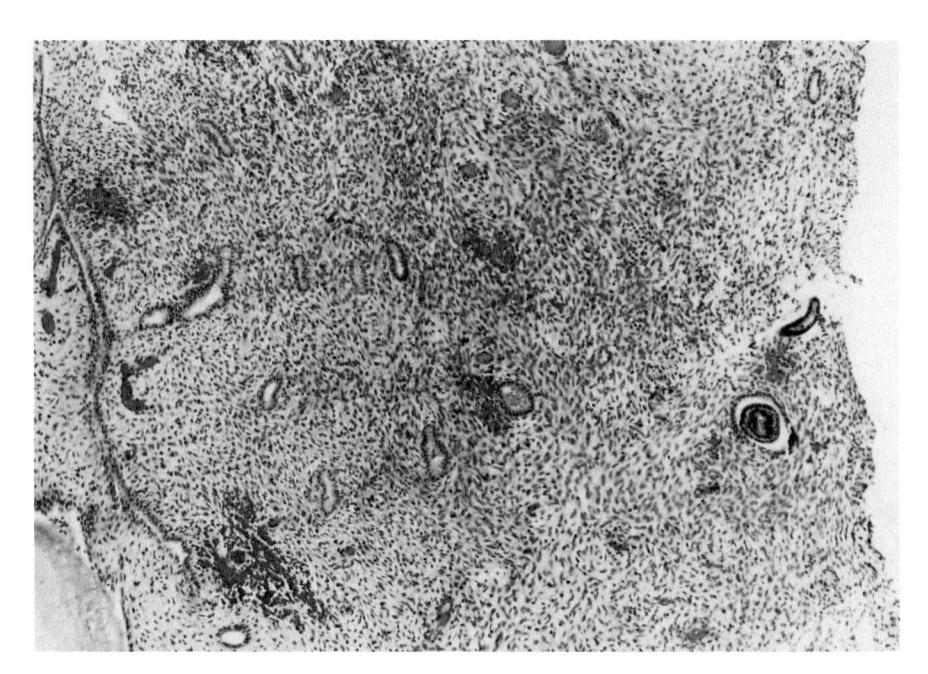

Figure 6-5. Oral contraceptive effect. Small inactive glands are seen in a dense stroma. The stroma is sometimes diffusely decidualized.

ism ranging from disordered proliferation, through the range of hyperplasias, and even carcinoma. The addition of progesterone to estrogen replacement may also result in a variety of patterns. In younger perimenopausal or recently postmenopausal women, a near-normal morphology may be seen. Other patterns encountered in estrogen- and progesterone-treated women include atrophy, weakly proliferative endometrium, disordered proliferation, mixed proliferative and secretory changes, and weakly secretory endometrium (Figs. 6-2, 6-6). In the absence of a provided clinical history, the pathologist is often confronted with an endometrial biopsy that fits no known straightforward diagnosis, but is not malignant. Diagnosis in a vacuum is often suboptimal (or to quote one pathology resident, "garbage in, garbage out!").

Progestational Therapy in Dysfunctional Uterine Bleeding

Progestational agents are often used to treat dysfunctional uterine bleeding, as well as in attempts to reverse simple or complex hyperplasia. In an endometrium sufficiently primed by estrogen, widespread decidualization of the stroma is initially seen. Glands may initially be hypersecretory, but over time become small and inactive (Fig. 6-7). With prolonged therapy, the entire endometrium becomes inactive.

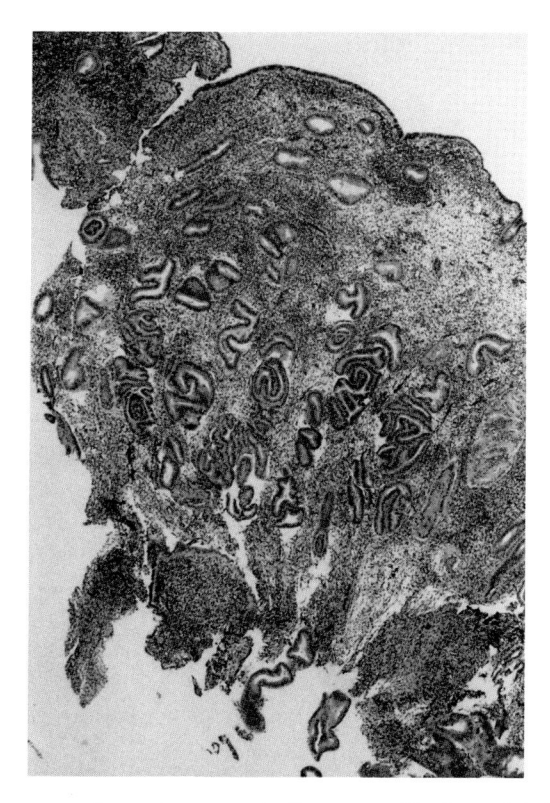

Figure 6-6. Hormonal replacement therapy. Endometrial samples from women receiving combination estrogen–progestin therapy often show foci of irregularly crowded glands, with a mixture of proliferative and secretory features. This "confused" endometrium is difficult to interpret in the absence of a clinical history.

If the underlying process is hyperplastic, the architecture of the hyperplasia may remain, with superimposed secretory effect, so-called secretory hyperplasia. Here the glands may resemble secretory glands, but there is increased gland/stroma ratio (Fig. 6-8). Similarly, carcinomas may show superimposed secretory effect, termed *secretory carcinoma of the endometrium* (see Chapter 10). A total or partial response of endometrial hyperplasia to progesterone may also occur, in which case either normal endometrial patterns or a mixture of hyperplasia and progesterone effect may be seen (Fig. 6-9).

Therapy For Endometriosis

Danazol and continuous therapy with GnRH agonists exert an antigonadotropic effect, leading to an inactive or atrophic endometrium (Fig. 6-10).[7]

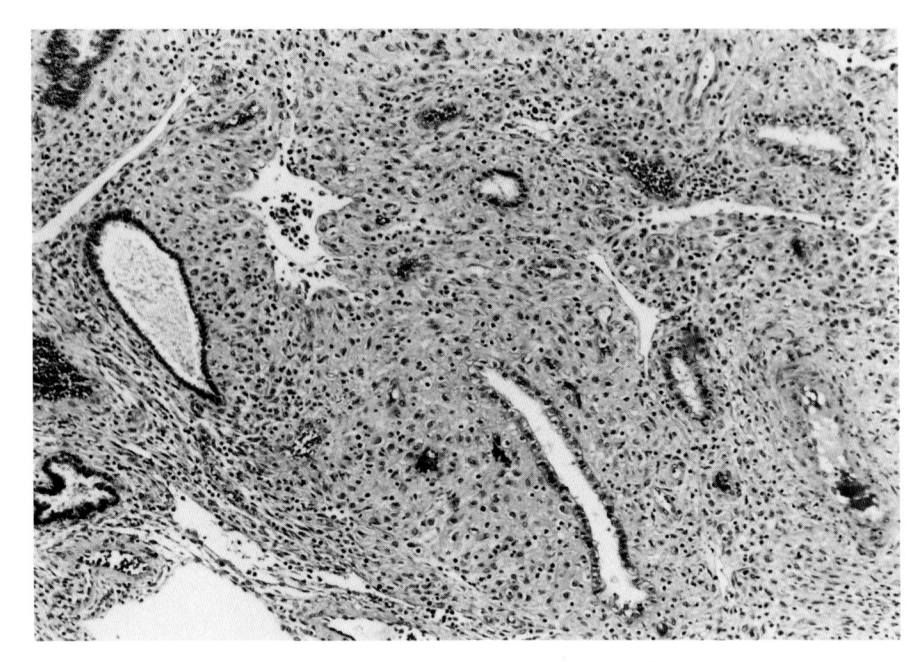

Figure 6-7. Inactive glands in a diffusely decidualized stroma are seen in this biopsy from a patient treated with a progestin.

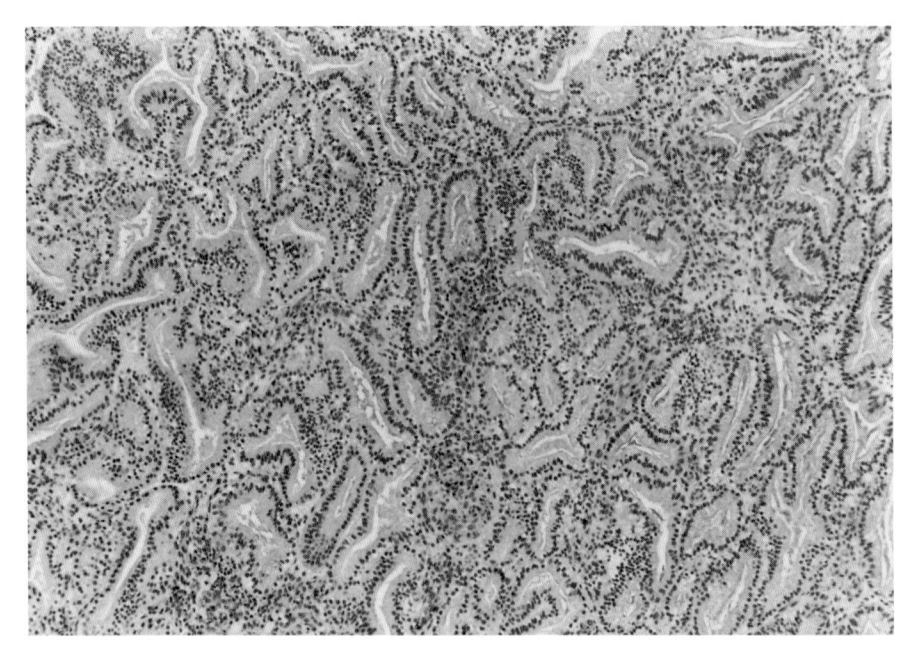

Figure 6-8. Secretory hyperplasia. The architecture is consistent with complex hyperplasia, but the glands show secretory features. This is usually a transient effect caused by superimposition of progesterone effect, endogenous or exogenous, on a preexisting hyperplasia.

Effects of Endogenous Hormonal Therapy

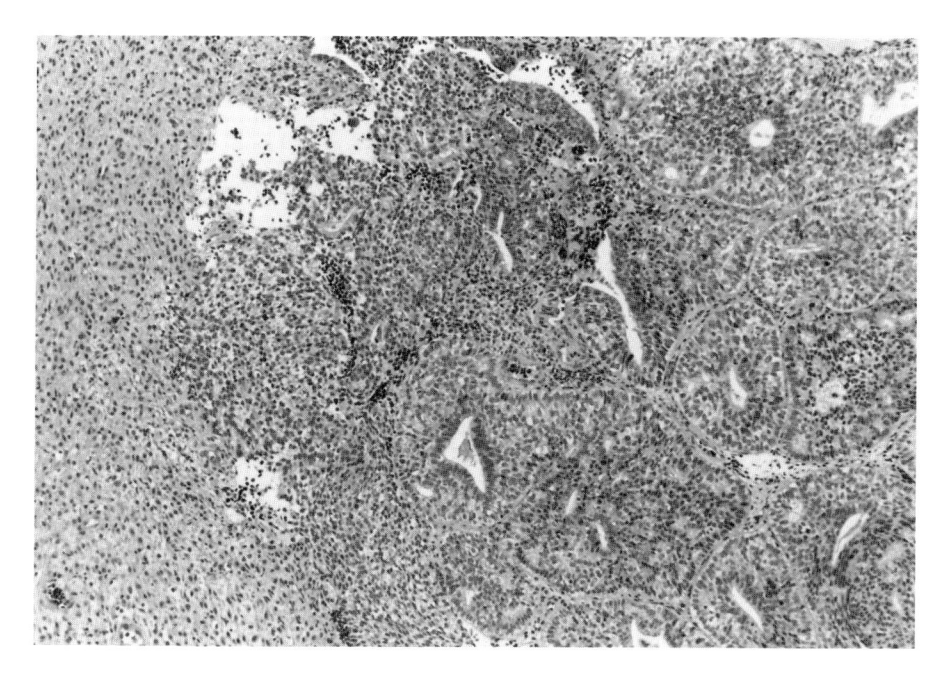

Figure 6-9. Superimposed progestational effect on an area of complex hyperplasia. Adjacent fragments showed areas of frank adenocarcinoma, and other areas showing pure progesterone effect, as demonstrated in Fig. 6-7.

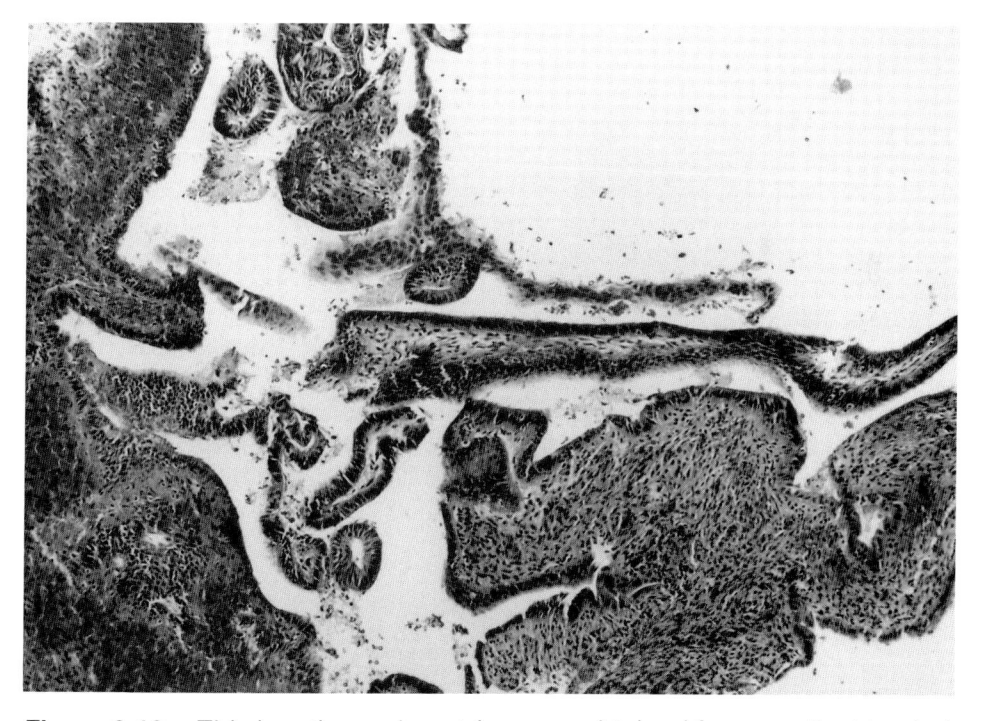

Figure 6-10. This inactive endometrium was obtained from a patient treated with a GnRH agonist.

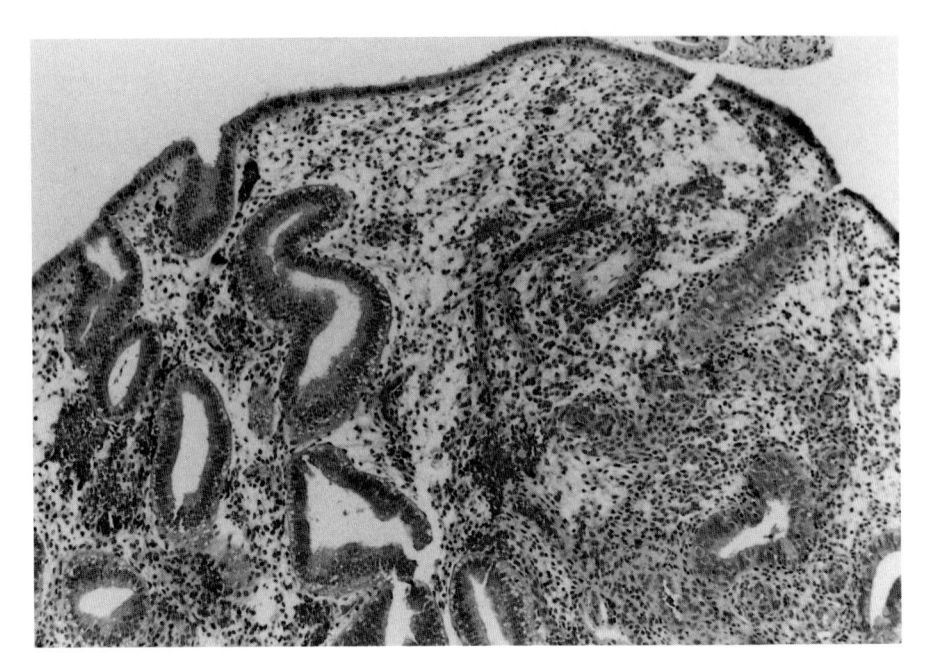

Figure 6-11. Glandular–stromal asynchrony. The glands are suggestive of day 17–18, while the stroma meets the dating criteria for day 22–23.

Ovulation Induction Therapy

Ovulation induction may result in normal endometrial patterns; however, irregularities have been described. Ovulation induction with Pergonal (HMG)/HCG can result in glandular–stromal asynchrony. Glandular maturation may lag or be irregular, and there may be premature spiral arteriole development.[8] A picture consistent with day 17–18 glands and day 22–23 stroma is often seen (Fig. 6-11). Benda[9] has described characteristic changes in the secretory endometrium seen in women treated with clomiphene (Clomid). Early secretory changes include straighter glands with scanter secretions, and markedly distinct crisp subnuclear vacuoles (Figs. 6-12, 6-13). Later in the cycle, the secretory glands show low cuboidal epithelium, with rare hypersecretory glands; decidualized stromal cells are sometimes smaller (Fig. 6-14). Lumenal secretions appeared inspissated.

Tamoxifen Therapy

Tamoxifen, in widespread use for its antiestrogenic effect in breast cancer therapy, has received a great deal of attention recently, due to its estrogenic effect on the postmenopausal endometrium. In addition to the usual spectrum of hyperestrogenic endometrial patterns, characteristic polyps with cystic glands and densely fibrous stroma have been described (Fig. 6-15).[10]

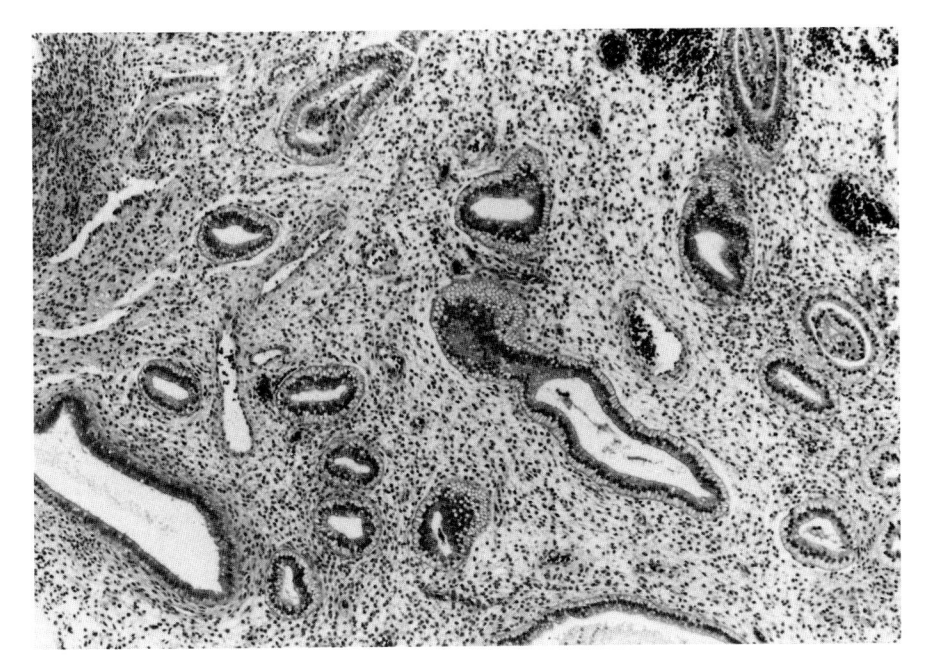

Figure 6-12. Early secretory endometrium after clomid therapy. Glands are straighter than expected, with exaggerated, crisp subnuclear vacuoles. (The author would like to thank Dr. J. Benda for supplying the sections of Clomid-treated endometrium shown in this figure.)

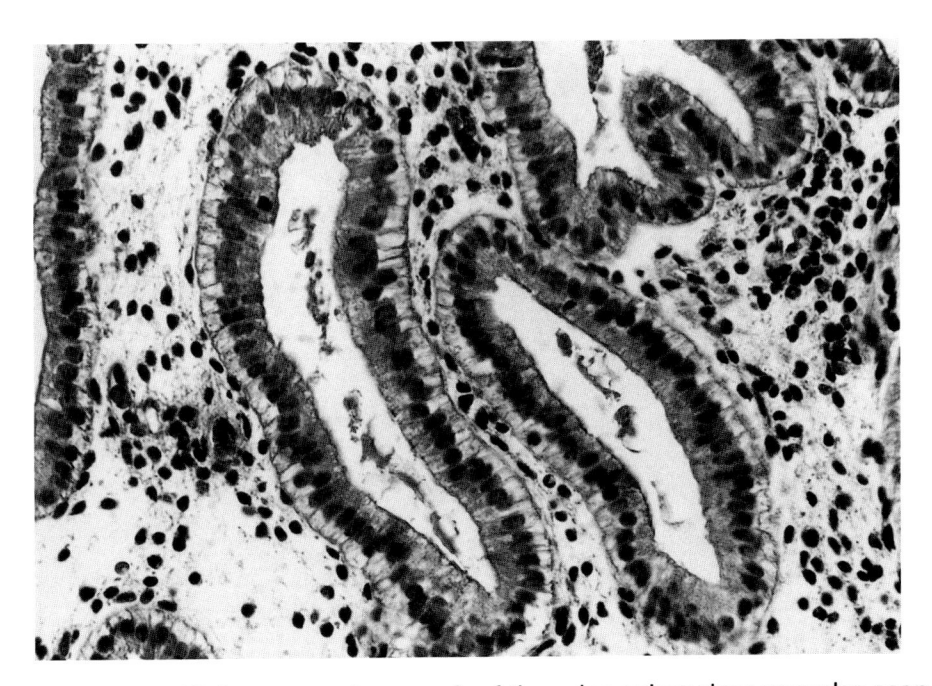

Figure 6-13. High-power micrograph of the crisp subnuclear vacuoles seen during the early secretory period with Clomid therapy. (The author would like to thank Dr. J. Benda for supplying the sections of Clomid-treated endometrium shown in this figure.)

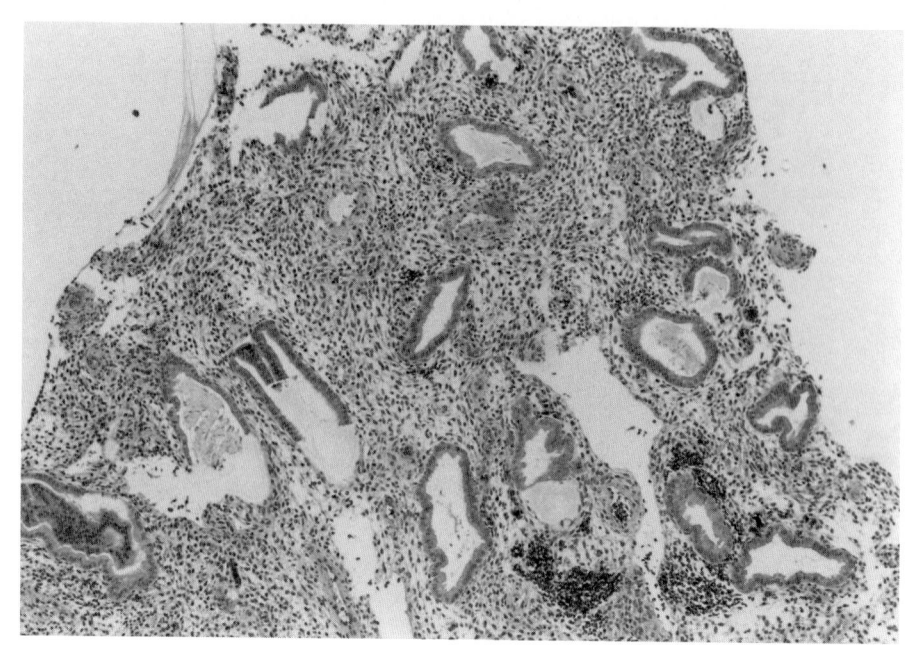

Figure 6-14. Late secretory endometrium after Clomid therapy. Straighter than expected secretory glands are lined by low cuboidal epithelium. Predecidual cells may be smaller than in a spontaneous cycle. (The author would like to thank Dr. J. Benda for supplying the sections of Clomid-treated endometrium shown in this figure.)

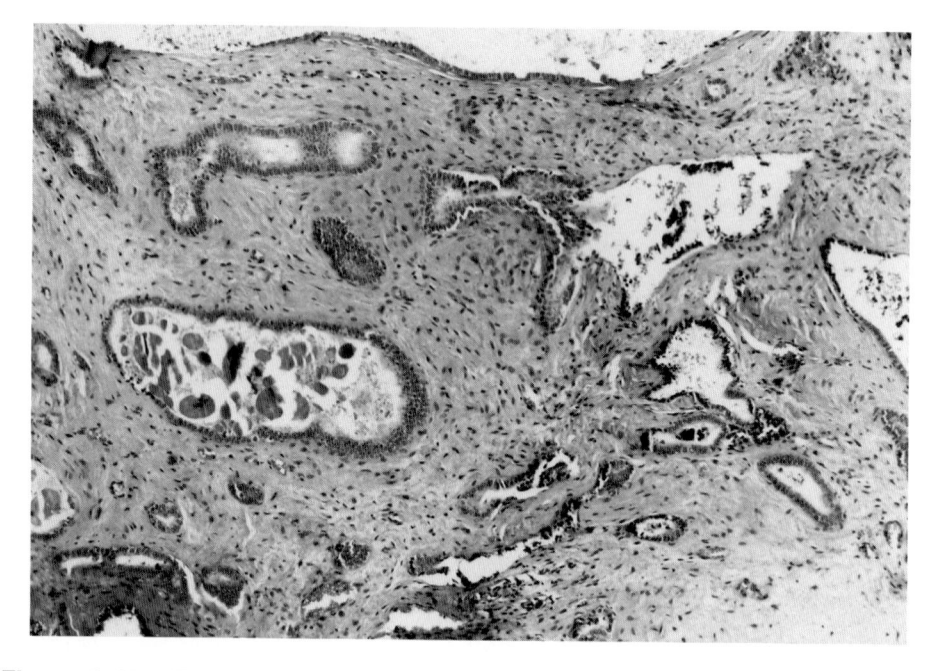

Figure 6-15. This section from an endometrial polyp from a patient on tamoxifen therapy shows the markedly fibrotic stroma and dilated glands sometimes seen in these polyps.

THE ENDOMETRIUM IN INFERTILITY— LUTEAL PHASE DEFECTS

The endometrial biopsy is often employed as part of an infertility workup. It can be useful in the assessment of organic intrauterine pathology that may interfere with fertility. In addition, the endometrial biopsy during an infertility workup may uncover morphology representative of the same hormonal imbalances that can cause DUB. In the absence of organic endometrial pathology, the main questions are whether ovulation has occurred, and, if so, whether there is a luteal phase defect.

Luteal phase defect is traditionally defined as a deficiency of progesterone production by the corpus luteum. Other authors[11] have suggested an intrinsic endometrial defect, with deficient or decreased number of progesterone receptors.

In infertility as in other areas, the evaluation of the endometrial histology in the absence of clinical information is fruitless at times, and a history is crucial for proper interpretation. Endometrial dating has traditionally been performed using the classic criteria of Noyes et al.[12] Correlation with the clinical endometrial date has been achieved in the past by counting backward from the next menstrual period, on the assumption that the luteal phase is a fixed 14 days. This is now known to be untrue, with variations in the length of the luteal phase present in women of normal fertility,[13] and the morphologic endometrial date correlates better with the LH surge.[14] It must also be recognized that morphologic endometrial dating is imprecise, with a high interobserver variability. Although the morphologic changes in the endometrium are more uniform around the time of ovulation,[14] most clinicians opt to biopsy later in the secretory phase, to get an overall view of the cumulative luteal phase.

A variety of patterns may be found in the endometrial sample of an infertility patient. The tissue may be completely normal and in-phase. An organic lesion may be detected. The spectrum of secretory and nonsecretory patterns seen with DUB may be seen. The morphologic expressions of luteal phase defects include weakly secretory endometrium, out-of-phase endometrium, dyssynchronous maturation, and irregular ripening.

Weakly secretory endometrium, as well as irregular ripening, as discussed, may be secondary to either poor corpus luteum function, or poor endometrial response, diffuse or focal.

Out-of-phase endometrium is morphologically normal secretory endometrium that has delayed maturation as compared with the expected chronologic date. Clinical evaluation of the expected endometrial date on the day of the biopsy must therefore be made. There is controversy over whether the criteria for diagnosing out-of-phase endometrium is met if there is a 2-day discrepancy, or only if a greater than 2-day discrepancy exists. Because of the sporadic occurrence of maturational lag in normally fertile women,[13] many clinicians require two successive out-of-phase cycles to diagnose luteal phase defect.

Dyssynchronous maturation with glands and stroma meeting different dating criteria is often seen in a background of ovulation inducing agents.

REFERENCES

1. Van Bogaert, LJ, Maldague P, et al: Endometrial biopsy interpretation—shortcomings and problems in current gynecologic practice. *Obstet Gynecol* 51:25–28, 1978.
2. Sobrinho LG, Kase N: Endocrinologic aspects of dysfunctional uterine bleeding. *Clin Obstet Gynecol* 13:400–415, 1970.
3. Dallenbach-Hellweg G: Special forms of hyperplasia. In *Histopathology of the endometrium*. Springer Verlag, Berlin, 1987, pp 129–130.
4. Israel R, Mishell DR, Labudovich M: Mechanisms of normal and dysfunctional uterine bleeding. *Clin Obstet Gynecol* 13:386–399, 1970.
5. Aksel S, Jones GS: Etiology and treatment of dysfunctional uterine bleeding. *Obstet Gynecol* 44:1–13, 1974.
6. Hendrickson MR, Kempson RL: The approach to endometrial diagnosis: a system of nomenclature. In *Surgical pathology of the uterine corpus*. WB Saunders, Philadelphia, 1980, pp 99–157.
7. Buckley CH, Fox H: The effect of therapeutic and contraceptive hormones on the endometrium. In *Biopsy pathology of the endometrium*. Raven Press, New York, 1989, pp 68–92.
8. Seif MW, Pearson JM, Ibrahim ZH, et al: Endometrium in in-vitro fertilization cycles: morphological and functional differentiation in the implantation phase. *Hum Reprod* 7:6–11, 1992.
9. Benda JA: Clomiphene's effect on endometrium in infertility. *Int J Gynecol Pathol* 11:273–282, 1992.
10. Nuovo MA, Nuovo GJ, McCaffrey RM, et al: Endometrial polyps in postmenopausal patients receiving Tamoxifen. *Int J Gynecol Pathol* 8:125–131, 1989.
11. Li TC, Cooke ID: Evaluation of the luteal phase. *Hum Reprod* 6:484–499, 1991.
12. Noyes RW, Hertig AT, Rock J: Dating the endometrial biopsy. *Fertil Steril* 1:3–25, 1950.
13. Langren B, Unden A, Diczfalusy E: Hormonal profile of the cycle in 68 normally menstruating women. *Acta Endocrinol* (Copenhagen) 94:89–98, 1980.
14. Johannisson E, Langren B, Rohr H, et al: Endometrial morphology and peripheral hormone levels in women with regular menstrual cycles. *Fertil Steril* 48:401–408, 1987.

7
Benign Organic Lesions of the Endometrium

Debra S. Heller, M.D.

ABNORMAL UTERINE BLEEDING

Abnormal patterns of uterine bleeding are among the most common problems seen in the gynecologist's office, and endometrial sampling is often employed in their investigation. After malignant and hyperplastic conditions have been ruled out, there is a long list of benign potential causes of abnormal uterine bleeding. These can be divided into organic causes of abnormal bleeding and dysfunctional uterine bleeding. Organic causes include lesions within the uterus or pelvis, conditions related to pregnancy, and some systemic conditions. The endometrial lesions in this category are the subject of this discussion (Table 7-1). Dysfunctional uterine bleeding (DUB), that is, bleeding due to hormonal irregularities, is covered in Chapter 6.

Organic lesions of the endometrium may present with abnormal uterine bleeding patterns, cause infertility, or be asymptomatic.

ENDOMETRITIS

Endometritis is classified as acute or chronic based on the type of inflammatory infiltrate. The etiology may be apparent, but the cause is frequently nonspecific.

TABLE 7-1. Organic Causes of Abnormal Uterine Bleeding and Other Benign Organic Lesions of the Endometrium

---

Endometritis
   Acute endometritis, nonspecific
   Chronic endometritis, nonspecific
   Specific identifiable causes of endometritis
      Tuberculous endometritis
      Actinomyces
      Viral endometritis (herpes, cytomegalovirus)
      Pregnancy-related infections
      Uncommon infections and inflammations: e.g. pinworm, schistosomiasis, fungi, sarcoid, foreign body
Endometrial polyps
   Usual endometrial polyps
   Adenomyomatous polyps
   Atypical polypoid adenomyoma
Asherman's syndrome
Pregnancy-related conditions
Leiomyomas
Adenomyosis
Endometriosis
Systemic diseases with coagulation defects
Adenomatoid tumor

Acute Endometritis

In the absence of retained products of conception, acute endometritis is considerably less common than chronic endometritis. Acute endometritis may be secondary to bacteria, including *Neisseria gonorrhea, Chlamydia,* or *Actinomyces.* Diagnostic criteria are strict, because a nonpathologic infiltrate of polymorphonuclear leukocytes, as well as stromal granulocytes, which resemble polymorphonuclear leukocytes, is present at certain times in the normal menstrual cycle. In order to be diagnostic for acute endometritis, the specimen must have microabscess formation, characterized by collections of polymorphonuclear leukocytes in gland lumina and stroma. There is destruction of glandular epithelium by this infiltrate (Fig. 7-1).

Chronic Endometritis

The hallmark of chronic endometritis is plasma cell infiltration of the endometrial stroma (Fig. 7-2). Plasma cells are not a component of normal endometrium. Other less specific changes include lymphocyte infiltration, the formation of lymphoid follicles, hemosiderin deposition, necrosis, and vascular ectasia.[1] Secretory endometrium cannot be reliably dated in the presence of

Endometritis

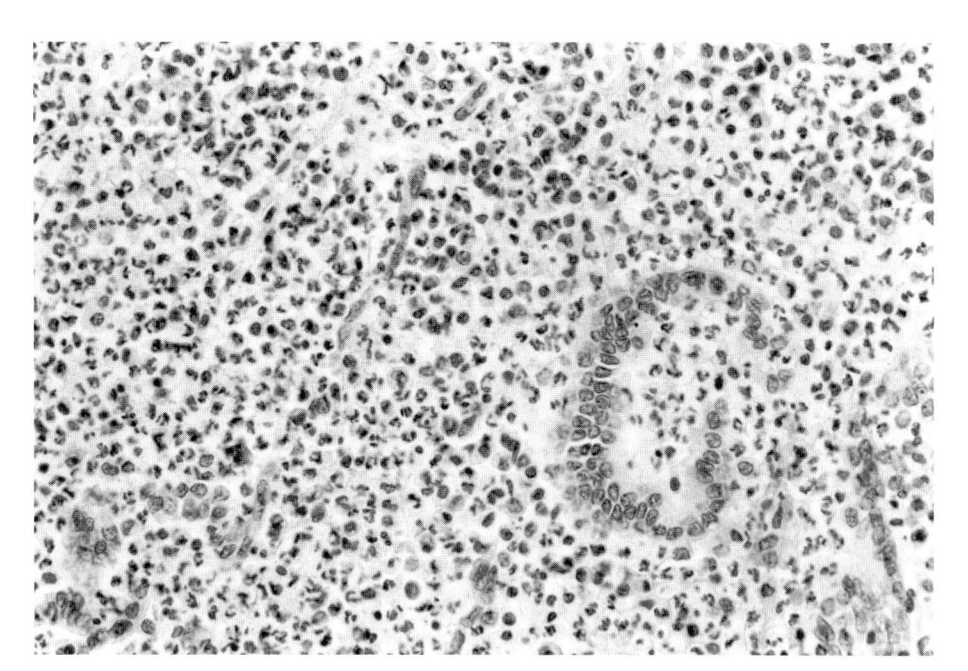

Figure 7-1. As polymorphonuclear leukocytes may be present in normal endometrium, the diagnosis of acute endometritis rests on the finding of microabscesses, seen here in endometrial stroma and destroying a gland.

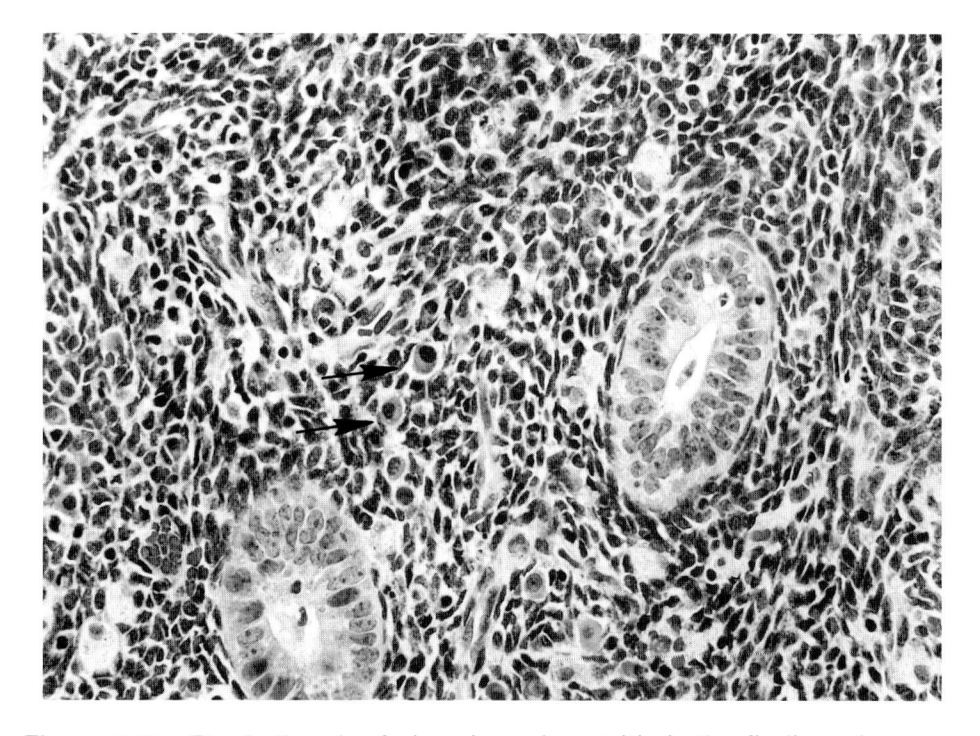

Figure 7-2. The hallmark of chronic endometritis is the finding of plasma cells (arrows).

chronic endometritis. Chronic endometritis may be secondary to an identifiable etiology such as an IUD, or may be due to unknown causes.

In a study on chronic endometritis by Rotterdam,[1] in 53% of patients chronic endometritis was associated with either postabortal or postpartum conditions, IUD use, or pelvic inflammatory disease; 26% of cases were secondary to conditions obstructing menstrual flow such as leiomyomata or endometrial polyps; 4.5% had cervical intraepithelial neoplasia grade III (CIN III) as their only gynecologic pathology; and in 16.5% of cases, no etiology was found.

Greenwood and Moran[2] described morphologic features of the endometrium that correlated with plasma cell infiltrates and were easier to identify. These included superficial stromal edema, increased stromal density, and a pleomorphic stromal inflammatory infiltrate composed predominantly of lymphocytes in the absence of premenstrual changes or other endometrial lesions. The authors pointed out the utility of their criteria, since plasma cells are frequently hard to detect. The first two of these criteria can be detected at low power, arousing suspicion of chronic endometritis, and allowing for a more directed search for plasma cells.

Less common forms of chronic endometritis include infections secondary to cytomegalovirus (CMV)[3] or herpes simplex[4] (Fig. 7-3). Classic viral inclusions are the most helpful in making the diagnosis, but may be difficult to detect in CMV infection. Another rare form of chronic endometritis is xanthogranulomatous endometritis (Fig. 7-4), usually encountered after pyo-

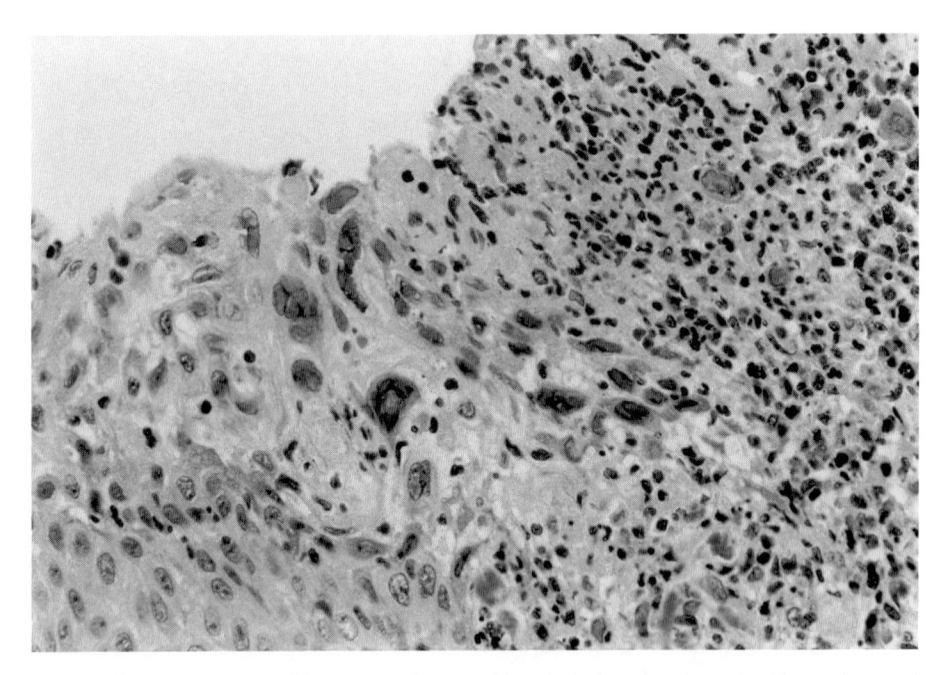

Figure 7-3. Endometritis secondary to Herpes simplex is rare. Here the typical multinucleated cells with glassy intranuclear inclusions are seen in a cervical biopsy, a more common site of infection in the female genital tract.

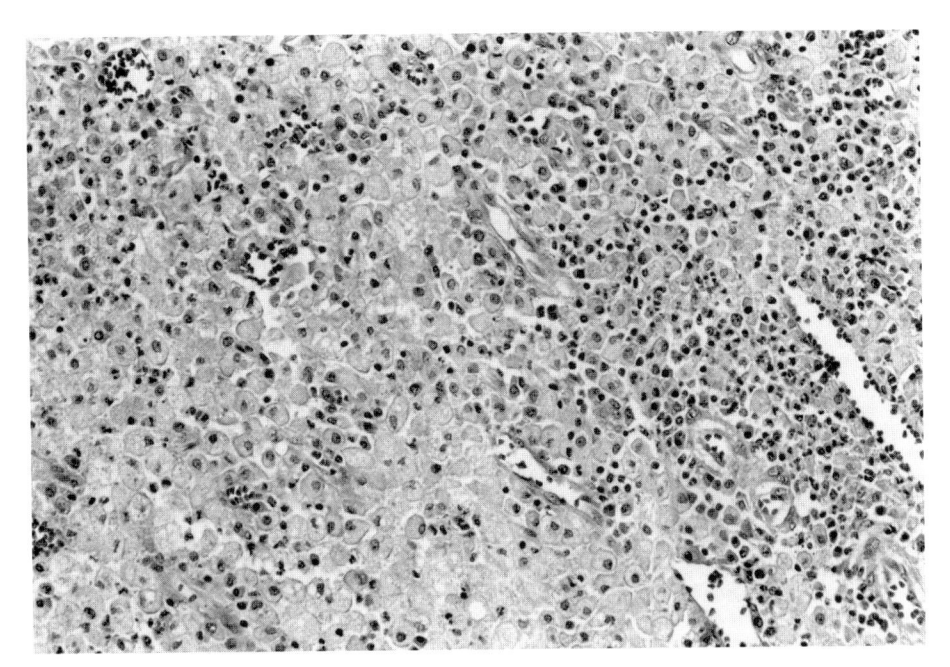

Figure 7-4. Endometrial stroma is infiltrated by foamy macrophages in xanthogranulomatous endometritis.

metra or hematometra.[5] Here the endometrial stroma is infiltrated by foamy or hemosiderin-laden macrophages.

Granulomatous Endometritis

Rarely, granulomatous inflammation of the endometrium may occur with fungi such as *Blastomyces, Coccidioides,* and *Cryptococcus,* as well as with *Enterobius* infection, schistosomiasis, foreign bodies, and sarcoidosis.[5] The overwhelming majority of cases of granulomatous endometritis, however, are secondary to tuberculosis.

Tuberculous Endometritis

Genital tract tuberculosis probably occurs secondary to hematogenous spread. It predominantly affects the fallopian tubes, and less often, the endometrium.[7] Infertility, either primary or secondary, is the main symptom, which may lead to endometrial sampling. Other symptoms include amenorrhea, menstrual irregularities, and abdominal pain.[8] Histologically, the finding of epithelioid granulomas with Langhans' giant cells is suggestive but not diagnostic of tuberculosis (Fig. 7-5). Central caseous necrosis is less common than in pulmonary tuberculosis,[7] and the granulomas may coalesce. The definitive diagnosis rests on the demonstration of acid-fast bacilli, either by

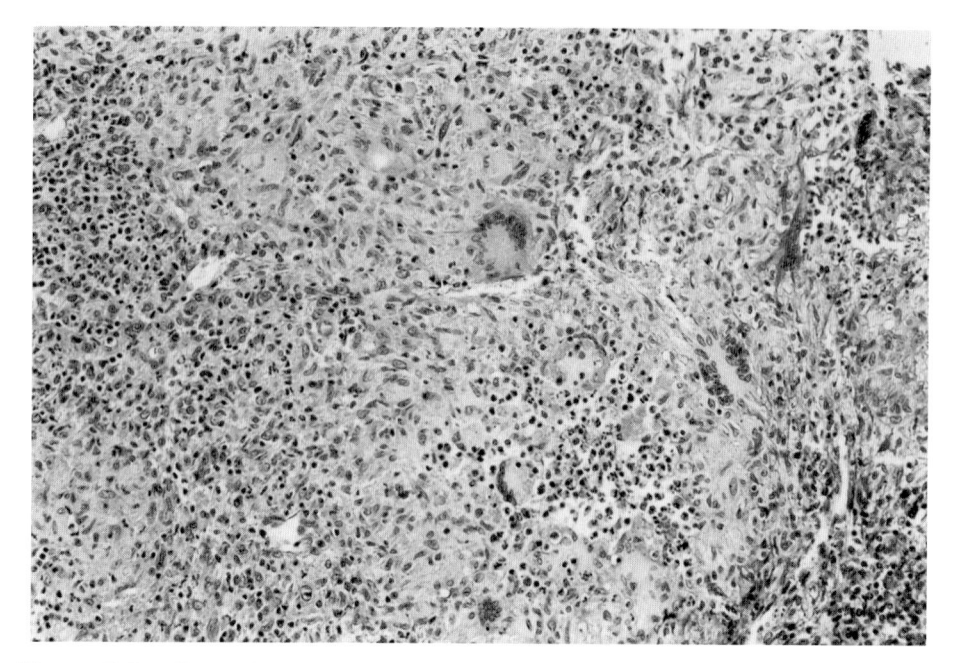

Figure 7-5. Granulomatous endometritis secondary to tuberculosis. Several Langhans' giant cells are seen among the epithelioid cells of this granuloma. Caseation is not present.

special tissue stain or by culture. It should be noted that tissue stains for acid-fast bacilli are notoriously insensitive, even in the face of culture-proven disease.

Actinomyces

Endometrial infection with *Actinomyces* is associated with IUD and pessary usage,[9] and is usually associated with an acute inflammatory infiltrate. While definitive diagnosis rests on culture or immunohistochemistry,[5] the typical "sulfur granules" may be recognized on pap smear, endocervical, or endometrial curettings (Fig. 7-6A,B), and can be reliably identified in most cases. These "sulfur granules" are actually colonies of the organisms with a peripheral radial organization.

LEIOMYOMAS

The endometrium overlying submucosal leiomyomas can show pressure atrophy and necrosis, or may lag behind the remaining endometrium in development, potentially yielding a false impression of luteal phase defect on

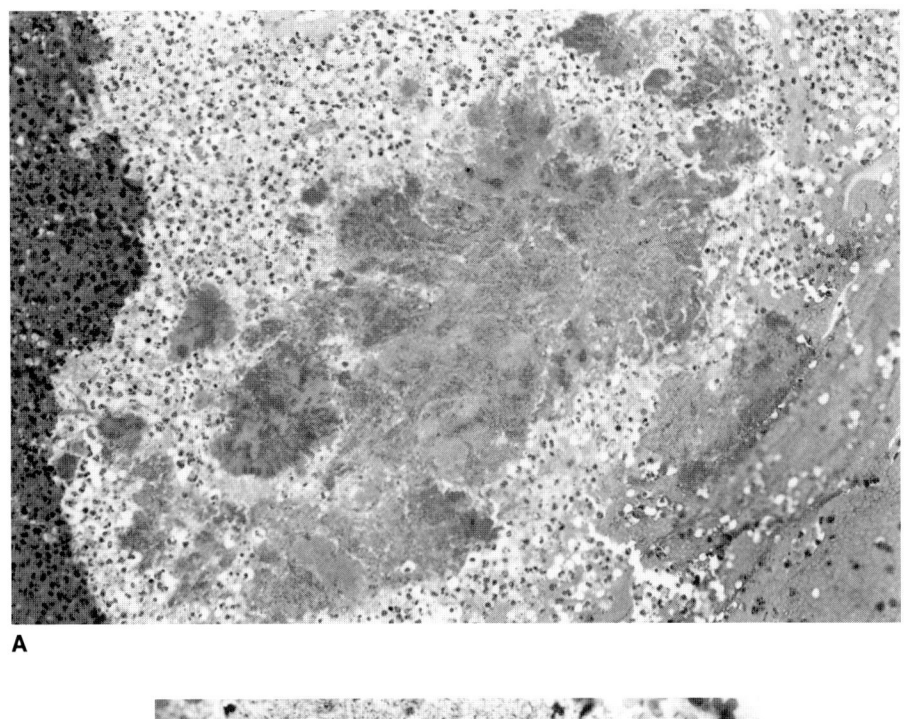

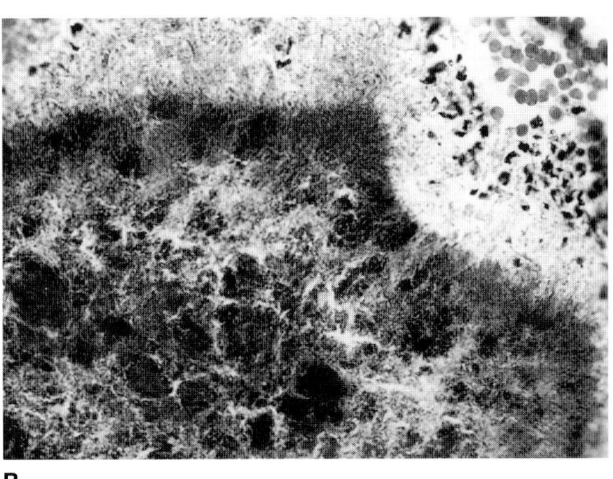

Figure 7-6. (A) Actinomyces is often seen in curettings among inflammatory debris, appearing smudgy. (B) If well preserved, the radial configuration of the colony can be appreciated.

endometrial sampling. Fragments of the leiomyoma may be present in the curettage specimen[5] (see Chapter 4).

ADENOMYOSIS AND ENDOMETRIOSIS

While not conditions of the endometrium itself, these lesions can be associated with abnormal bleeding. Endometrial sampling would not be diagnostic for these problems.

ASHERMAN'S SYNDROME

Asherman's syndrome, the formation of intrauterine adhesions after a traumatic curettage, almost always occurs after a pregnancy-related event. It can cause amenorrhea, hypomenorrhea, and infertility. If there is minimal scarring, menses may be normal. Endometrial sampling in Asherman's syndrome generally obtains scant tissue, and may show inactive endometrial glands, fibrotic stroma, scar tissue, and myometrium, although normal endometrium may also be seen.[10]

PREGNANCY-RELATED CAUSES OF UTERINE BLEEDING

See Chapter 11.

ENDOMETRIAL POLYPS

Endometrial polyps are frequently encountered, and are often the cause of abnormal bleeding. Less common polypoid lesions include atypical polypoid adenomyoma, discussed below, and adenofibroma (see Chapter 10).

Typical Endometrial Polyps

Endometrial polyps are composed of endometrial glands in a fibrotic stroma containing thick-walled blood vessels. Occasionally, the stroma contains abundant smooth muscle, and this is called an *adenomyomatous polyp* (Fig. 7-7). The endometrial glands may be in-phase with the rest of the endometrium, but are more often out-of-phase. The glands are more responsive to

Endometrial Polyps

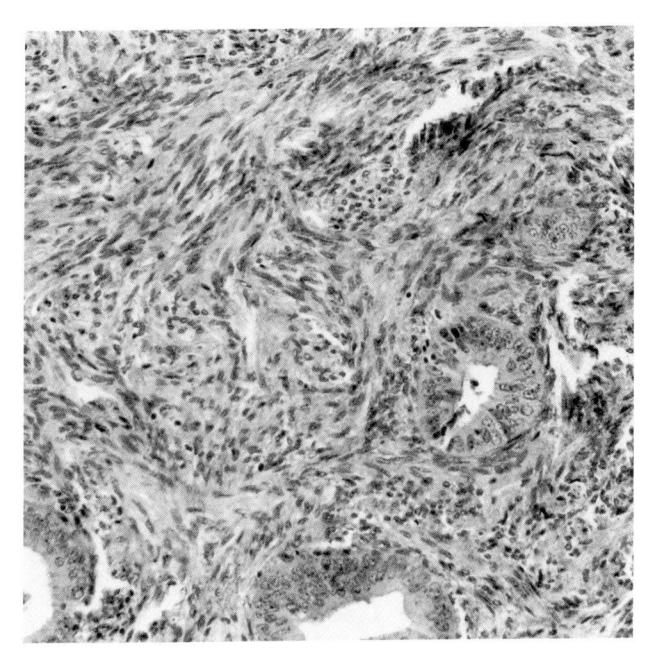

Figure 7-7. This adenomyomatous polyp shows prominent smooth muscle in the stroma.

estrogen than progesterone, so polyps are more likely to show proliferative rather than secretory activity. The glands are often irregular and stellate, and varying degrees of hyperplasia and even carcinoma may occur. Alternatively, in postmenopausal women, the glands may show cystic atrophic changes. For diagnostic purposes, the ideal polyp is polypoid in shape, with a surface epithelial lining all around, and has a recognizable stalk containing thick-walled blood vessels (Fig. 7-8). Unfortunately, endometrial polyps frequently fragment on curettage,[11] making pathologic diagnosis difficult, particularly with in-phase endometrial glands. It is not uncommon for the clinician to diagnose a polyp on hysteroscopy, and then have the pathologist be unable to confirm this diagnosis.

Atypical Polypoid Adenomyoma

An unusual variant of endometrial polyp is the atypical polypoid adenomyoma (APA), a lesion usually occurring in premenopausal women.[12,13] Irregular atypical endometrial glands are present in a benign smooth muscle stroma in this polypoid lesion (Fig. 7-9). The glands show markedly atypical nuclei, mitotic activity, and frequently squamous metaplasia.[13] These findings may be misinterpreted as adenocarcinoma with myometrial invasion, but there are certain distinguishing features. The smooth muscle bundles in APA are

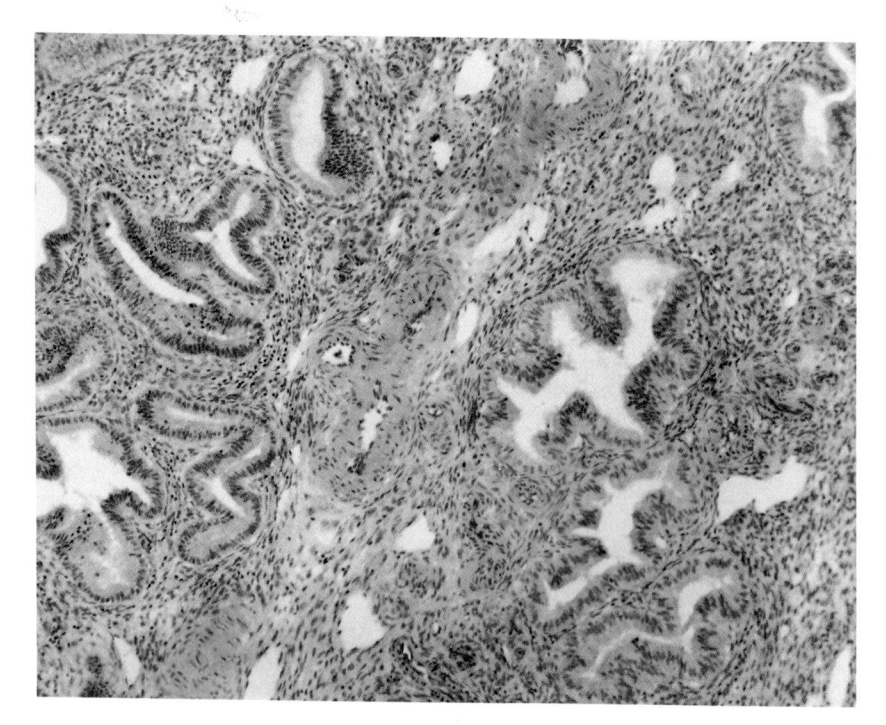

Figure 7-8. The stalk of this endometrial polyp contains thick-walled blood vessels. Glands are irregular, often with a stellate configuration.

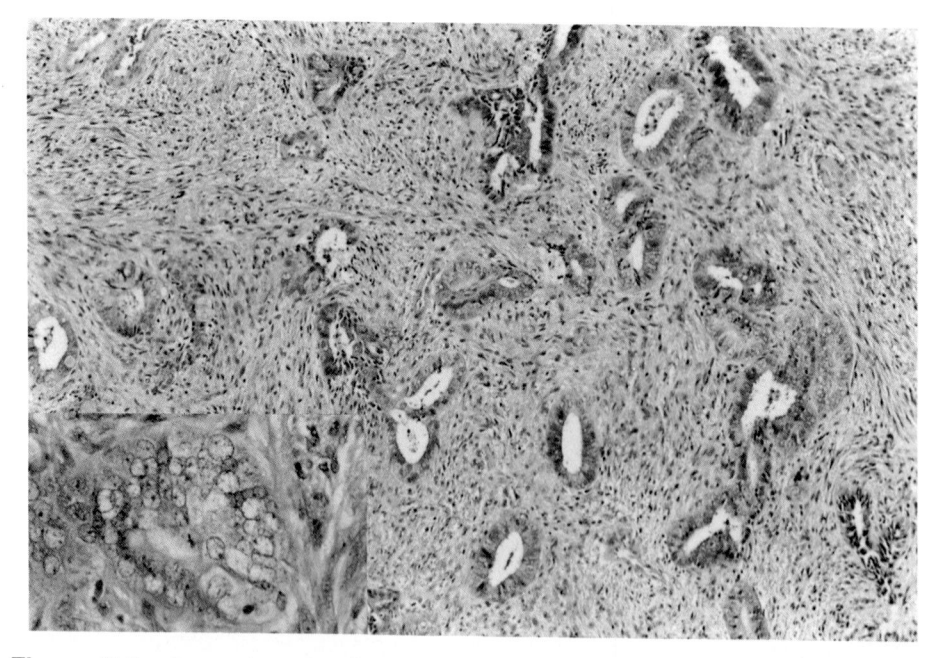

Figure 7-9. Irregular glands are embedded in a benign smooth muscle stroma in atypical polypoid adenomyoma. Note marked nuclear atypia in the glandular epithelium (inset).

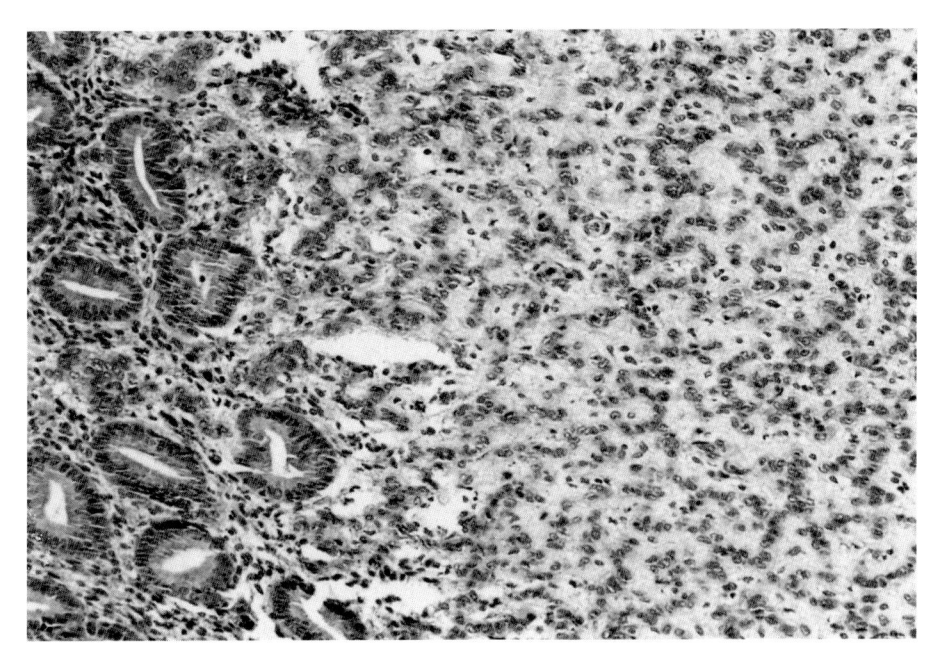

Figure 7-10. An adenomatoid tumor, composed of small anastomosing epithelial cells, is present within this endometrial specimen.

more cellular than in normal myometrium, and chunks of myometrium invaded by endometrial adenocarcinoma are rarely seen on curettage.[12] In a hysterectomy, the polypoid nature of the lesion can be appreciated. APA must also be distinguished from adenomyosis, which contains endometrial stroma as well as glands, and in the case of a mitotically active smooth muscle component, from malignant mixed Müllerian tumor. Atypical polypoid adenomyomas do not metastasize, but can be persistent. Some cases have been cured by single curettage, but others have required repeat procedures, and in the absence of a desire to preserve fertility, hysterectomy may be the better option.[12]

ADENOMATOID TUMOR

Usually incidental findings, adenomatoid tumors most often occur in the fallopian tube, but can occur subserosally in the uterus. Rarely, there can be an intraendometrial component to the lesion (Fig. 7-10), causing diagnostic difficulty if obtained on a curettage specimen.[14] The epithelioid and signet ring cell infiltrate can be mistaken for a metastatic adenocarcinoma or vascular lesion; however, positive alcian blue and keratin stains, and negative mucicarmine, PAS (periodic acid Schiff), and Factor VIII stains may be helpful in making the distinction.[14]

REFERENCES

1. Rotterdam H: Chronic endometritis. A clinicopathologic study. *Pathol Ann* 13:209–231, 1978.
2. Greenwood SM, Moran JJ: Chronic endometritis: morphologic and clinical observations. *Obstet Gynecol* 58:176–184, 1981.
3. Wenckebach GF, Curry B. Cytomegalovirus infection of the female genital tract. *Arch Pathol Lab Med* 100:609–612, 1976.
4. Schneider V, Behm F, Mumaw V: Ascending herpetic endometritis. *Obstet Gynecol* 59:259–262, 1982.
5. Buckley CH, Fox H: *Biopsy pathology of the endometrium.* Raven Press, New York, 1989, pp 105–131.
6. Hendrickson MR, Kempson RL: *Surgical pathology of the uterine corpus.* Philadelphia, Saunders, 1980, 215–246.
7. Nogales-Ortiz F, Tarancón I, Nogales FF: The pathology of female genital tuberculosis—a 31 year study of 1436 cases. *Obstet Gynecol* 53:422–428, 1979.
8. Bazaz-Malik G, Maheshwari B, Lal N: Tuberculous endometritis: a clinicopathological study of 1000 cases. *Br J Obstet Gynecol* 90:84–86, 1983.
9. Bhagavan GS, Gupta PK: Genital actinomycosis and intrauterine contraceptive devices—cytopathologic diagnosis and clinical significance. *Hum Pathol* 9:567–578, 1978.
10. Dallenbach-Hellweg G: Histopathology of the Endometrium. Springer-Verlag, Berlin, 1987, pp 199.
11. Van Bogaert LJ: Clinicopathologic findings in endometrial polyps. *Obstet Gynecol* 71:771–773, 1988.
12. Young RH, Treger T, Scully RE: Atypical polypoid adenomyoma of the uterus. A report of 27 cases. *Am J Clin Pathol* 86:139–145, 1986.
13. Mazur M: Atypical polypoid adenomyomas of the endometrium. *Am J Surg Pathol* 5:473–482, 1981.
14. Carlier MT, Dardick I, Lagace AF, et al: Adenomatoid tumor of the uterus: presentation in endometrial curettings. Int J Gynecol Pathol 5:69–74, 1986.

8
Endometrial Metaplasias

Debra S. Heller, M.D.

Müllerian epithelium is multipotential, and metaplastic changes (change from one tissue type to another) can occur in both the epithelial, and less commonly the stromal components of the endometrium, usually in association with nonsecretory endometrial patterns. Epithelial endometrial metaplasias are seen more frequently in hyperplastic and malignant endometria than in normal tissue, reflecting their association with estrogenic stimulation.[1] They are more common in the postmenopausal period. Epithelial metaplasias can also be seen in the setting of inflammation. Recognition of endometrial metaplasias is important to avoid overdiagnosis of neoplasia, particularly if the metaplastic areas are architecturally complex. The distinction between metaplasia and neoplasia can be particularly confusing on curettage.

EPITHELIAL METAPLASIAS OF THE ENDOMETRIUM

Squamous Metaplasia

Squamous epithelium can be present in the endometrium under several circumstances. In 1885, Zeller was the first to describe a series of cases of benign squamous metaplasia of the endometrium, calling the condition "psoriasis uterina."[2] Squamous metaplasia of the endometrium has been reported with estrogen excess, vitamin A deficiency, chronic endometritis, tuberculosis, syphilis, radiation, foreign bodies, and pyometra.[2,3] An unusual benign condition, ichthyosis uteri (literally "fish-skin uterus"), in which squamous metaplasia replaces the entire surface endometrium, was encountered in the past after intrauterine steam treatment for endometritis. With the merciful abandonment of this therapeutic modality, icthyosis uteri is rare,[4] and usually is seen in the setting of pyometra.[5] Benign squamous epithelium in the endometrium may also rarely occur as replacement of the superficial epithelial layer by a cervical condyloma.[6]

Malignant conditions associated with squamous differentiation in the endometrium include primary adenocarcinoma of the endometrium with squamous differentiation (metaplasia), the exceedingly rare primary squamous cell carcinoma of the endometrium, and upward spread of a cervical squamous cell carcinoma. (For a discussion of squamous differentiation in the setting of malignancy, see Chapter 10).

Squamous metaplasia of the endometrium is common, and may appear as mature, well-differentiated, cytologically benign keratinized squamous epithelium, or as immature squamous epithelial nodules, referred to as *morules* (Figs. 8-1, 8-2).

Squamous morules are cytologically benign and rarely contain mitoses. They are commonly associated with endometrial hyperplasia, a condition that has been termed *adenoacanthosis*.[7] Morules can coalesce into sheets, with or without areas of mature squamous metaplasia, which can cause diagnostic difficulty (Fig. 8-2). Endometrial hyperplasia with morular squamous metaplasia can be mistaken for the more serious atypical hyperplasia, or even endometrial adenocarcinoma, leading to unnecessary surgical intervention. In a series of 10 premenopausal patients with the diagnosis of

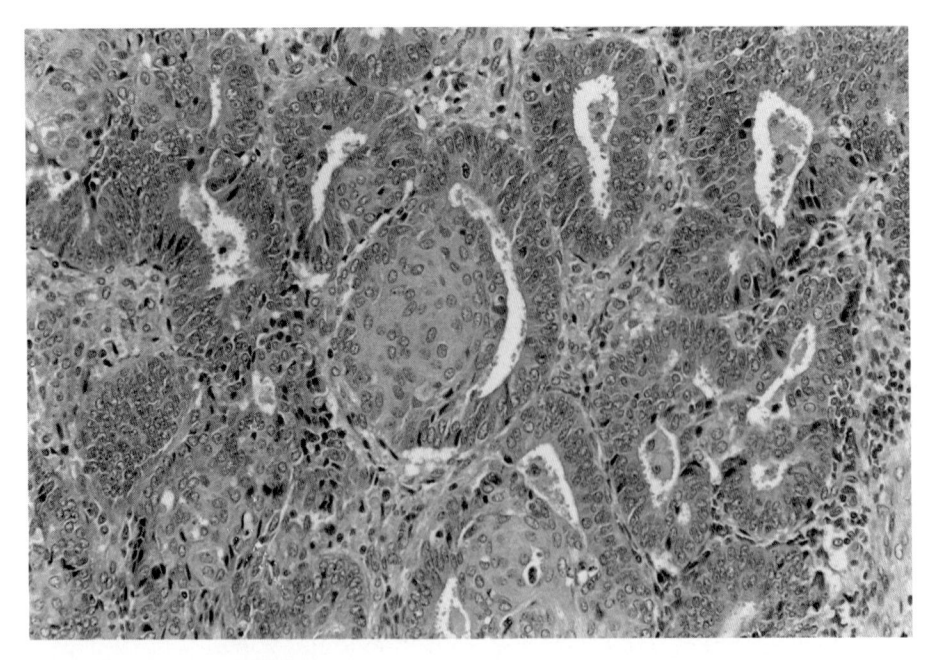

Figure 8-1. Immature squamous morules are seen in glandular lumens in this hyperplastic endometrium.

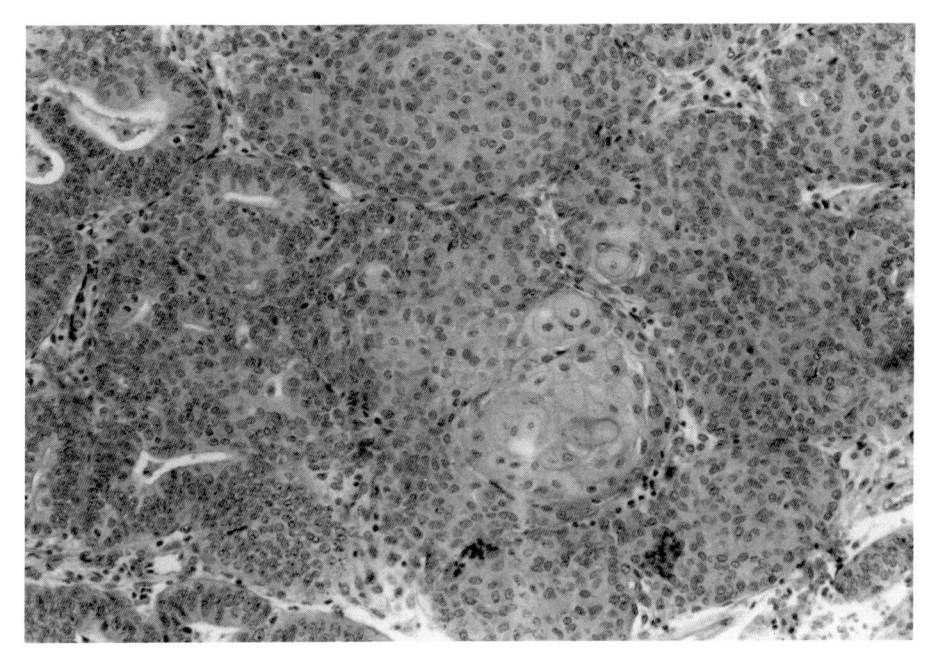

Figure 8-2. Mature squamous metaplasia is seen in the center of this field, surrounded by extensive morular (immature squamous) metaplasia. Although carcinoma may be present in this endometrium, extensive squamous metaplasia in and of itself is not diagnostic for malignancy.

adenoacanthosis, Crum et al found that the lesion was potentially reversible with conservative therapy.[7] However, while not diagnostic of carcinoma in and of itself, the finding of large masses of squamous metaplasia on biopsy may be associated with an unsampled carcinoma.

The differential diagnosis of squamous morules includes solid and nodular endometrial patterns. These include poorly differentiated carcinoma or sarcoma, endometrioid carcinoma with squamous differentiation, metastatic carcinoma, smooth muscle metaplasia of endometrial stroma, stromal nodular aggregates secondary to endometrial breakdown, lymphoid nodules, and granulomatous inflammation. The benign cytologic features of squamous metaplasia help distinguish it from malignancies. In endometrial adenocarcinoma with squamous differentiation, the glandular elements must meet the criteria for malignancy. The other entities are usually sufficiently distinctive histologically to prevent confusion; however, immunohistochemistry may be of assistance in some of these cases.

Mature squamous metaplasia may be confused with a primary endometrial squamous cell carcinoma or upward extension of a cervical carcinoma.[8] Squamous malignancies would be more likely to show nuclear atypia and mitotic activity. As pure squamous cell carcinoma of the endometrium is rare, the more likely site of a malignant purely squamous cell carcinoma would be the cervix, but clinical localization is obviously necessary.

Ciliated Cell (Tubal) Metaplasia

Ciliated cell metaplasia is exceedingly common, and individual epithelial cells often exhibit this change in normal proliferative endometrium (see Fig. 5-1). When the number of ciliated cells increases sufficiently to replace significant amounts of glandular or surface epithelium, the change is referred to as *ciliated cell metaplasia* (Fig. 8-3). This occurs particularly in states of estrogen excess.

The cells of ciliated cell metaplasia are cytologically benign, and resemble the ciliated cells of fallopian tube mucosa; hence the synonym *tubal metaplasia*. The metaplastic cells contain abundant, often eosinophilic, cytoplasm, and a perinuclear clearing may be seen. Mitotic figures are rare. The cells are arranged with their broader ciliated surface apically, with their narrower side against the basal lamina. The cells may occur in a single layer, or they may stratify, forming papillary projections.[8] In hyperplastic endometria, papillary formations of ciliated cell metaplasia may lead to an overdiagnosis of carcinoma. The benign nuclei and cilia help make the distinction, as cilia are exceedingly rare in endometrial carcinoma.[8]

Eosinophilic Metaplasia

Another epithelial metaplasia occurring in the endometrium is eosinophilic metaplasia. The cells of eosinophilic metaplasia resemble the eosinophilic

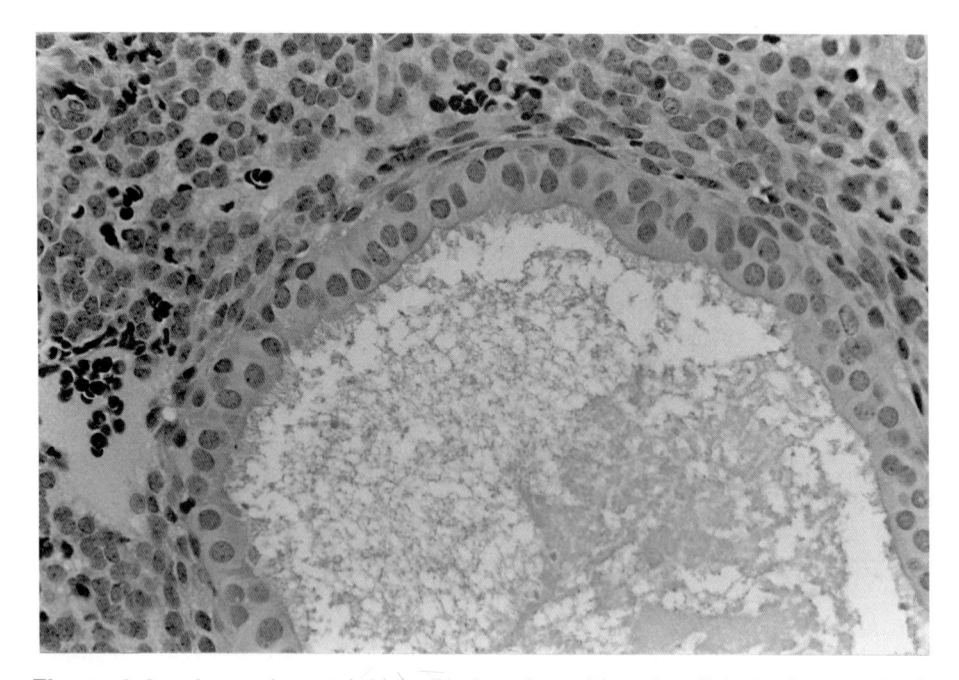

Figure 8-3. An endometrial gland showing ciliated cell (tubal) metaplasia.

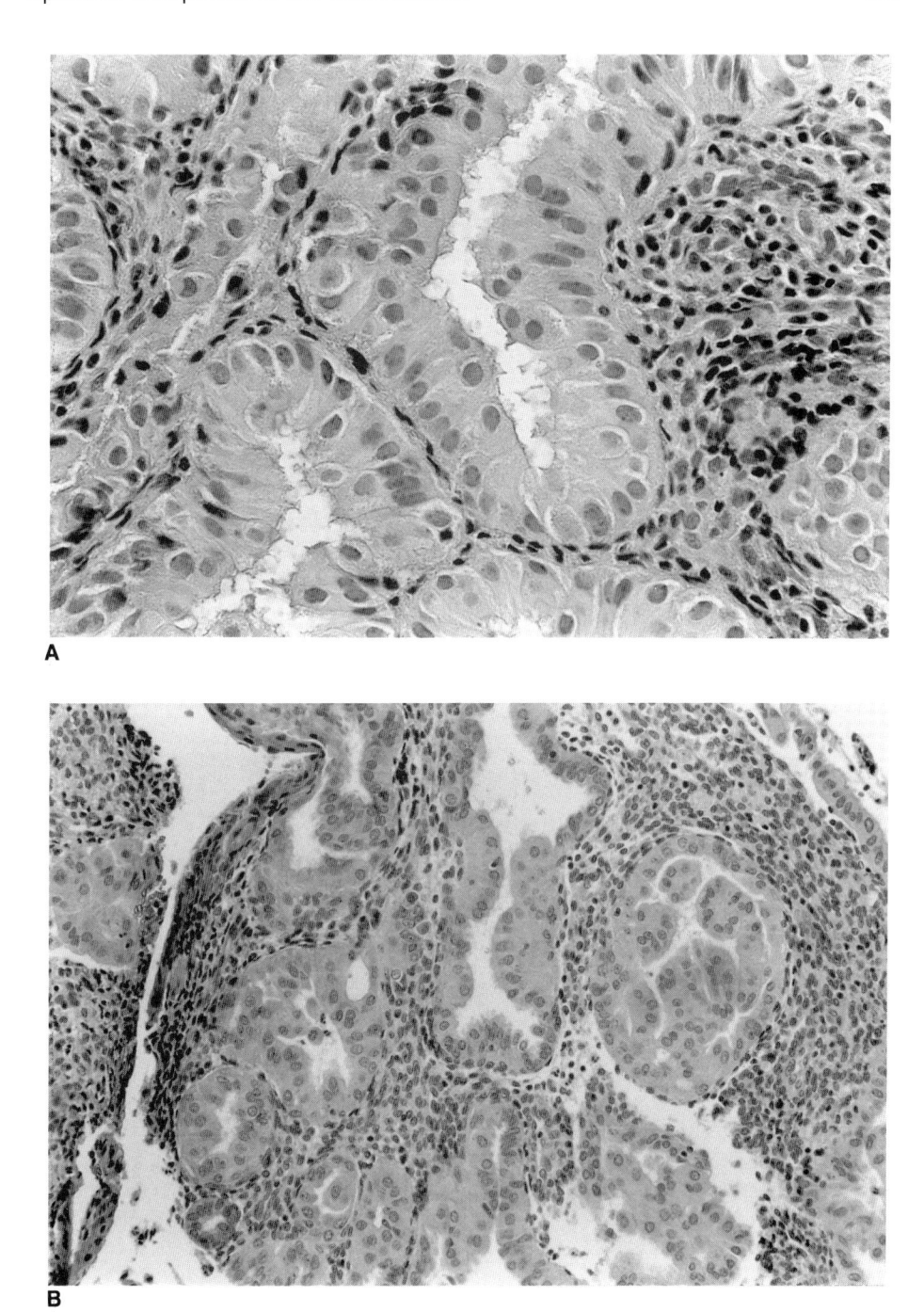

Figure 8-4. (A) Eosinophilic metaplasia of the endometrium. Glandular epithelium is replaced by cells with abundant eosinophilic cytoplasm. Tufting (B) should not be interpreted as malignancy.

cells seen in ciliated cell metaplasia, but without the cilia (Fig. 8-4A). Eosinophilic metaplasia has been found to be the most common metaplasia confused with carcinoma, due to the potentially shared feature of eosinophilic cytoplasm.[9] The tendency of eosinophilic metaplasia to show areas of tufting, and of stratification with cribriforming, adds to the diagnostic confusion (Fig. 8-4B). The focality of the cribriforming and lack of cytologic atypia help make the distinction from carcinoma.

Papillary Syncytial Metaplasia

This endometrial change is usually seen on the surface epithelium of the endometrium, and may be a degenerative effect rather than a true metaplasia. It consists of papillary projections of benign epithelial cells with poorly defined cellular borders. The papillae are devoid of fibrovascular cores, and are often infiltrated by acute inflammatory cells (Fig. 8-5). This change may be mistaken for endometrioid adenocarcinoma if the syncytia give a solid appearance, or as uterine papillary serous carcinoma.[8] The lack of cytologic atypia and of fibrovascular cores in papillary syncytial metaplasia help make the distinction.[8]

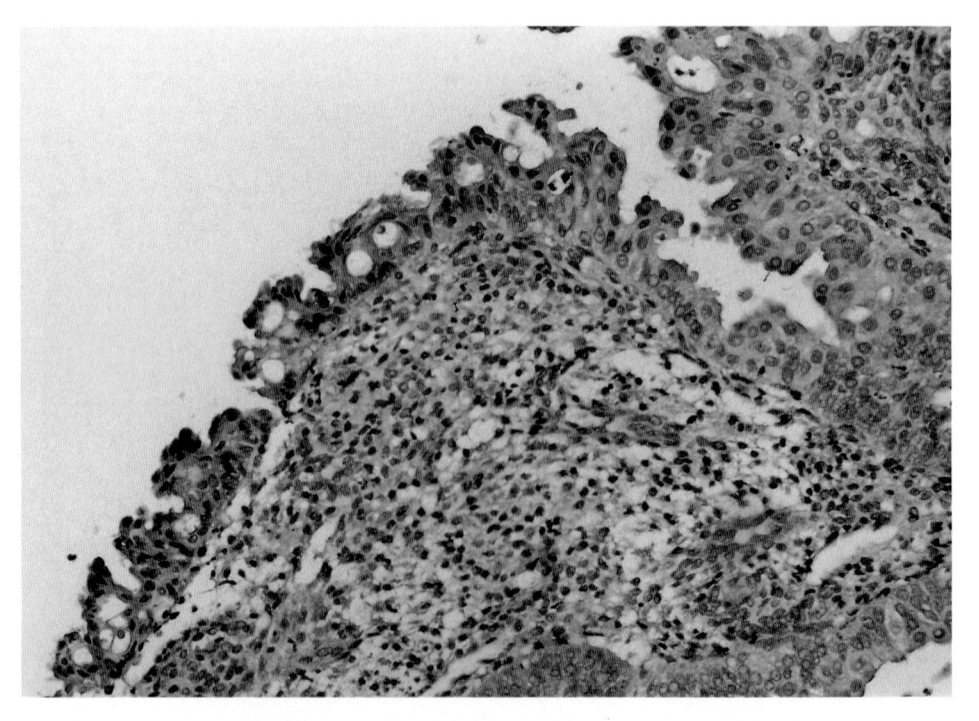

Figure 8-5. Papillary syncytial metaplasia on the endometrial surface. Note lack of atypia and lack of fibrovascular cores.

Mucinous Metaplasia

In mucinous metaplasia the endometrial glandular cells may resemble the mucinous cells of the endocervix (Fig. 8-6A), although the stroma is endometrial rather than endocervical. A variant, intestinal metaplasia, has been described, in which goblet cells occur[5] (Fig. 8-6B). Mucinous metaplasia occurs mainly in postmenopausal women, where it is usually focal. When it is diffuse, mucometra may occur.[5] Mucinous metaplasia may be confused with mucinous adenocarcinoma of the endometrium, mucinous adenocarcinoma of the endocervix, metastatic mucinous adenocarcinoma, or endocervical microglandular hyperplasia.[8] Differential diagnosis may be difficult because of lack of cytologic atypia in many mucinous carcinomas. Overall consideration of both architecture and cytologic features is required, and at times the distinction between benign and malignant mucinous change may not be possible on curettings alone (see Chapter 10).

Clear Cell Metaplasia and Hobnail Metaplasia

These are uncommon epithelial changes. In hobnail metaplasia, the apical surface of the cells is broader than the basal surface. The nuclei bulge into the free surface, supposedly resembling the hobnails used to shoe horses. Although the change may be mistaken for the hobnail cells sometimes seen in clear cell adenocarcinoma, the architecture and the lack of cytologic atypia should clearly differentiate them.[8]

The abundant clear cytoplasm of clear cell metaplastic cells contains glycogen and, to a lesser degree, mucin.[9] Clear cell metaplasia may be confused with the clear cell pattern of clear cell adenocarcinoma of the endometrium, but lacks the nuclear atypia of carcinoma.

Both hobnail and clear cell metaplasia may be mistaken for the Arias–Stella reaction. The metaplasias are usually seen in nonsecretory patterns, while the Arias–Stella reaction is associated with the presence of other gestational changes, such as hypersecretory endometrium, decidua, and even chorionic villi in the case of an intrauterine gestation. In addition, although lacking mitotic activity, the cells in the Arias–Stella reaction exhibit nuclear atypia, which is absent in the metaplasias.

STROMAL METAPLASIAS

These uncommon changes may be mistaken for the mesenchymal component of a malignant mixed mesodermal tumor (MMMT), however, stromal metaplasias are cytologically benign.

Rarely, benign mature cartilage may be seen in the endometrium, and this may represent either a stromal metaplastic change, or embedded fetal

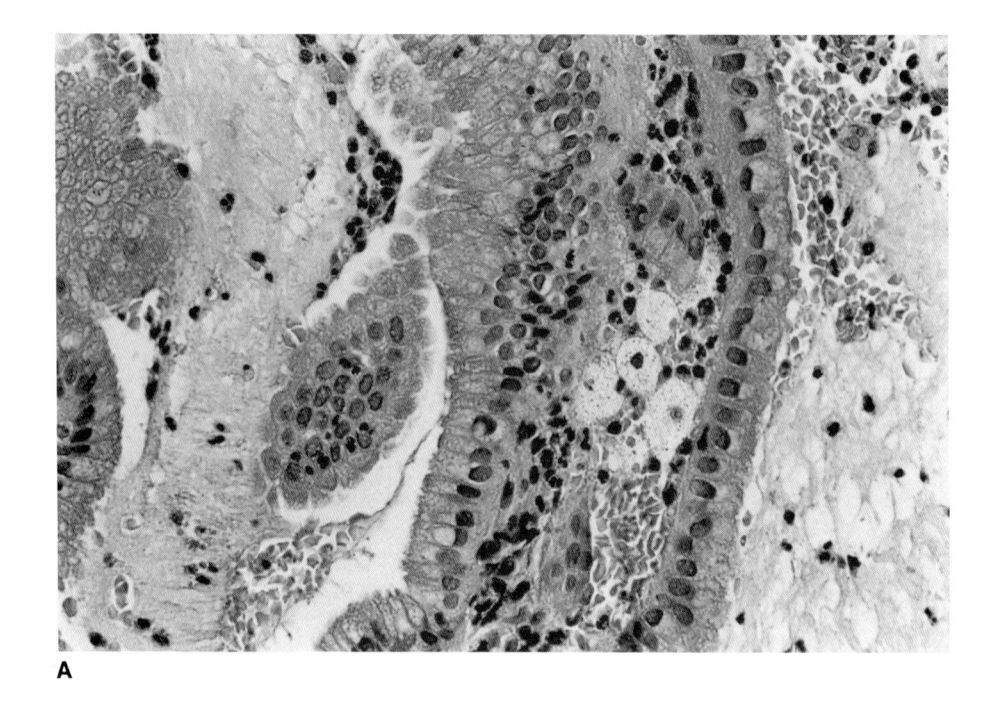

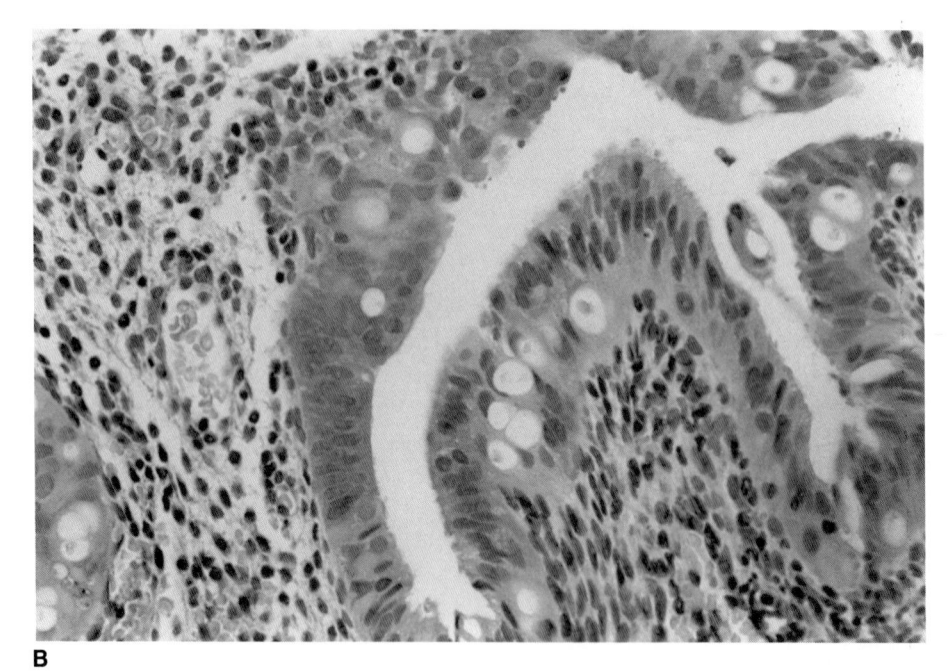

Figure 8-6. (A) Mucinous metaplasia. The glandular epithelium is replaced by cells resembling endocervical lining cells. A few stromal foam cells are seen. (B) Goblet cells are present in intestinal metaplasia of the endometrium, an uncommon variant of mucinous metaplasia.

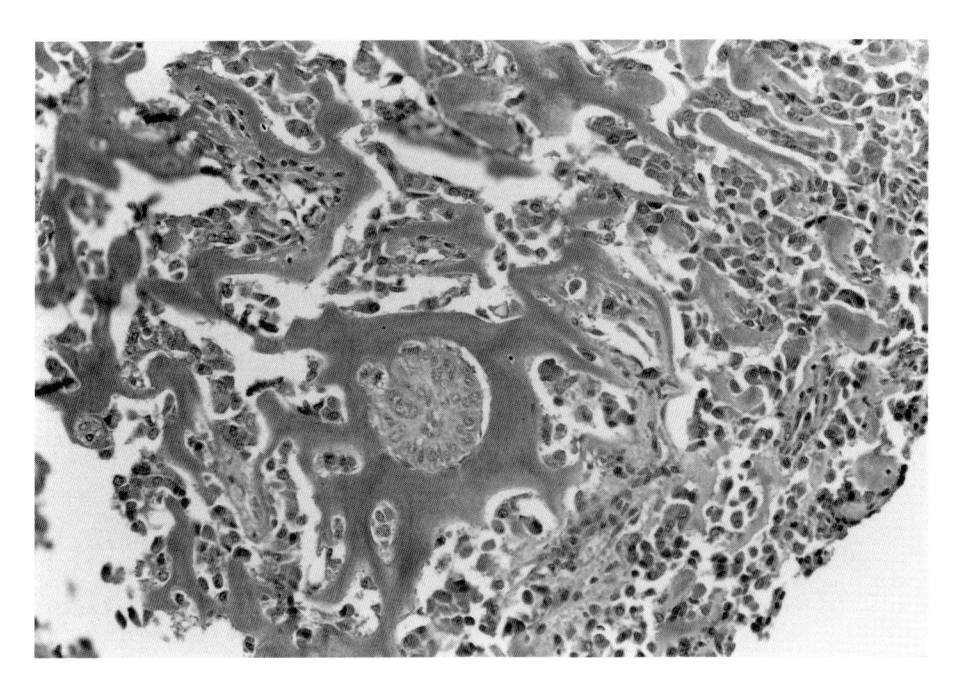

Figure 8-7. Osseous metaplasia of the endometrium. Note the endometrial gland trapped within osseous material.

remnants. A lack of a history of pregnancy and the presence of a transitional zone favor a metaplastic change.[5]

Osseous metaplasia occurs in a background setting of recurrent abortions and infection[5] (Fig. 8-7). Retained fetal parts may also occasionally be responsible for bone in the endometrium.

Benign nodules of smooth muscle may be seen in endometrial stroma, and must not be misconstrued as stromal nodules. The distinction is significant, because as Buckley and Fox[5] stress, although stromal nodules are benign, their presence requires that low-grade endometrial stromal sarcoma be ruled out.[5] Immunohistochemical stains for smooth muscle may help make the distinction.

Glial tissue in the endometrium is felt to be usually of fetal origin,[1] but rarely a case of immature teratoma arising in the uterus has been encountered.[8]

Stromal Foam Cells

Not a true metaplasia, stromal foam cells are probably transformed stromal cells that accumulate lipid in states of estrogen excess, developing an abundant vacuolated cytoplasm (Fig. 8-8).[1]

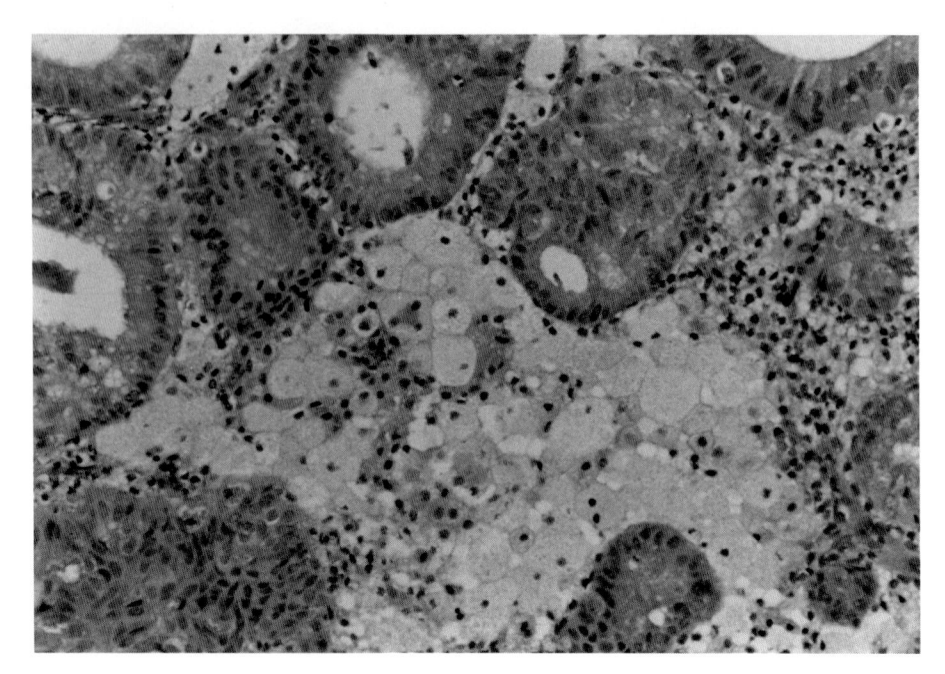

Figure 8-8. Stromal foam cells are frequently associated with hyperestrogenic states.

ASSOCIATION OF CARCINOMA AND THE EPITHELIAL METAPLASIAS OF THE ENDOMETRIUM

While the association of squamous metaplasia with endometrial carcinoma is well recognized, the association of other epithelial metaplasias with carcinoma also occurs. In a study of stage I adenocarcinomas of the endometrium,[10] 13 out of 60 samples initially diagnosed as carcinoma on curettage were reclassified as some form of hyperplasia, and of these, 11 also contained metaplastic changes. Of the remaining 47 patients, 15 had metaplasia, often of more than one type, coexisting with their carcinoma. These authors found mucinous, papillary, eosinophilic, tubal, and clear cell metaplasias in addition to squamous metaplasia. In this series, both tubal and eosinophilic metaplasias were noted to be more common than squamous metaplasia. The authors concluded that epithelial metaplasia must be viewed with concern when obtained on an in-office biopsy of a postmenopausal or perimenopausal patient because of the association with carcinoma. In this setting, they feel that a more thorough sampling should be considered.[10]

REFERENCES

1. Dallenbach-Hellweg G: *Histopathology of the endometrium,* 4th ed. Springer-Verlag, Berlin, 1987, pp 30, 124, 214–223.

References

2. Baggish M, Woodruff J: The occurrence of squamous epithelium in the endometrium. *Obstet Gynecol Surv* 22:69–115, 1967.
3. Kanbour A, Stock J: Squamous cell carcinoma in situ of the endometrium and fallopian tube as superficial extension of invasive cervical carcinoma. *Cancer* 42:570–580, 1978.
4. Kurman R, Norris H: Endometrial carcinoma. In Kurman R (ed): *Blaustein's pathology of the female genital tract,* 3rd ed. Springer-Verlag, New York, 1987, p 354.
5. Buckley CH, Fox H: *Biopsy pathology of the endometrium.* Raven Press, New York, 1989, pp 130–148.
6. Venkataseshan V, Woo T: Diffuse viral papillomatosis (condyloma) of the uterine cavity. *Int J Gynecol Pathol* 4:370–377, 1985.
7. Crum C, Richart RM, Fenoglio CM: Adenoacanthosis of the endometrium—a clinicopathologic study in premenopausal women. *Am J Surg Pathol* 5:15–20, 1981.
8. Henderson MR, Kempson RL: Surgical pathology of the uterine corpus. Saunders, Philadelphia, 1980, pp 158–214.
9. Hendrickson MR, Kempson RL: Endometrial epithelial metaplasias: proliferations frequently misdiagnosed as adenocarcinoma—report of 89 cases and proposed classification. *Am J Surg Pathol* 4:525–542, 1980.
10. Andersen WA, Peyton TT, Fechner RE, et al: Endometrial metaplasia associated with endometrial carcinoma. *Am J Obstet Gynecol* 157:597–604, 1987.

9
Endometrial Hyperplasias and Their Distinction from Adenocarcinomas

Rex Bentley, M.D.

Endometrial hyperplasia has been recognized as a precursor to endometrial carcinoma for nearly a century. Several types of studies have confirmed this association (for reviews, see Refs. 1–4). Synchronous studies have documented that 18–46% of women with endometrial carcinoma have coexisting endometrial hyperplasia. Retrospective studies have shown that up to three-fourths of women with endometrial carcinoma had hyperplasia in previous biopsies. Finally, back-dated prospective studies have retrospectively examined patients with endometrial hyperplasia who received repeat endometrial sampling and clinical evaluation after prolonged follow-up periods. A high incidence of subsequent endometrial cancer has been repeatedly demonstrated (3–80%, depending on the initial severity of hyperplasia) with an interval to carcinoma of 1–14 years. In part because of variations in nomenclature and treatment, an exact figure for the rate of progression of untreated endo-

The author would like to thank Ms. Rose Casey for her excellent secretarial support, Mr. Steven Conlon for photographic assistance, and Dr. Stanley Robboy for his insightful comments on this chapter.

metrial hyperplasia to carcinoma cannot be determined. It is important to realize, however, that many patients with hyperplasia will not progress to carcinoma, and likewise, many patients with endometrial carcinoma have no detectable prior or concurrent hyperplasia. A truly prospective trial investigating the natural history of endometrial carcinoma is unlikely to be performed, since it would now be considered unethical to withhold treatment from these patients.

EPIDEMIOLOGY

The epidemiology of endometrial carcinoma has been more extensively documented than endometrial hyperplasia, but it is generally felt that the risk factors and the populations affected are similar. Thus, risk factors include obesity, nulliparity, diabetes, hypertension, functioning ovarian tumors, and exogenous estrogen administration.[5] The identification of these risk factors may ultimately prove useful for screening purposes; for example, diabetic asymptomatic peri- and postmenopausal women have a fivefold higher incidence of endometrial hyperplasia compared to a hypertensive control group.[6] Exogenous estrogens have been strongly associated with endometrial hyperplasia; lower estrogen doses and the addition of progestins markedly reduce the incidence of hyperplasia, which can be as high as 57% after only 1 year of unopposed estrogen therapy.[7] The common thread in all these risk factors is increased or prolonged estrogen exposure, whether of endogenous or exogenous origin.

CLINICAL FEATURES

The typical presentation of endometrial hyperplasia regardless of age is abnormal bleeding from the uterus, often in association with anovulatory cycles. The vast majority of patients are peri- or postmenopausal, but hyperplasia can also occur in young women or even teenagers, where it is more often associated with abnormalities of the ovary including granulosa cell tumors, thecomas, polycystic ovarian disease, or other disorders leading to increased endogenous estrogens or anovulation. Although most patients are symptomatic, screening biopsies of asymptomatic peri- and postmenopausal women have shown that hyperplasia in women without symptoms is not rare with a prevalence of 1.3–5.2%.[6,8] Cytologic screening using cervical and/or vaginal cytologies or direct endometrial sampling is insensitive and unreliable for screening purposes.[5] When positive, however, cytology is important. Generally, techniques that obtain tissue for histologic evaluation such as biopsy or curettage are preferable to cytologic techniques.

GROSS FINDINGS

The uterus may be somewhat enlarged. Usually, the endometrium appears lush and generally increased in thickness, but is otherwise unremarkable. The increased endometrial thickness can be detected by ultrasound (see Chapter 2). Occasionally the hyperplastic epithelium may form a polypoid mass (hyperplastic polyp), but these are usually sessile and relatively small, in contrast to endometrial polyps, which are often pedunculated. In a curettage specimen, the only clue to the diagnosis may be an unusually large volume of endometrium recovered. This may be especially striking if the patient is postmenopausal and would normally have very scanty endometrium. This observation is obviously of minimal significance if the patient is receiving estrogen replacement therapy.

MICROSCOPIC FINDINGS

The hallmark of all hyperplasias is an increase in the amount of glandular tissue relative to stroma, with concomitant architectural and sometimes cytologic changes as outlined below. Since only a minority of patients with hyperplasia develop carcinoma, many older studies tried to subclassify or grade hyperplasias in an attempt to identify those patients at highest risk for progression of their disease. No uniform system was widely adopted, and by the late 1970s there existed a confusing array of terms such as "adenomatous hyperplasia," "atypical hyperplasia," "atypical adenomatous hyperplasia," and "carcinoma in situ," which were used differently by different authors (reviewed in Ref. 1). In part to address this problem, the International Society of Gynecological Pathologists (ISGP) and the World Health Organization (WHO) have proposed a classification scheme based largely on the work of Kurman and Norris.[9,10] This classification scheme has been followed in the recent AFIP fascicle[5] and in several major textbooks of gynecologic pathology.[4,11]

In the ISPG/WHO classification scheme, architectural and cytologic features of the endometrium are independently evaluated. The architecture is classified as either simple or complex, and the cytologic features as atypical or not atypical. "Adenomatous" is accepted as a synonym for complex.

Simple Hyperplasia

The WHO category of simple hyperplasia includes lesions that were formerly termed "cystic hyperplasia" and "mild adenomatous" hyperplasia. In simple hyperplasia, the glandular volume relative to stroma is increased, but the glands are not yet markedly crowded. In comparison to normal proliferative endometrium (Figs. 9-1, 9-2) the glands lose their regular orientation toward

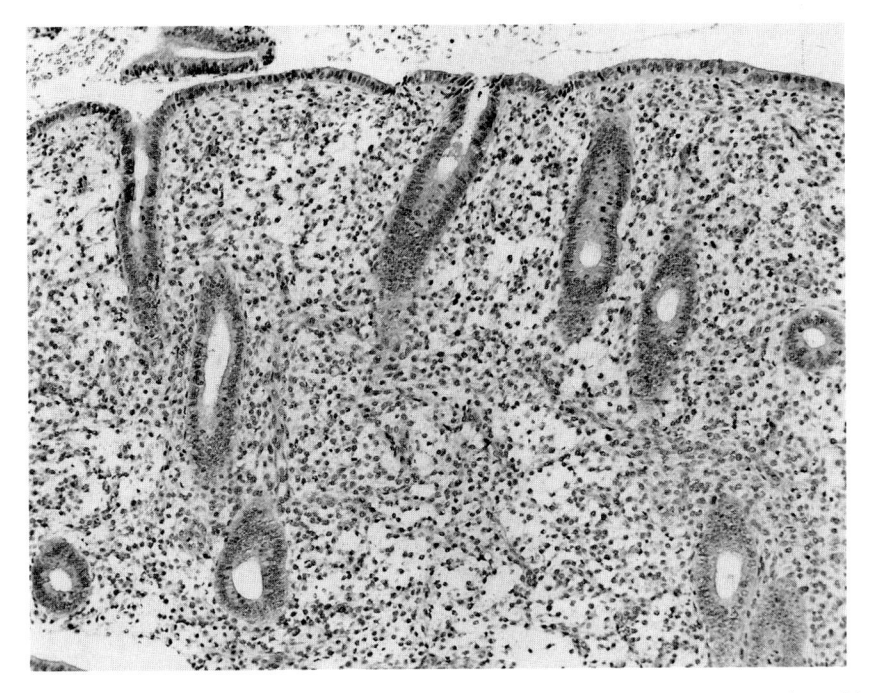

Figure 9-1. Normal proliferative endometrium, perpendicular section. Note the uniform size of the glands, the parallel walls, and the orientation of the glands toward the surface. (Endometrial curetting, 100×.)

the surface and become more randomly oriented. The gland size varies from small and round to cystically dilated and slightly irregular in outline (Figs. 9-3, 9-4). The glands are usually lined by a proliferative-type epithelium. A small percentage of hyperplasias of all types can show secretory changes, typically in the form of well-developed subnuclear and supranuclear vacuoles, but stromal pseudodecidualization has not been described except with exogenous hormones.[2] Secretory hyperplasia, like secretory carcinoma, is usually a transient pattern seen during the secretory phase of the menstrual cycle, but it can also be seen in postmenopausal patients. In cystic hyperplasia, the stroma may be abundant with little or no apparent glandular crowding (Fig. 9-4). Occasional outpouchings or serrated gland borders can be seen, but if these are extensive, the diagnosis becomes that of complex hyperplasia. The differential diagnosis of simple hyperplasia is usually between a disordered proliferative or atrophic endometrium on one hand, and complex hyperplasia on the other. Cystic atrophy and cystic hyperplasia can be differentiated by the activity of the epithelial cells. In hyperplasia, these are columnar, often pseudostratified (Fig. 9-5), and mitotically active, while in atrophy they are low columnar to cuboidal and lack mitotic activity (Fig. 9-6). Many pathologists distinguish between simple hyperplasia and disordered proliferative endometrium or persistent proliferative endometrium (Fig. 9-7) with the implication that disordered proliferative endometrium has

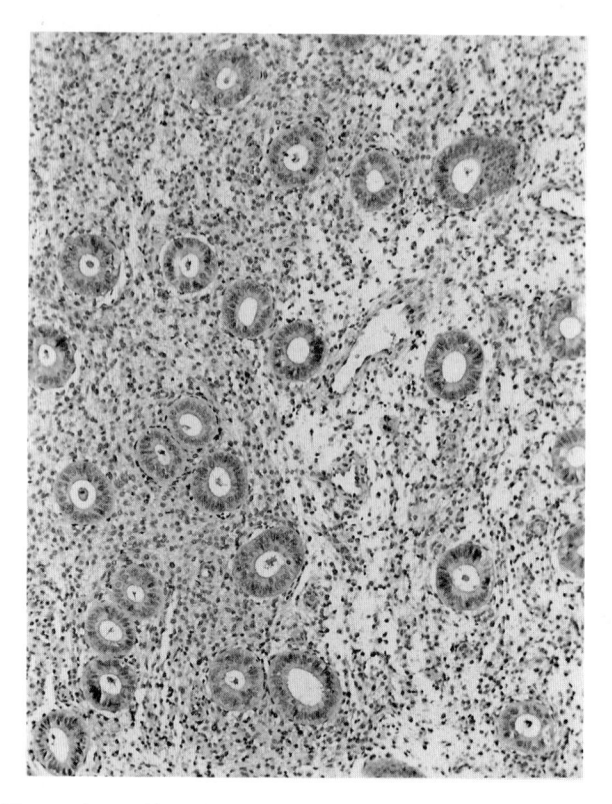

Figure 9-2. Normal proliferative endometrium, cross section. In comparison to the perpendicular section, the glands appear more numerous. They are round and uniform in size, however, and should not be mistaken for hyperplasia. (Endometrial curettings, 100×.)

no preneoplastic potential.[3] As disordered proliferative endometrium is often nearly indistinguishable from hyperplasia on curettings,[2] both conditions are often considered as simple hyperplasia since both have minimal malignant potential and can be treated similarly.[10]

Complex Hyperplasia

Complex hyperplasia is defined as having back-to-back glands with markedly irregular and serrated glandular outlines. Gland outpouchings and "buds" are frequent (Figs. 9-8 through 9-10). Stratification of glandular cell nuclei is usually present (Figs. 9-5, 9-9) but is not of diagnostic significance; stratification can be seen in any hyperplasia.[10] Most cases of what were previously termed moderate or severe "adenomatous hyperplasia" are in this category. Although complex hyperplasia is described as having back-to-back glands, it is important to realize that a thin rim of stroma should separate the glands, as illustrated in the original study of Kurman and Norris.[2,10] The complete absence of stroma is pathognomonic for the diagnosis of adenocarcinoma

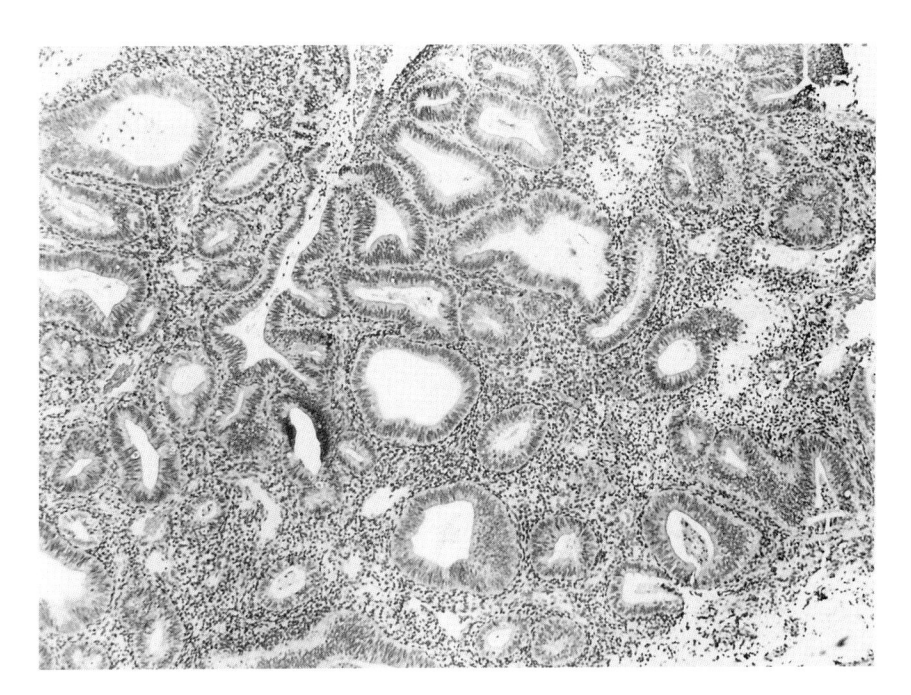

Figure 9-3. Simple hyperplasia. There is an increase in the ratio of endometrial glands to stroma, giving a somewhat more crowded appearance to the endometrium. The glands are less uniform in size and shape than in normal proliferative endometrium. There is also a mild degree of nuclear pseudostratification. (Endometrial curetting, 68×.)

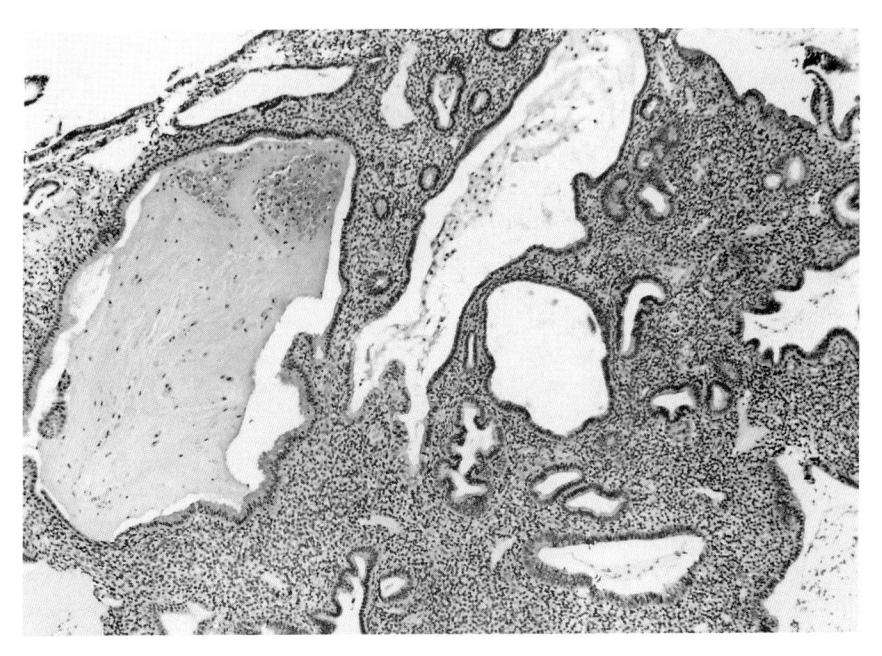

Figure 9-4. Simple hyperplasia, cystic type. When simple hyperplasia has numerous large cystically dilated glands such as seen here, it is often termed *cystic hyperplasia*. As in all simple hyperplasias marked crowding of the glands is not seen. (Endometrial curettings, 68×.)

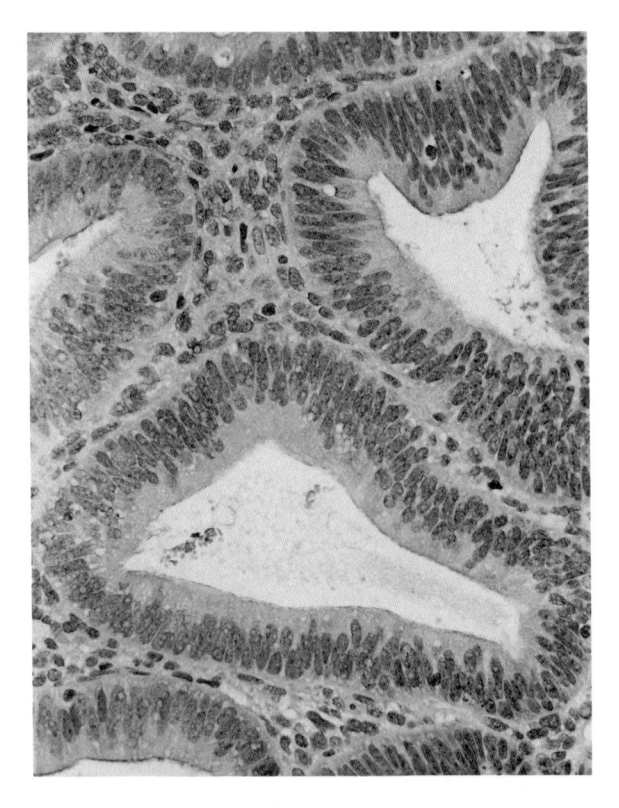

Figure 9-5. Nuclear pseudostratification in complex hyperplasia. Nuclear pseudostratification is a common feature in all endometrial hyperplasias, and is often a prominent feature of complex hyperplasia. Moderate pseudostratification can be seen in this high-power view of complex hyperplasia. Note the resemblance to adenomatous polyps in the gastrointestinal tract. (Endometrial curettings, 320×.)

Figure 9-6. Cystic atrophy. Although at low power cystic hyperplasia and cystic atrophy may appear similar, at high power there are distinct differences. In this high-power view of cystic atrophy, the epithelial cells are markedly flattened to low cuboidal and lack mitotic activity. Contrast this appearance to Fig. 9-4. (Hysterectomy, 400×.)

Figure 9-7. Persistent proliferative (anovulatory) endometrium. This example of persistent proliferative endometrium from a young woman with polycystic ovaries shows slight irregularity to the glandular outlines at the bottom of the field with a mild variability in gland size. In the center of the field is a dilated, thin-walled vascular space (arrow). Although not seen here, fibrin thrombi are commonly present in these vessels. Basement membrane thickening, another feature of this lesion, is seen focally (arrowheads). These changes are included by some under the term *disordered proliferative endometrium*. (Endometrial curettings, 130×.)

Microscopic Findings

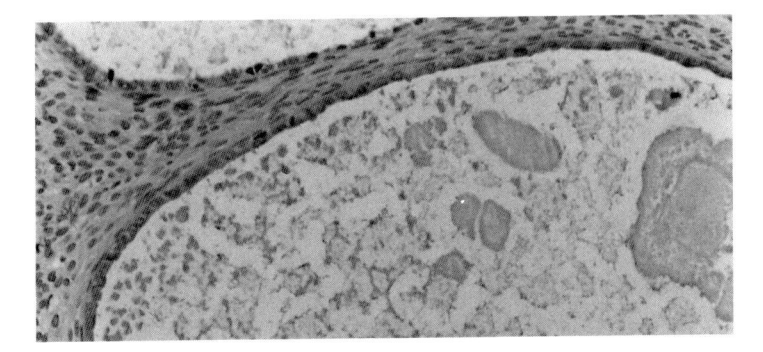

Figure 9-6.

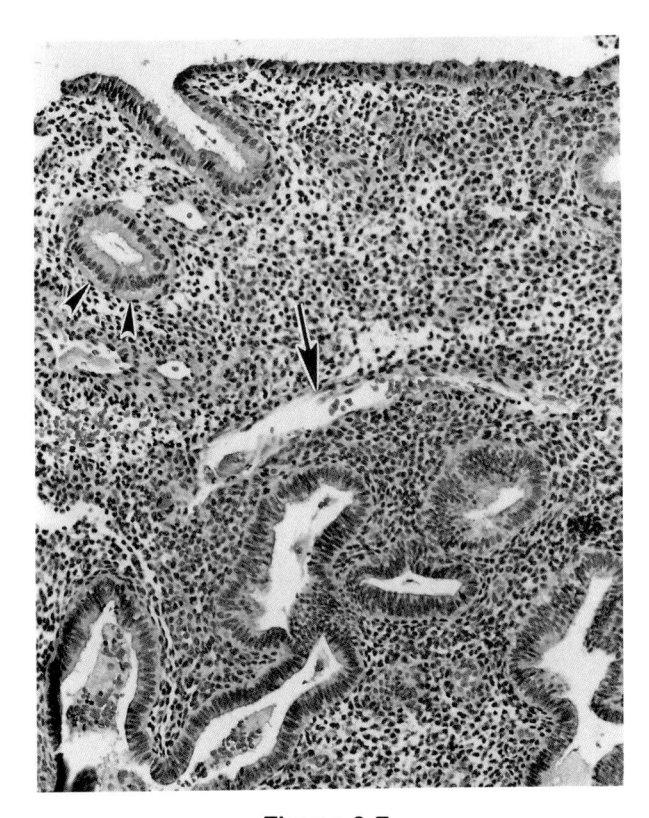

Figure 9-7.

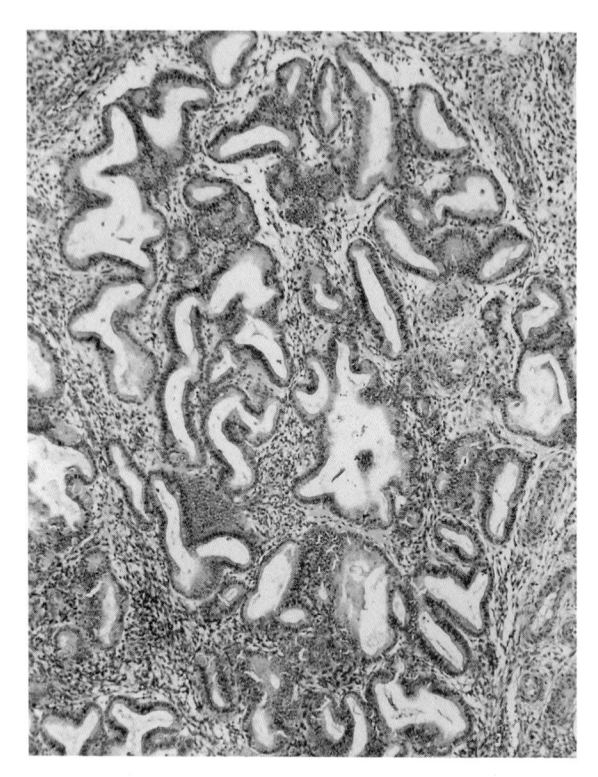

Figure 9-8. Complex hyperplasia. This low-power view of complex hyperplasia shows marked glandular crowding, approaching back-to-back in some areas. In addition, the glandular outlines are more complex than in simple hyperplasia, with papillary infoldings, "buds," and glands that appear branched. In biopsies or curettings, it is important to identify these changes in areas with intact stroma, as artifactual loss of stroma can give a strikingly similar appearance. (Endometrial curettings, 68×.)

Figure 9-9. Complex hyperplasia. A higher-power view of another case of complex hyperplasia in which the glandular architecture is strikingly complex. No cytologic atypia is present, however. (Endometrial curettings, 170×.)

Figure 9-10. Complex hyperplasia with squamous metaplasia. In this example of complex hyperplasia, the glands are markedly crowded but are mostly round in outline, lacking the architectural complexity seen in Fig. 9-9. The presence of squamous metaplasia (arrows) in complex hyperplasia can make the glandular pattern appear misleadingly "busy" and confluent, and can lead to a mistaken impression of carcinoma. (Hysterectomy, 250×.)

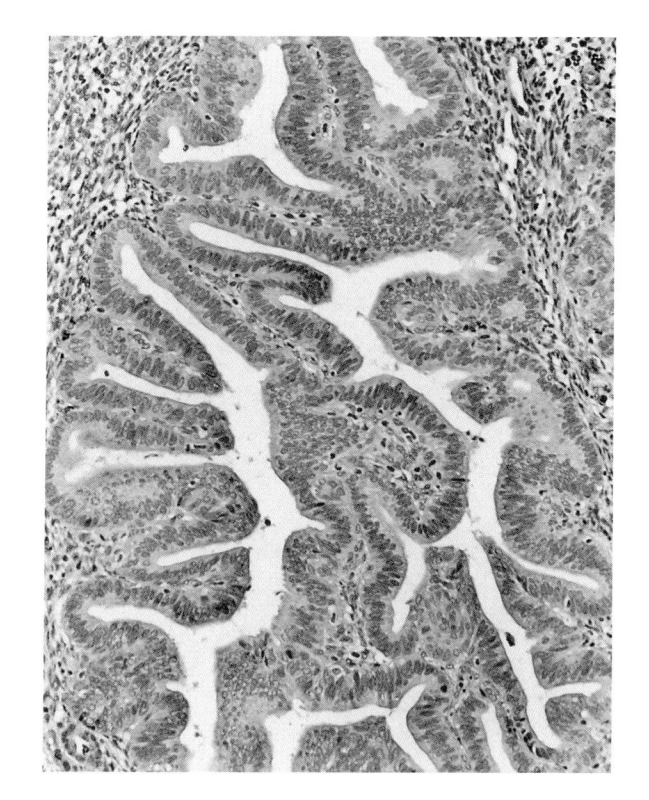

Figure 9-9.

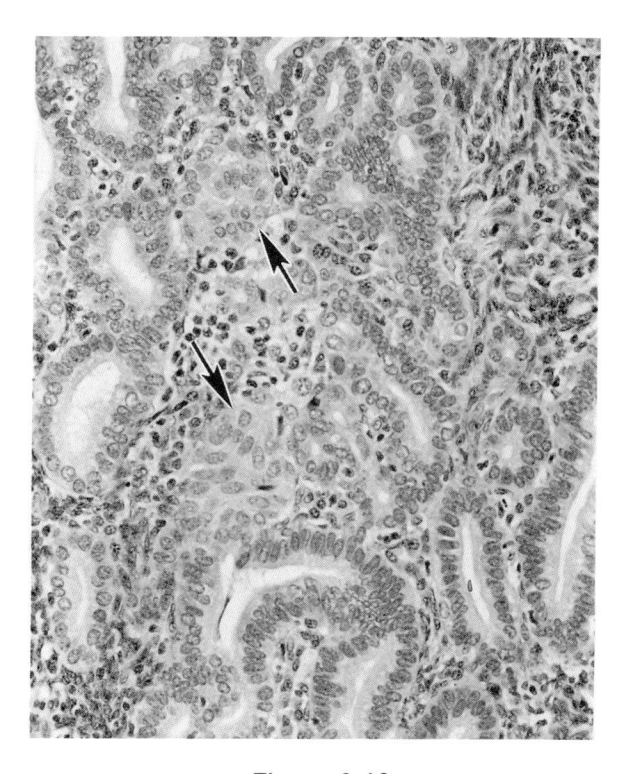

Figure 9-10.

123

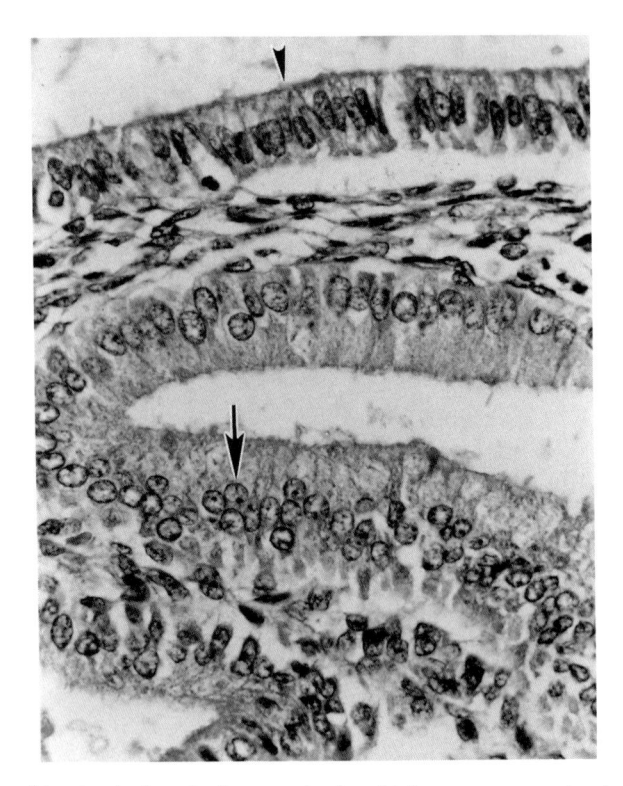

Figure 9-11. Atypical simple hyperplasia. At low power, atypical simple hyperplasia is identical in appearance to simple hyperplasia without atypia. In this high-power view of atypical simple hyperplasia, scattered groups of glands have rounded nuclei, cleared chromatin, and small nucleoli (arrow). In this example, there is little nuclear stratification. Although not readily apparent in this black-and-white photograph, the atypical cells have an abundant and eosinophilic cytoplasm. These changes represent the mildest form of cytologic atypia. The arrowhead indicates a normal adjacent gland for comparison. (Hysterectomy, 520×.)

(see below). The WHO accepts "adenomatous" as a synonym for this pattern of hyperplasia, but "complex" is considered preferable as it avoids confusion with the previous definitions.

Atypical Hyperplasia

After the hyperplasia is classified as either simple or complex by architectural pattern, it is evaluated for the presence or absence of cytologic atypia. This concept has been the most controversial and the most difficult to apply reproducibly in clinical material. There is general agreement that the definition includes increased nuclear size, nuclear rounding, clearing and clumping of chromatin, loss of nuclear polarity, and the presence of nucleoli (Figs. 9-11 through 9-13). Other useful features include abundant cytoplasm with

Microscopic Findings

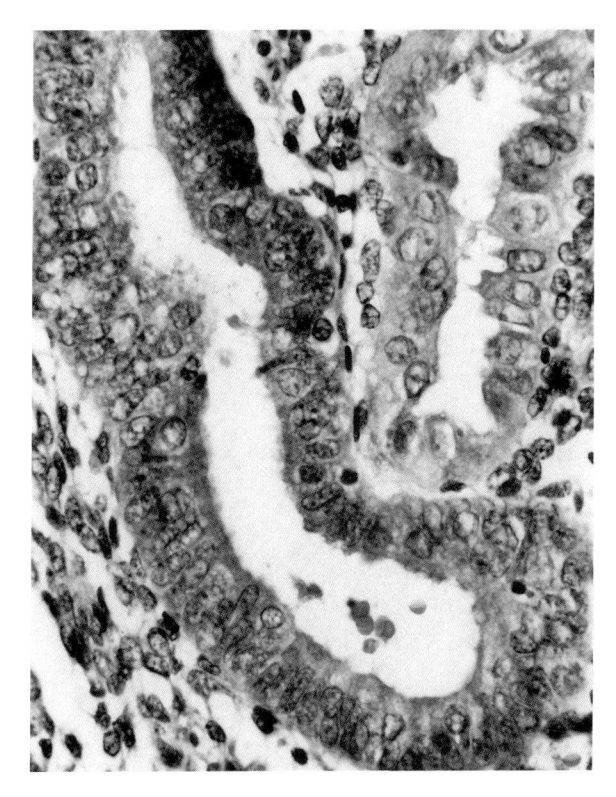

Figure 9-12. Atypical complex hyperplasia. At low power, atypical complex hyperplasia is identical in appearance to complex hyperplasia without atypia. Atypia is much more common in complex hyperplasia than in simple hyperplasia and is more frequently severe when present. In this high-power view, the smaller gland shows severely atypical cytologic changes with enlarged nuclei, chromatin clumping and clearing, and prominent nucleoli. The nuclei are round having lost their normal cigar-shaped profiles, and they have lost any regular orientation toward the lumen. The larger gland also shows cytologic atypia, but to a lesser degree. (Hysterectomy, 520×.)

dense eosinophilia.[12] Mitotic activity is not a criteria for atypia, and does not help to distinguish atypical hyperplasia from nonatypical hyperplasias.[5,13] Glandular stratification is used by some pathologists as a criterion[2,12] even though the one study that has specifically addressed this point failed to demonstrate prognostic significance for this feature.[10] This is an important difference, since many of these highly stratified lesions, which would have previously been designated as "severe adenomatous hyperplasia," are now classified as complex hyperplasia without atypia when stratification is not accepted as a criteria for atypicality. Many pathologists are uncomfortable in downplaying the significance of these lesions, which in the older literature were associated with a high risk of concurrent or future adenocarcinoma.[14,15] Most gynecologic pathologists have seen occasional biopsies that would be classified as complex hyperplasia without atypia but that at hysterectomy

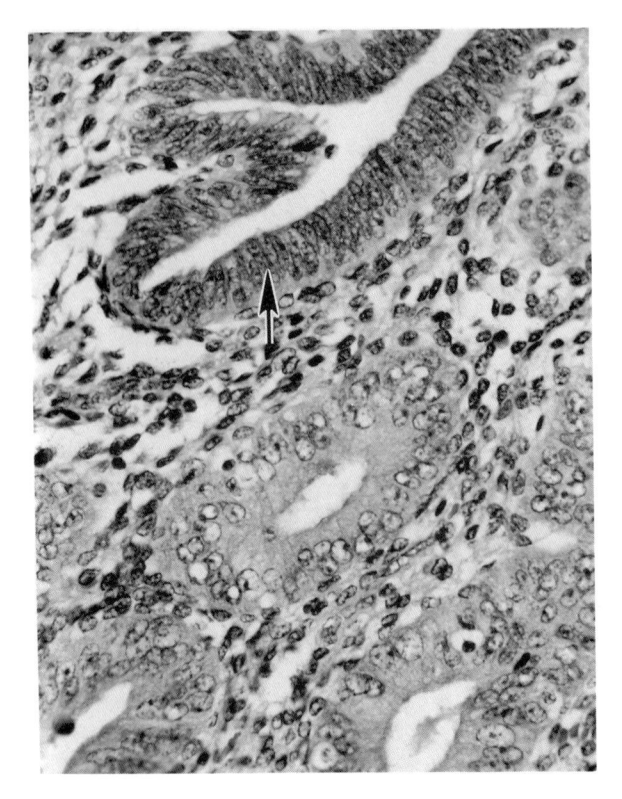

Figure 9-13. Atypical complex hyperplasia. Another high-power view of atypical hyperplasia showing essentially the same features as Fig. 9-12. As evidenced by the nonatypical adjacent glands (arrow), atypia is usually a focal rather than a diffuse finding. (Hysterectomy, 400×.)

prove to be well-differentiated carcinomas by virtue of myometrial invasion, despite their lack of definite cytologic atypia as defined by Kurman and Norris. Fortunately, these cases are infrequent.

RISK OF PROGRESSION TO ENDOMETRIAL CARCINOMA

The natural history of endometrial hyperplasia has been difficult to assess (for reviews, see Refs. 1–3). There has never been, and undoubtedly never will be, a truly prospective study documenting the natural history of untreated endometrial hyperplasia. The classification scheme recommended by the WHO/ISGP is based largely on the backdated prospective study of Kurman et al.[10] These authors identified 170 patients with hyperplasia in

TABLE 9-1. Natural History of Endometrial Hyperplasia

Classification of hyperplasia	Number of patients	Progression to carcinoma (%)
		Individual groups
Simple hyperplasia	93	1%
Complex hyperplasia	29	3%
Simple atypical	13	8%
Complex atypical hyperplasia	35	29%
		Combinations of groups
Simple or complex hyperplasias	122	2%*
Atypical hyperplasias	48	23%*

*$P = .01$.
Source: Modified from Ref. 10.

whom a hysterectomy was not performed for at least 1 year after the original biopsy. Although these patients were considered "untreated" for the purposes of the study, many in fact received hormonal treatments. Overall, only 2% of the nonatypical hyperplasias progressed to carcinoma, while 23% of the atypical lesions progressed (Table 9-1). It should be noted, however, that many of their results did not reach statistical significance. Only 13 cases were classified as atypical simple hyperplasia, and the 8% progression rate represents but a single patient out of the entire group of 13. This figure is not statistically different from either the atypical complex *or* the nonatypical hyperplasias. Despite the limited data, cytologic atypia was stressed as the key feature in assessing risk for subsequent carcinoma.[10] This concept was in keeping with several earlier studies[1] and has been borne out in several subsequent studies;[3,16] it has now become generally accepted.[2,4,5]

An additional very important feature of atypical hyperplasia is the relatively high incidence of *concurrent* carcinomas of the endometrium. Of all patients who show atypical hyperplasia on biopsy or curettage, 17–25% will be found to have carcinoma in their hysterectomy specimens even if the hysterectomy is performed immediately.[9,12] This apparent discordance is due to a combination of sampling artifact and to the difficulty in finding reliable morphologic indicators of malignancy in the superficial and disrupted endometrial samples obtained by biopsy or curettage (see below). This uncertainty requires that most patients with atypical hyperplasia be treated as if they had well-differentiated endometrial carcinoma, where hysterectomy is the treatment of choice. The possible exception to this is endometrial carcinoma in very young women, where even well-differentiated carcinoma can sometimes be successfully treated without hysterectomy.[17] In addition, the high rate of concurrent carcinomas (17–25%) suggests that "progession" in atypical hyperplasia (23%) may in fact represent persistence of residual unsuspected carcinoma.

CARCINOMA IN SITU

Carcinoma in situ (CIS) of the endometrium has long been sought as an intermediary in the development of carcinoma because of the parallel with CIS of the cervix and other sites. By definition, an adenocarcinoma in situ is a lesion in which the glandular cells have undergone malignant change but have yet to penetrate basement membrane and invade stroma. Many lesions that were once classified as CIS are now classified as atypical hyperplasia in the WHO/ISPG classification scheme. Others have used the phrase to signify groups of five or six glands having the cytologic features of malignancy. This diagnosis seems unwarranted for a lesion that may regress and is responsive to hormonal treatment in many patients. Furthermore, the diagnosis has proved poorly reproducible. For these reasons, the WHO/ISPG does not recommend carcinoma in situ of the endometrium as a diagnostic category, a view that is shared by most pathologists.[1,2,5,11]

DISTINGUISHING ATYPICAL ENDOMETRIAL HYPERPLASIA FROM WELL-DIFFERENTIATED ADENOCARCINOMA

The ability to distinguish between atypical hyperplasia and well-differentiated adenocarcinoma continues to be of major importance, since it theoretically identifies those patients at risk for invasive disease. The root of the problem in developing histologic criteria for carcinoma is that so few well-differentiated carcinomas recur that it is difficult to correlate microscopic features with adverse prognosis. Thus, there is no "gold standard" for determining malignancy in clinicopathologic studies. Most recent studies of this issue have attempted to define carcinoma by the presence of histologically ominous features. The most convincing histologic feature of malignancy is myometrial invasion. This feature is unfortunately rarely encountered in biopsy or curettage specimens,[12,18] and the normally irregular endometrial–myometrial border can make evaluation of myometrial invasion difficult even when it is present. A second feature diagnostic of invasion is stromal desmoplasia. While not proving myometrial invasion, this feature does identify tumors that have invaded endometrial stroma, and are presumably capable of invading other tissues as well. Kurman and Norris[9] rely on the presence of "stromal invasion" for the distinction. They define stromal invasion as the presence of at least 1 of the patterns shown in Table 9-2 (Figs. 9-14 through 9-17). Feature 1 (stromal desmoplasia, Fig. 9-14) directly indicates stromal invasion. Small foci showing features 2, 3, or 4 can be seen in hyperplasias and so cannot be directly indicative of stromal invasion, although may be associated with it. Thus, stromal invasion is inferred from the quantity of these features with 2.1 mm as an arbitrary minimum for a diagnosis of carcinoma. In 204 patients with atypical hyperplasia or carci-

TABLE 9-2. Criteria for Distinguishing Adenocarcinoma from Atypical Hyperplasia

Kurman and Norris[9]

Fibrous, desmoplastic reaction in the stroma
Confluent glandular bridges and aggregates of glands lacking intervening stroma*
Branching, complex papillary epithelial lined processes*
Squamous cell proliferations replacing glands and forming solid sheets*

Tavassoli and Kraus[12]

Nuclei large, variable size
Nuclear outlines irregular
Nuclear membranes irregular
Nucleoli large, irregular, spiculated
Cytoplasm scant, pale, amphophilic
Loss of nuclear polarity
Cribiform pattern
Intraglandular "bridging" without stromal support
Gland profiles irregular, size variable

Hendrickson, et al.[18]

Architectural features
  Confluent complex glands with little intervening stroma; often a villoglandular pattern
  Gland-within-gland pattern with many papillary infolding and bridges, often resulting in a complex filigree pattern
  Appearance of cellular stratification, at least focally
Cytologic features
  Nucleomegaly
  Chromatin clearing
  Prominent nucleoli
  Mitotic figures
When *both* cellular stratification and nuclear abnormalities are lacking, the case is not accepted as well-differentiated endometrial adenocarcinoma.

*Must occupy a minimum of 2.1 mm in diameter.
Source: Modified from Refs. 9, 12, and 18.

noma identified retrospectively, use of these criteria in curettings had moderate predictive value for the ultimate findings in the hysterectomy specimens. Carcinoma was found in the resected uterus of 50% of the endometria classified as well-differentiated endometrial carcinoma, but was seen in only 17% of the endometria classified as atypical hyperplasia. More importantly, however, these criteria segregated out those patients with a low risk of invasion. Although 17% of the patients classified as atypical hyperplasia had adenocarcinoma in their subsequent hysterectomy specimens, these cancers were all confined to the endometrium or were only superficially invasive. All of the deeply invasive tumors were found in patients who had stromal invasion

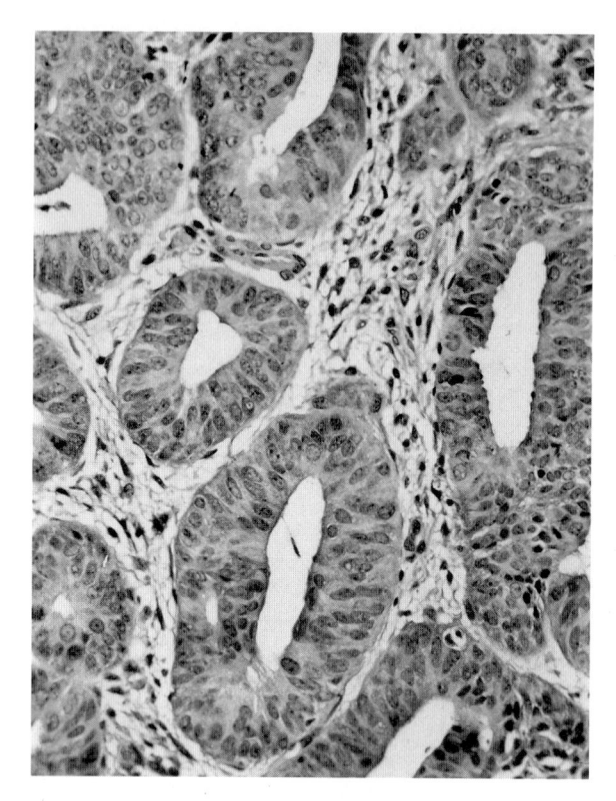

Figure 9-14. Well-differentiated adenocarcinoma, stromal invasion. The stroma between these highly atypical glands is replaced by edematous fibroblastic tissue typical of the desmoplastic response to invasive cancer. (Endometrial curettings, 250×.)

Figure 9-15. Well-differentiated adenocarcinoma, glandular confluence and cribiform pattern. This example of well-differentiated carcinoma shows complete loss of stroma between glands, leading to glandular confluence and a "cribiform," or gland-within-gland pattern. Some authors feel this pattern is diagnostic of carcinoma only if it measures 2.1 mm or more in diameter (see text). (Hysterectomy, 170×.)

Figure 9-16. Well-differentiated adenocarcinoma, extensive papillary pattern. An extensive papillary pattern is seen in this well-differentiated adenocarcinoma. Elsewhere in this hysterectomy specimen there was typical endometrioid carcinoma. Papillary metaplasia, a benign process, can mimic this pattern, but is always a focal finding and is never this extensive. (Hysterectomy, 52×.)

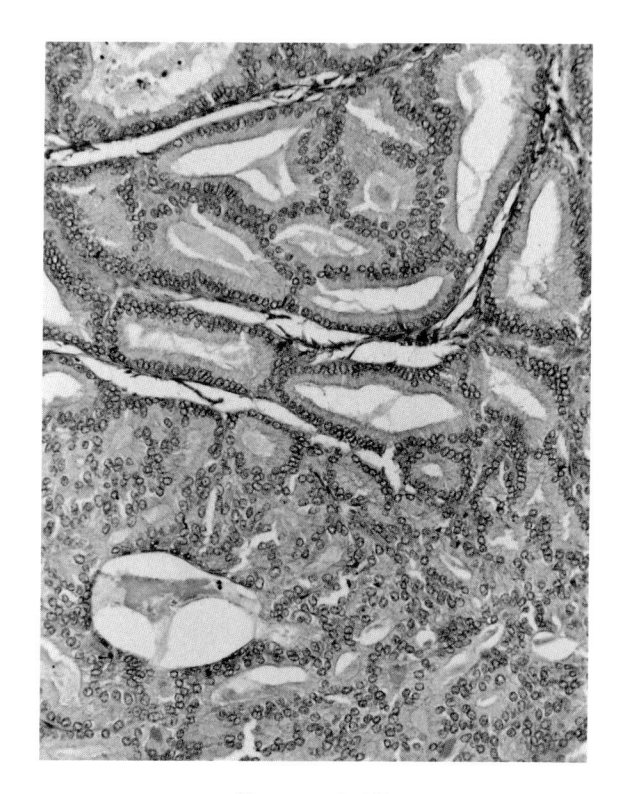

Figure 9-15.

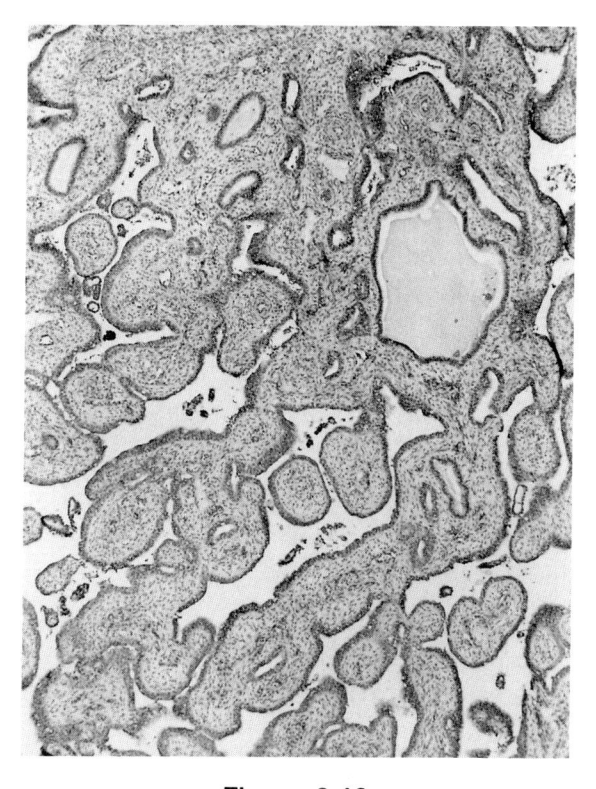

Figure 9-16.

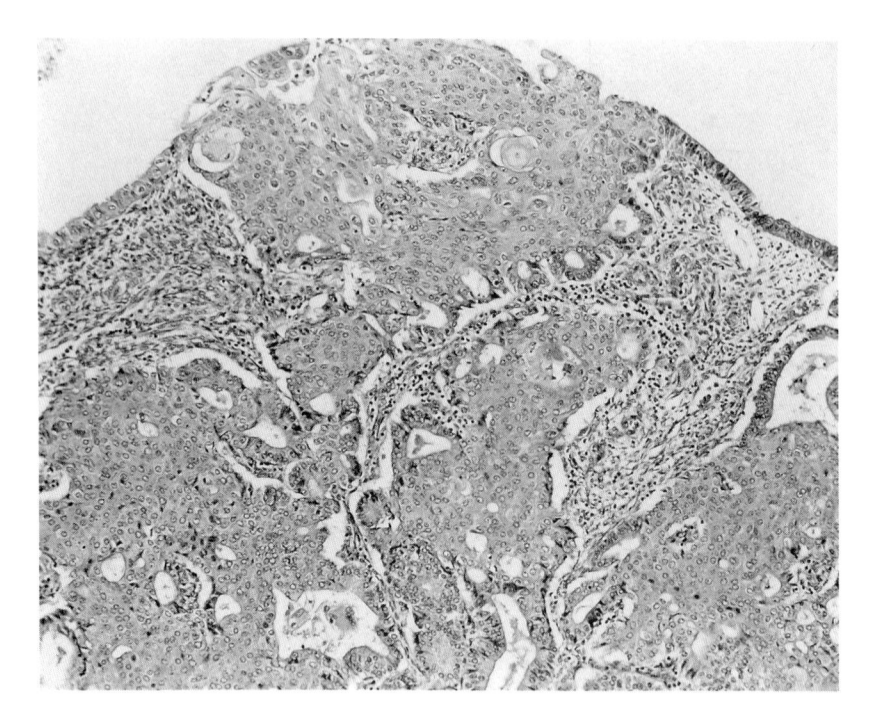

Figure 9-17. Well-differentiated adenocarcinoma with squamous metaplasia. This is an example of well-differentiated adenocarcinoma by virtue of the extensive squamous metaplasia, measuring over 2.1 mm in size according to the criteria of Kurman et al. This criteria is not universally accepted (see text), and this lesion could also be classified as an atypical hyperplasia. No typical carcinoma was seen elsewhere in this specimen, nor was there myometrial invasion. (Hysterectomy, 100×.)

(and hence carcinoma) in their curettings. Nevertheless, this relatively high incidence of carcinoma in patients classified as having atypical hyperplasia has led to criticism on the grounds that some potentially serious cancers would be missed in a large series of patients.[18] Indeed, the one other group that has used these criteria to separate carcinoma from hyperplasia reported a deeply invasive carcinoma (to within 0.3 cm of serosa) in the hysterectomy specimen of a woman who had atypical hyperplasia on biopsy and curettage.[19] In addition, the utilization of squamous metaplasia as a criterion has been controversial and is not accepted by some pathologists.[2] However, these criteria are the most reproducible of the well-known proposals and clearly distinguish the majority of cases accurately, even when applied by other groups.[19]

Other proposed criteria rely heavily on cytologic evaluation, which are not a part of the Kurman et al criteria and are more subjective in their application. The two most widely quoted proposals are those of Tavassoli et al[12] and Hendrickson et al;[18] these are summarized in Table 9-2. The predictive value of the criteria proposed by Tavassoli and Kraus were not prospectively stud-

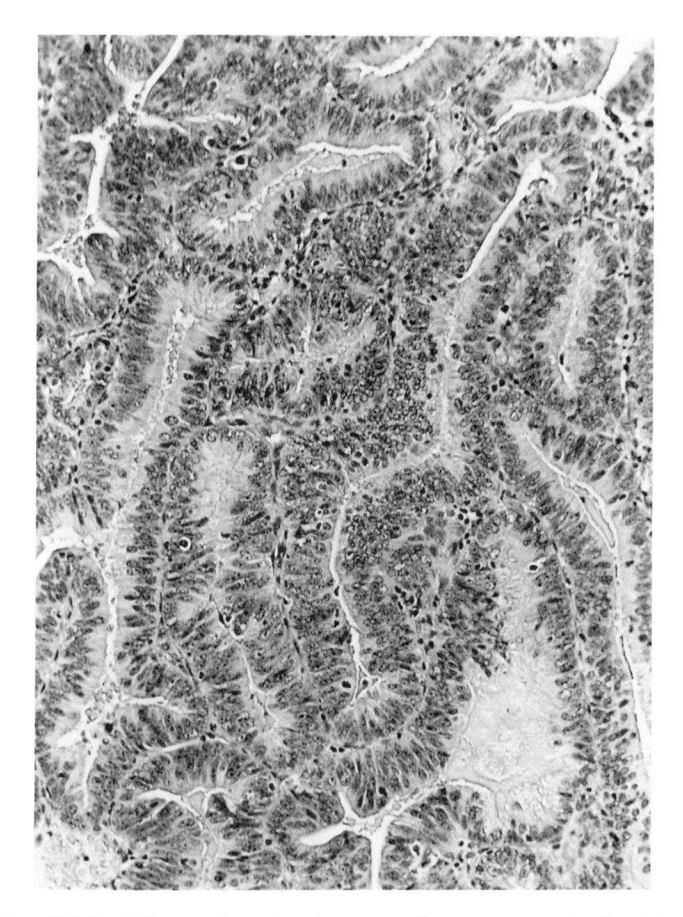

Figure 9-18. Well-differentiated adenocarcinoma vs. atypical hyperplasia. In this field, the severe cytologic atypia, stratification, and crowding would lead to a diagnosis of adenocarcinoma using the criteria of Kempson et al, but not using the criteria of Kurman and Norris, as this change measured less than 2.1 mm. (Endometrial curettings, 170×.)

ied, but they represent commonly used criteria.[2] Hendrickson et al[18] present a thoughtful and rational approach to this problem and present preliminary criteria based on the findings in 50 endometrial cancers that were very well differentiated but clearly showed at least focal myometrial invasion. These preliminary criteria are relatively subjective but have been thought to be potentially superior to those of Kurman and Norris by some reviewers.[4] Unfortunately, a definitive follow-up to this preliminary work has yet to appear. Some cases that meet the criteria of Hendrickson et al for carcinoma do not clearly meet the criteria proposed by Kurman and Norris (Fig. 9-18).

Finally, the presence of foam cells in the endometrial stroma has been widely viewed as associated with carcinoma (Fig. 9-19). While foam cells occur more frequently in carcinoma and atypical hyperplasia, they are nonspecific and can be seen in benign processes. Nevertheless, their presence

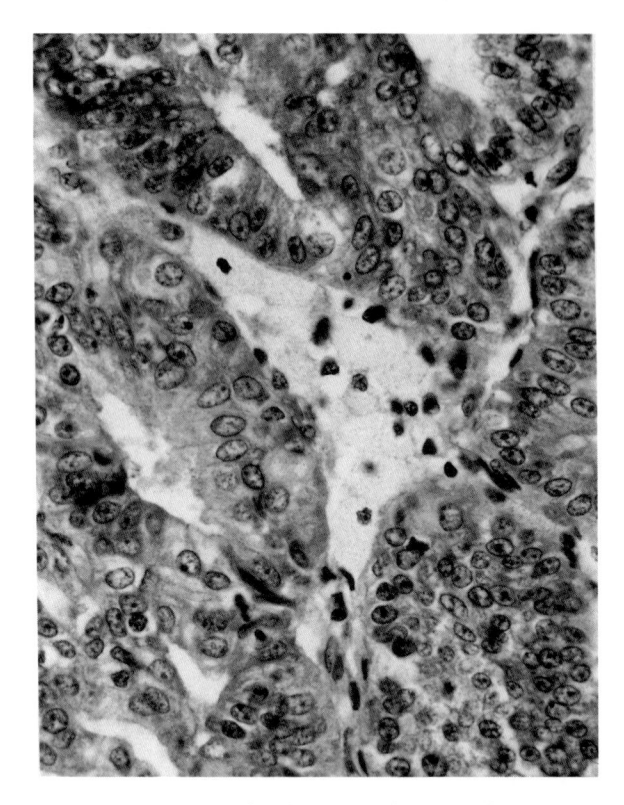

Figure 9-19. Well-differentiated adenocarcinoma, foam cells. In the center of the field is a collection of foam cells in the stroma separating the glands of a well-differentiated adenocarcinoma. Foam cells are thought to result from necrosis of the stroma, and are more frequent in carcinomas. (Hysterectomy, 520×.)

should provoke a search for evidence of an underlying neoplastic or preneoplastic lesion.

THERAPY

Therapy for endometrial hyperplasia must be tailored to the age and preferences of the patient.[20] In some institutions, postmenopausal women are often encouraged to undergo hysterectomy. If contraindicated, simple or complex hyperplasia can be treated with moderate doses of progestins followed by repeat endometrial sampling to document response. Hysterectomy should be strongly recommended to all patients with atypical hyperplasia in the postmenopausal group, as 28% of women in this age group will have residual carcinoma found at hysterectomy.[10]

Perimenopausal women with simple or complex hyperplasia can be given progestins with a high success rate, with repeat sampling every 3 months until the lesion resolves. Atypical hyperplasia should be treated by hysterectomy whenever possible, again because of the high rate of concurrent adenocarcinoma in this age group.

In contrast, younger women with hyperplasia who wish to retain childbearing capability can often be managed with progestins, ovulation induction, or artificial cycles even when biopsies show atypical hyperplasia. Before deciding on conservative therapy, the endometrium must be thoroughly sampled to rule out invasive carcinoma. Even if no carcinoma is found in curettings, approximately 10% of patients in this age group will have residual carcinoma. These carcinomas are typically well differentiated and minimally invasive.[10] Furthermore, some of these carcinomas are responsive to hormonal treatment in younger women.[17]

SUMMARY

Endometrial hyperplasia is well established as a precursor to many cases of endometrial adenocarcinoma. Recent classifications organize hyperplasias according to their architectural pattern (simple or complex) and by the presence or absence of cytologic atypia. The presence of cytologic atypia confers a high risk of progression to carcinoma, particularly when associated with complex architecture, as well as a high chance of an unsuspected coexisting carcinoma. The distinction of atypical hyperplasia from well-differentiated adenocarcinoma is possible in the majority of cases by attention to proposed morphologic criteria, but in some cases there will be a discrepancy between biopsy and hysterectomy findings.

REFERENCES

1. Scully RE: Definition of precursors in gynecologic cancer. *Cancer* 48:531–537, 1981.
2. Silverberg SG: Hyperplasia and carcinoma of the endometrium. *Semin Diag Pathol* 5:135–153, 1988.
3. Huang SJ, Amparo EG, Fu YS: Endometrial hyperplasia: histologic classification and behavior. *Surg Pathol* 1:215–229, 1988.
4. Clement PB, Scully RE: Endometrial hyperplasia and carcinoma. In Clement PB, Young RH (eds): *Tumors and tumorlike lesions of the uterine corpus and cervix*. Churchill Livingstone, New York, 1993.
5. Silverberg SG, Kurman RJ: *Tumors of the uterine corpus and gestational trophoblastic disease*. Armed Forces Institute of Pathology, Washington, DC, 1992, pp 18–34.
6. Grönroos M, Salmi TA, Vuento MH, et al: Mass screening for endometrial cancer directed in risk groups of patients with diabetes and patients with hypertension. *Cancer* 71:1279–1282, 1993.
7. Gelfand MM, Ferenczy A: A prospective 1-year study of estrogen and progestin in postmenopausal women: effects on the endometrium. *Obstet Gynecol* 74:398–402, 1989.

8. Archer DF, McIntyre-Seltman K, Wilborn WW, et al: Endometrial morphology in asymptomatic postmenopausal women. *Am J Obstet Gynecol* 165:317–322, 1991.
9. Kurman RJ, Norris HJ: Evaluation of criteria for distinguishing atypical endometrial hyperplasia from well-differentiated carcinoma. *Cancer* 49:2547–2559, 1982.
10. Kurman RJ, Kaminski PF, Norris HJ: The behavior of endometrial hyperplasia: a long-term study of "untreated" hyperplasia in 170 patients. *Cancer* 56:403–412, 1985.
11. Kurman RJ, Norris NJ: Endometrial hyperplasia and metaplasia. In Kurman RJ (ed): *Blaustein's pathology of the female genital tract.* Springer-Verlag, New York, 1987.
12. Tavassoli F, Kraus FT: Endometrial lesions in uteri resected for atypical endometrial hyperplasia. *Am J Clin Pathol* 70:770–779, 1978.
13. Pirog EC, Czerwinski W: Diagnostic and prognostic significance of the mitotic index in endometrial adenocarcinoma. *Gynecol Oncol* 46:337–340, 1992.
14. Gusberg SB, Kaplan AL: Precursors of corpus cancer IV: adenomatous hyperplasia as stage 0 carcinoma of the endometrium. *Am J Obstet Gynecol* 87:662–678, 1963.
15. Sherman AI, Brown S: The precursors of endometrial carcinoma. *Am J Obstet Gynecol* 135:947–956, 1979.
16. Ferenczy A, Gelfand M: The biologic significance of cytologic atypia in progestogen-treated endometrial hyperplasia. *Am J Obstet Gynecol* 160:126–131, 1989.
17. Lee KR, Scully R: Complex endometrial hyperplasia and carcinoma in adolescents and young women 15 to 20 years of age. *Int J Gynecol Pathol* 8:201–213, 1989.
18. Hendrickson MR, Ross JC, Kempson RL: Toward the development of morphologic criteria for well-differentiated adenocarcinoma of the endometrium. *Am J Surg Pathol* 7:819–838, 1983.
19. King A, Ibrahim MS, Wagner RJ. Stromal invasion in endometrial adenocarcinoma. *Am J Obstet Gynecol* 149:10–14, 1984.
20. DiSaia PJ, Creasman WT: Endometrial hyperplasia/estrogen therapy. In *Clinical gynecologic oncology,* 4th ed. Mosby Yearbook, St Louis, 1993.

10
Endometrial Malignancies

Debra S. Heller, M.D.

ENDOMETRIAL CARCINOMA

Endometrial carcinoma is the most common invasive neoplasm of the female genital tract.[1] The majority of endometrial carcinomas are of the endometrioid or "usual" type, and the following discussion will refer to this type unless otherwise specified.

Estrogen excess, either exogenous or endogenous, has been directly implicated in the etiology of some endometrial carcinomas, as well as in the hyperplasias. Other associated factors include obesity, hypertension, diabetes, and a history of low fertility and anovulatory cycles.[1]

Distinguishing Well-Differentiated Endometrial Adenocarcinoma from Atypical Hyperplasia

While the histologic diagnosis of endometrial carcinoma usually poses no difficulty, the distinction between atypical hyperplasia and well-differentiated endometrial adenocarcinoma can be difficult, particularly in curettings. The concept of endometrial carcinoma in situ (CIS) has been proposed, but has not gained widespread acceptance. The distinction between atypical hyperplasia and carcinoma often has no effect on the treatment of healthy postmenopausal patients, who usually undergo hysterectomies in either case. The difficulty arises in the younger patient desirous of fertility, or the patient who is a poor surgical risk. Here the distinction is more critical, as the gynecologist is more likely to attempt medical management of the lesion in the face of a benign diagnosis.

Various criteria have been proposed to distinguish well-differentiated endometrial adenocarcinoma from atypical hyperplasia, and this has led to a great deal of confusion in the literature. Most authors base the distinction on their definition of stromal invasion. Suggested distinguishing architectural features presumptive of stromal invasion have included glandular crowding, cribriform glandular patterns, lack of intervening stroma, stromal desmoplasia, and stromal necrosis.[2,3]

Kurman and Norris require that areas meeting their criteria for stromal invasion occupy at least 2.1 mm (half of a low-power field measuring 4.2 mm) to be predictive of a biologically significant cancer in the uterus,[3] a point not agreed on by all authors.[4]

The sole reliance on architecture without attention to cytologic features has been criticized by Hendrickson et al.[5] Kurman and Norris later added frankly malignant cells or high-grade tumor as evidence of malignancy on curettage, even in the absence of demonstrable stromal invasion.[2] If large masses of squamous metaplastic tissue are obtained on biopsy, this is not diagnostic in and of itself for carcinoma, but may be associated with an unsampled malignancy.

Diagnosis of Endometrial Carcinoma

The diagnosis of endometrial carcinoma is usually made on an endometrial biopsy or curettage performed for either postmenopausal bleeding or irregular bleeding in the perimenopausal period. The pathologist must first determine whether carcinoma is present, and whether it is of primary endometrial origin, if this can be determined. If it is an endometrial adenocarcinoma, the grade should be stated in the report, recognizing that some of the histologic variants are not graded in the same manner (see section on grading). If the neoplasm is one of the variants of usual endometrioid adenocarcinoma, this should be stated in the report, and absence of this statement implies that the tumor is endometrioid (Table 10-1).

It must be stressed that the grade assigned to the curettage specimen may not be the same as that given at the time of hysterectomy, as endometrial sampling is not always representative.

Clinicians will often request that the uterus be opened in the operating room at the time of hysterectomy, for either gross or frozen-section assessment of the degree of myometrial invasion. The current International Federation of Gynecology and Obstetrics (FIGO) staging of endometrial carcinoma is surgical, and intraoperative assessment of the degree of myometrial invasion is sometimes used to determine whether to perform lymph node sampling. The final pathology report of the hysterectomy specimen should state the diagnosis of carcinoma, the type if not endometrioid, the tumor grade, and the degree of myometrial invasion. Myometrial invasion is more usefully expressed in percentages, rather than in the vague "within the inner half." Vascular and lymphatic space involvement should be mentioned if present (Fig. 10-1), as well as any tumor spread to the adjacent organs.

TABLE 10-1. A Classification of Endometrial Carcinoma

Endometrioid, or "usual" adenocarcinoma
Variants of Endometrioid Adenocarcinoma
  "Villoglandular" pattern
  Secretory pattern
  Ciliated cell pattern
Endometrial adenocarcinoma with squamous differentiation
Mucinous adenocarcinoma
Clear cell adenocarcinoma
Uterine papillary serous carcinoma (UPSC)
Squamous cell carcinoma
Mixed-cell-type carcinoma
Undifferentiated carcinoma
  Small cell carcinoma
  Glassy cell carcinoma
  Other
Carcinoma metastatic to the endometrium

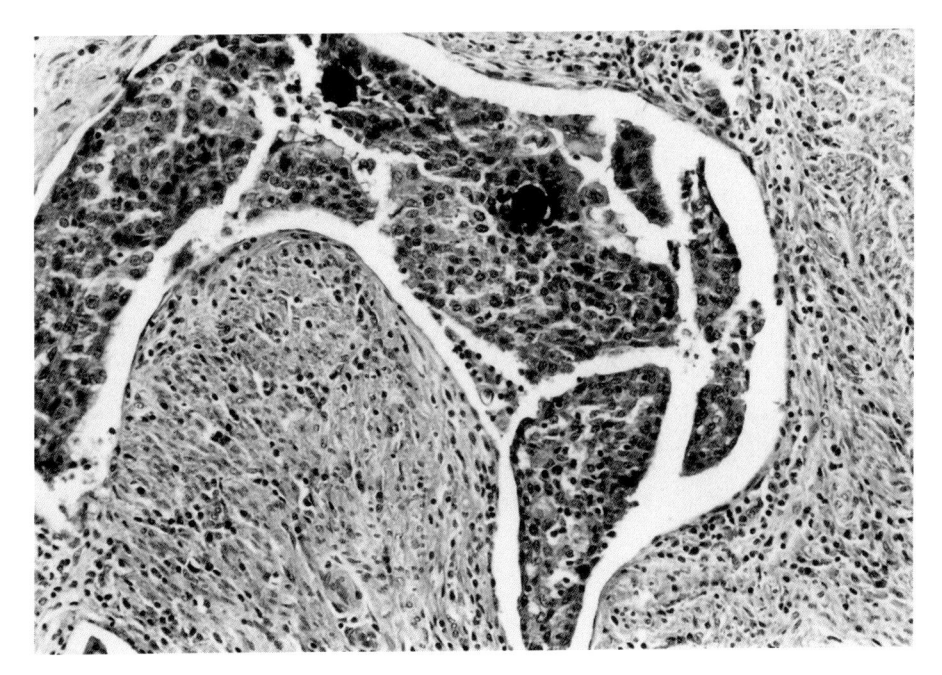

Figure 10-1. Endometrial carcinoma involving a myometrial lymphovascular space.

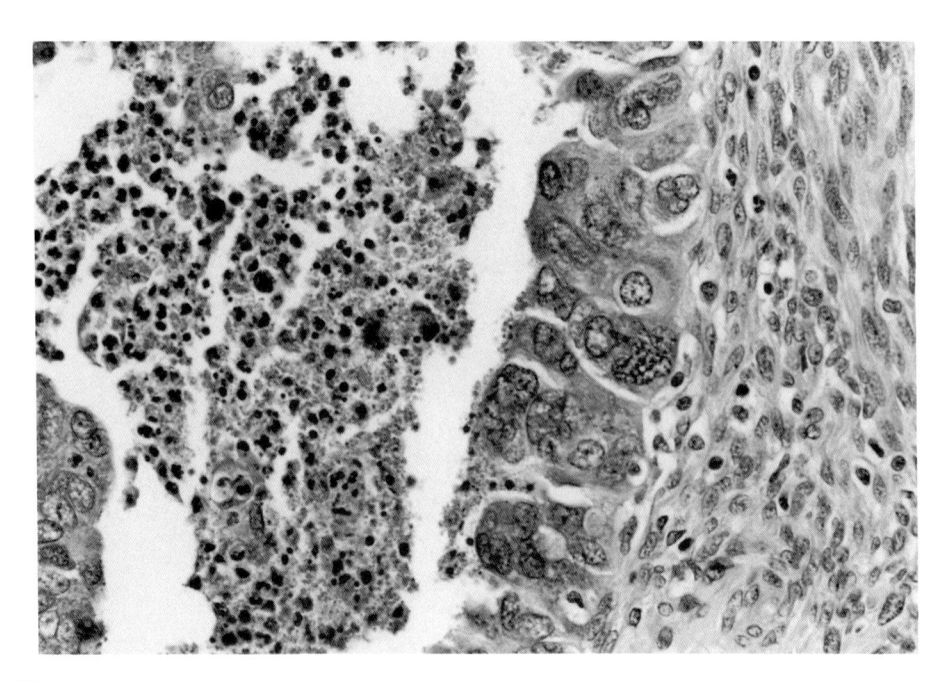

Figure 10-2. Marked nuclear atypia with hyperchromatism and multinucleation is present in this malignant endometrial gland.

Grading Endometrial Carcinoma

While some studies have graded endometrial carcinomas by relying heavily on nuclear grading, the most widely utilized system of grading endometrial carcinoma is the FIGO system, an architectural evaluation based on the amount of the tumor that is solid.[7] In this classification, grade 1 tumors show less than or equal to 5% solid pattern, grade 2 tumors are 6–50% solid, and grade 3 tumors are over 50% solid. Solid sheets of mature or immature squamous elements should not be included in the grading assessment, which applies to the glandular element. Adenocarcinomas with squamous differentiation are graded on the nuclear grade of the glandular portion of the tumor. Significant nuclear atypia disproportionate to the architectural grade raises the grade by 1 (Fig. 10-2). Grading is predominantly by nuclear features in clear cell carcinoma, uterine papillary serous carcinoma, and in squamous cell carcinoma of the endometrium, which have more limited architectural patterns.[7]

Staging of Endometrial Carcinoma

The FIGO staging of endometrial adenocarcinoma has recently been revised to a surgically rather than clinically staged system, and is as follows:[7]

Stage Ia, grades 1, 2, or 3 (G123)—tumor limited to the endometrium
Stage Ib, G123—invasion to less than one-half of the myometrium

Stage Ic, G123—invasion to more than one-half of the myometrium
Stage IIa, G123—endocervical glandular involvement only
Stage IIb, G123—cervical stromal invasion
Stage IIIa, G123—tumor invades serosa and/or adnexa, and/or positive peritoneal cytology
Stage IIIb, G123—vaginal metastases
Stage IIIc, G123—metastases to pelvic and/or paraaortic lymph nodes
Grade IVa, G123—tumor invasion of bladder and/or bowel mucosa
Grade IVb—distant metastases including intraabdominal and/or inguinal lymph nodes

In this new staging system, the fractional curettage previously used to separate stage I from stage II is no longer valid.

HISTOLOGIC TYPES OF ENDOMETRIAL CARCINOMA

Endometrioid ("Usual") Adenocarcinoma

Endometrioid adenocarcinoma represents over 75% of all cases of endometrial adenocarcinoma.[1] The diagnosis rests predominantly on demonstration of stromal invasion by neoplastic glandular elements, as discussed above. The glands may show nuclear atypia as in atypical hyperplasia, but the nuclei may be surprisingly innocuous in appearance. Well-differentiated endometrial adenocarcinoma is composed of ≤5% solid elements, by FIGO grading. The lesion is one of glandular crowding, with back-to-back glands and cribriforming. Normal stroma is not present between the neoplastic glands; it is either absent, desmoplastic, or replaced by inflammatory cells (Figs. 10-3, 10-4). Mitotic figures are easily found in the malignant glands, and as mentioned, nuclear atypia is variable. Moderately differentiated endometrial adenocarcinoma contains 6–50% solid elements (Fig. 10-5), and poorly differentiated endometrial adenocarcinoma is composed of over 50% solid elements (Fig. 10-6). Sheets of cells with squamous differentiation are not to be considered as the solid elements in grading an endometrial carcinoma.

A pattern of delicate papillary projections of epithelium on thin fibrovascular stalks is sometimes encountered, architecturally reminiscent of the villous adenoma of the colon. Hendrickson and Kempson call this the "villoglandular" pattern[8] (Fig. 10-7). It is important not to confuse this entity with uterine papillary serous carcinoma, which is so much worse prognostically (Fig. 10-8A,B).

In postmenopausal women, the endometrium adjacent to an endometrial carcinoma may be atrophic, or hyperplastic. There is evidence to suggest that biologically there may be two distinct forms of endometrial carcinoma, one associated with estrogen excess, and one not.[1,9] Patients with type I tumors, associated with estrogen excess, frequently show some of the classic clinical factors associated with endometrial carcinoma and with hyperes-

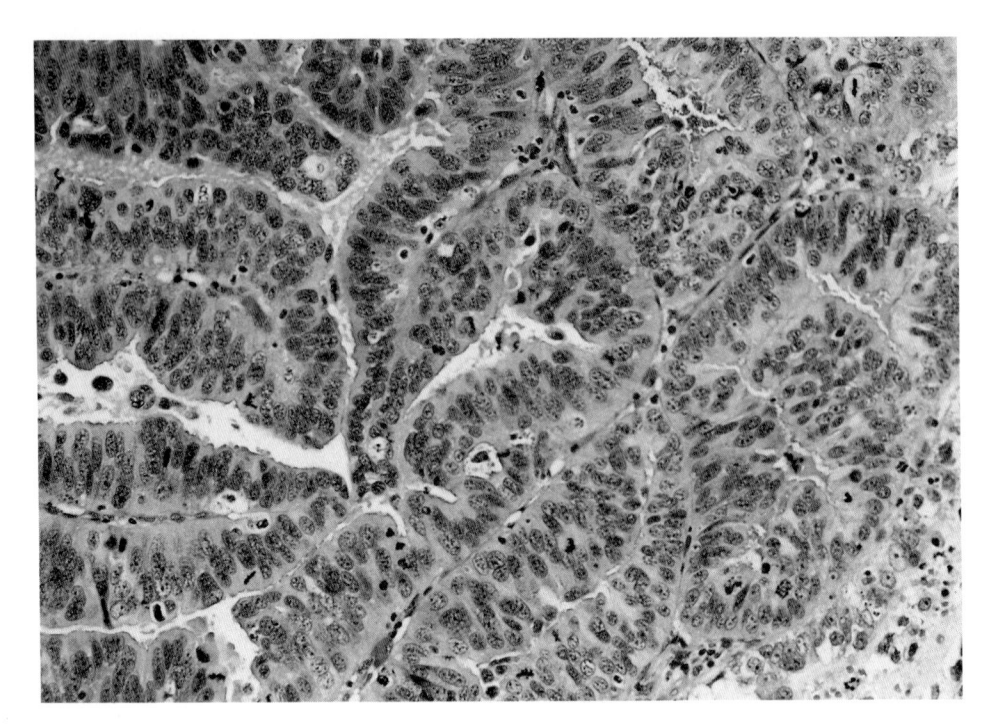

Figure 10-3. Well-differentiated endometrial adenocarcinoma showing back-to-back glands without intervening stroma.

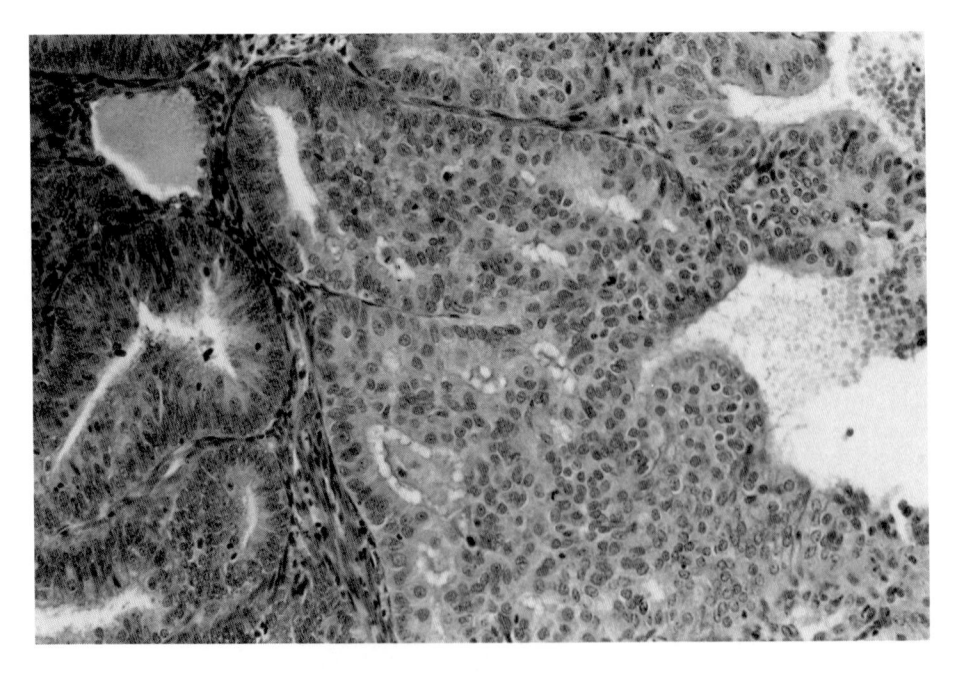

Figure 10-4. Well-differentiated endometrial adenocarcinoma showing cribriforming (gland-within-gland).

Histologic Types of Endometrial Carcinoma

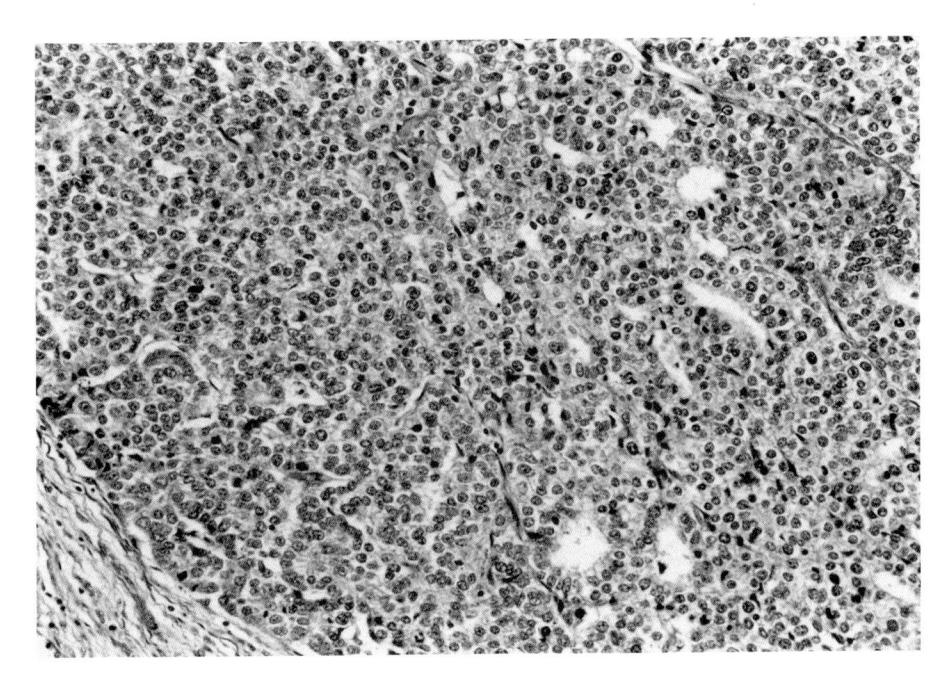

Figure 10-5. Moderately differentiated endometrial adenocarcinoma showing solid areas admixed with glandular ones.

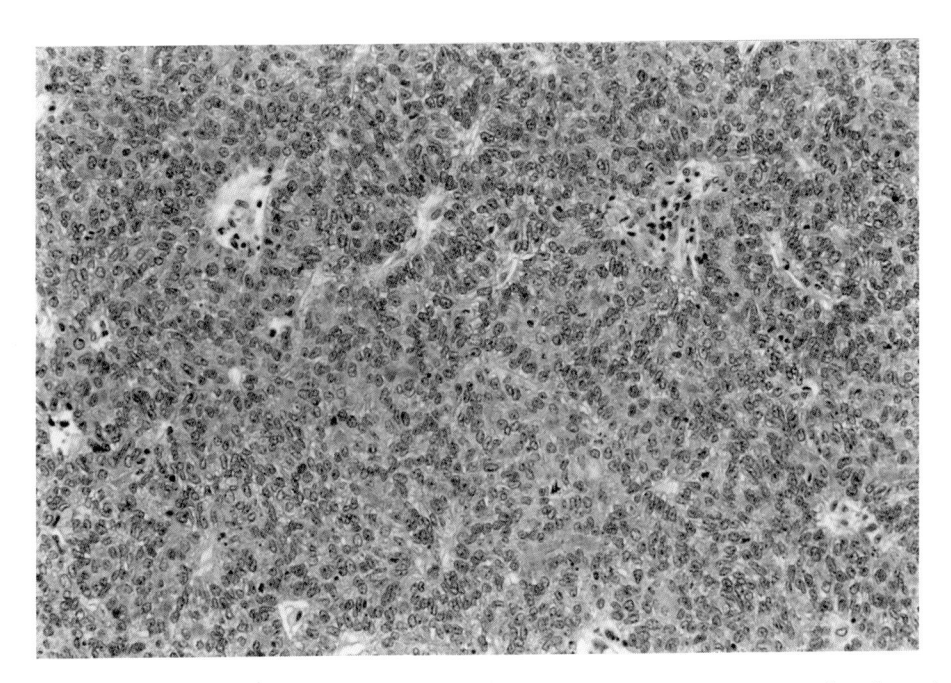

Figure 10-6. Poorly differentiated endometrial adenocarcinoma is almost totally solid.

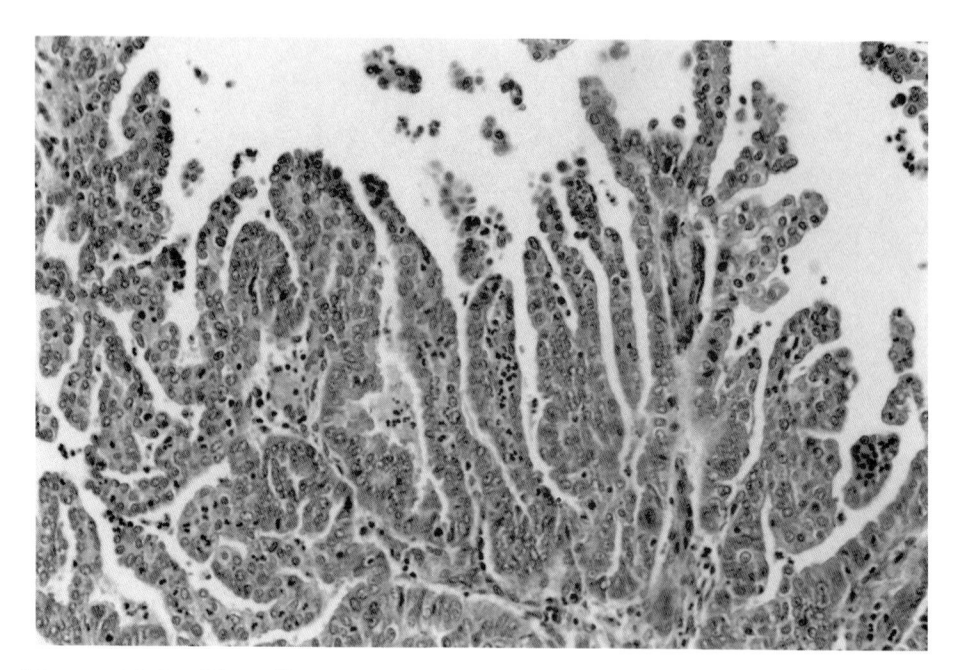

Figure 10-7. The villoglandular pattern of well-differentiated endometrial adenocarcinoma, with its delicate fibrovascular stalks and lesser atypia, should not be mistaken for uterine papillary serous carcinoma (see Fig. 10-8).

trogenism: obesity, anovulation and infertility, diabetes, and hypertension. They often have hyperplastic endometrium adjacent to their tumors. Patients with type I tumors are more often younger than women with type II carcinomas. They are more likely to be Caucasian, and their tumors are more often of lower grade and better prognosis. Type II endometrial adenocarcinoma, in contrast, occurs in women who do not have the standard endometrial carcinoma risk factors, are more often African-American, and tend to have higher-grade tumors with a worse prognosis.

Endometrial Adenocarcinoma with Squamous Differentiation

In the past, it was customary to separate "adenoacanthoma" from "adenosquamous carcinoma" of the endometrium, according to whether the squamous elements appeared benign or malignant. It was felt that adenosquamous carcinoma had a significantly worse prognosis than adenoacanthoma. It has been found, however, that better prognostication can be obtained by grading the glandular elements, and that the differentiation of the squamous elements usually parallels that of the glandular component.[10,11] Thus, it has been recommended that the diagnoses adenoacanthoma and adenosquamous carcinoma, often a cause for confusion, be dropped, and replaced by the single diagnosis "adenocarcinoma with squamous differentiation," with tumor grade based on the glandular component of the tumor[10,11] (Fig. 10-9).

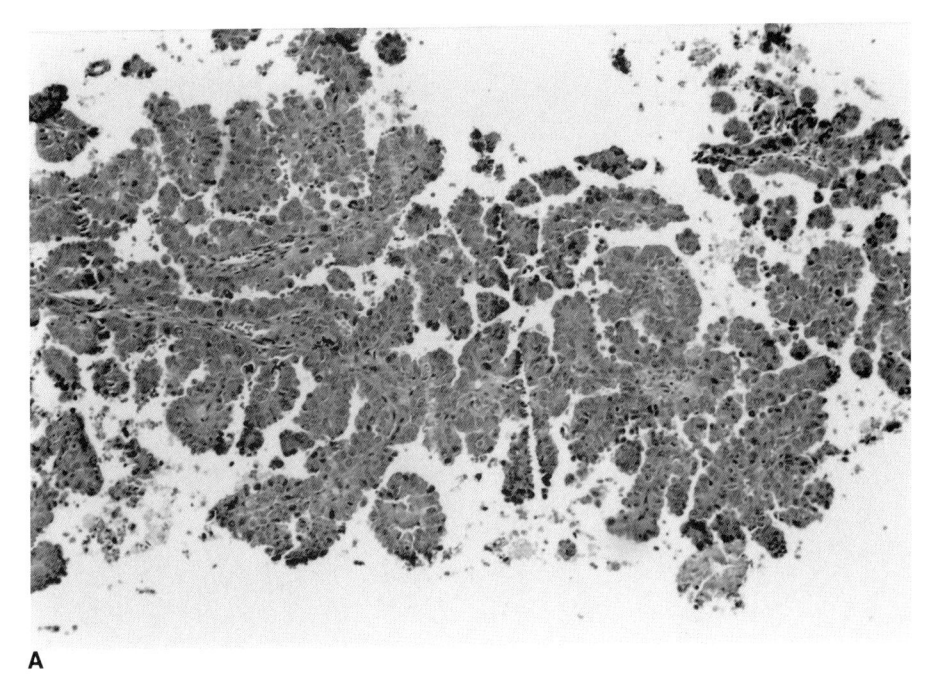

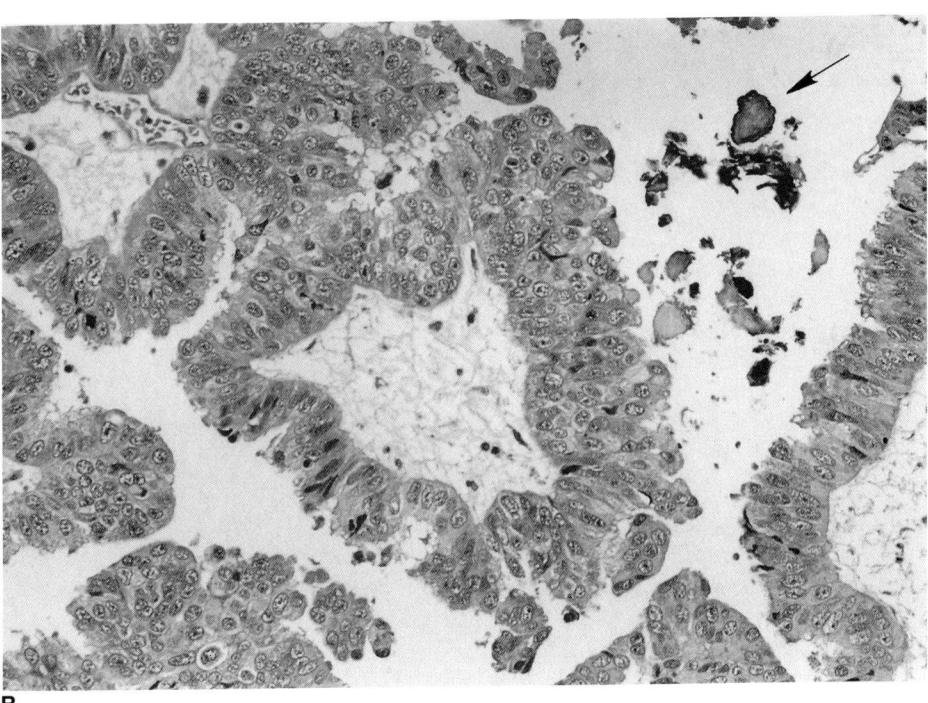

Figure 10-8. (A,B) Uterine papillary serous carcinoma resembles ovarian papillary serous carcinoma, with broad fibrovascular stalks lined by piled up, markedly atypical cells. Psammoma bodies are sometimes seen (Fig. 8-8B, arrow).

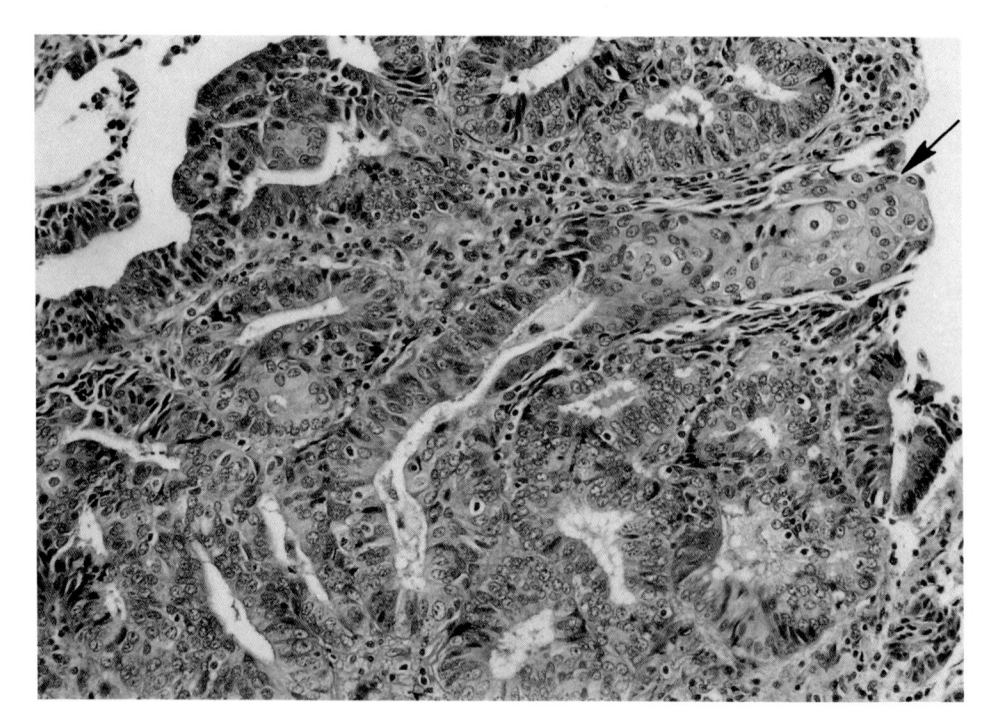

Figure 10-9. Well differentiated endometrial adenocarcinoma with squamous differentiation (arrow).

Prognosis of adenocarcinoma with squamous differentiation, as in conventional endometrial adenocarcinoma, relates to the age of the patient, tumor stage and grade, and depth of myometrial invasion.[10] Interestingly, in this study,[10] although the probability of nodal metastases was similar in tumors with or without squamous differentiation, the risk of death was significantly less in the tumors with squamous differentiation.

Secretory Carcinoma of the Endometrium

Secretory adenocarcinoma usually represents a well-differentiated endometrioid adenocarcinoma with superimposed progesterone effect, either endogenous or exogenous, although this is not always the case.[12] This pattern can be seen in the endometrial carcinomas of premenopausal as well as postmenopausal women. While it can be confused with clear cell adenocarcinoma because of the cytoplasmic vacuolization with high glycogen content, it should be distinguished from clear cell adenocarcinoma, which has a significantly worse prognosis. In secretory adenocarcinoma, the glandular architecture usually resembles that of a grade I endometrial adenocarcinoma, with the glands themselves reminiscent of secretory glands of cycle days 17–22.[13] Mitoses are uncommon, as is nuclear atypia, distinguishing features when considering a clear cell carcinoma. In secretory carcinoma, glandular

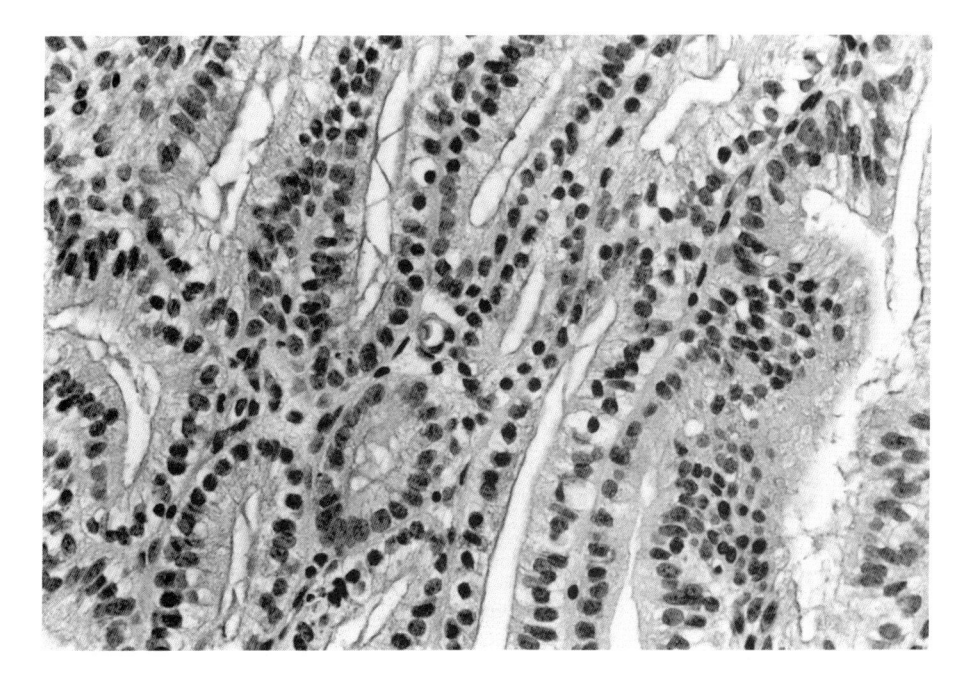

Figure 10-10. Secretory carcinoma of the endometrium. The glands show secretory features, but the architecture is that of a well differentiated adenocarcinoma of the endometrium.

cells may show piling up, and there is cytoplasmic vacuolization either above or below the nuclei (Fig. 10-10). Distinction from a mucinous adenocarcinoma is made by the presence of abundant mucopolysaccharides in the latter. The prognosis for secretory carcinoma is similar to that for usual endometrioid adenocarcinoma, and since most are grade I, the patients tend to have a good prognosis.[14]

Ciliated Cell Adenocarcinoma

Ciliated cells can be found in benign endometria, both normal and hyperplastic, as discussed in Chapter 8. Although ciliated cell malignancies do exist, the presence of proliferations of ciliated cells in a variety of organs leads the pathologist toward a benign diagnosis, since cilia are a sign of advanced cellular differentiation. Rare cases of endometrial adenocarcinoma largely composed of ciliated cells have been described.[15] These authors stress that most ciliated proliferations in the endometrium are benign, and that some of the benign proliferations can be architecturally complex, and be mistaken for carcinoma. Available follow-up of eight patients in this series indicates this neoplasm to be of low virulence, as none of the patients had local recurrences or metastases for a period of up to 8 years, even with myometrial invasion present in the hysterectomy specimen.

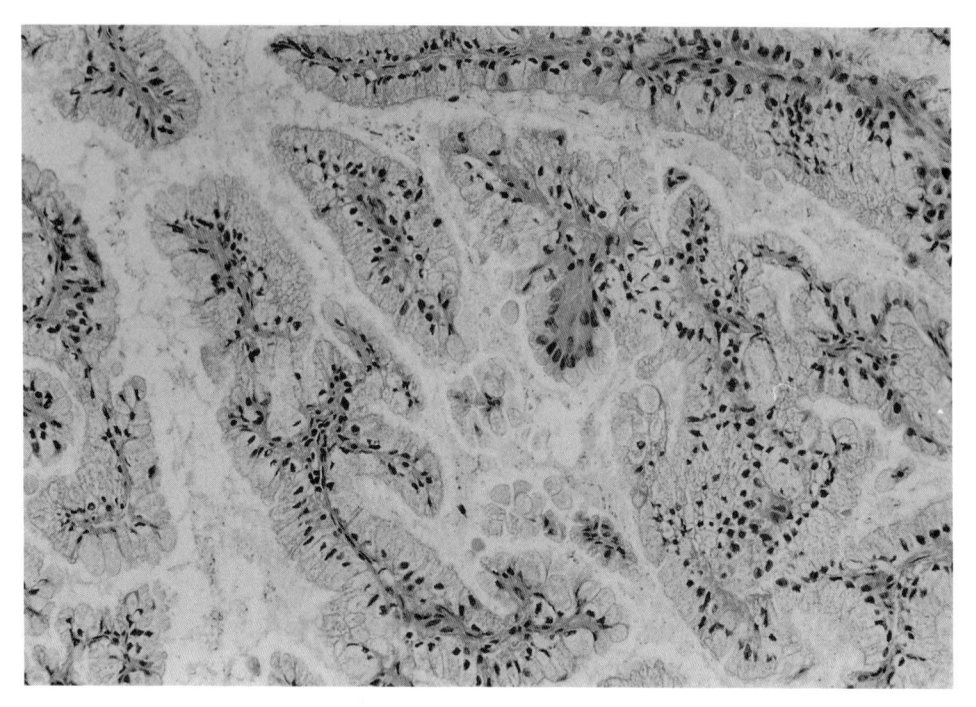

Figure 10-11. Mucinous adenocarcinoma of the endometrium.

Mucinous Adenocarcinoma

Pure mucinous carcinomas of the endometrium are rare, but a mucinous epithelial proliferation can make up a significant proportion of an endometrial adenocarcinoma. In this variant, the epithelial cells contain abundant mucin in the cytoplasm, which may be demonstrated with special stains. The pattern of the tumor resembles mucinous adenocarcinoma of the endocervix or ovary. Glands may be composed of cells with tall columnar mucinous cells with basal nuclei, or there may be more pseudostratification.[14] Distinction can be made from both clear cell adenocarcinoma and secretory adenocarcinoma by the fact that these two tumors contain abundant glycogen, while the mucinous adenocarcinoma contains abundant mucin. Mucinous carcinomas of the endometrium are usually well differentiated, with minimal mitotic activity or atypia (Fig. 10-11). The prognosis is the same as in usual endometrioid carcinoma.[14] Because of the difference in therapies, an extremely important distinction is between a mucinous adenocarcinoma of the endometrium, and one of the endocervix. While the main distinction is anatomic,[16] other methods of separating the two have been attempted (see subsequent discussion).

Clear Cell Adenocarcinoma

Clear cell adenocarcinoma of the endometrium is currently felt to be derived from Müllerian epithelium rather than from mesonephric remnants.[17] It is a disease almost exclusively of postmenopausal women.[12] Clear cell adenocarcinoma occurs more commonly in the ovary than the endometrium, and has also been well documented in the vagina and cervix, particularly with intrauterine diethylstilbestrol (DES) exposure.

Clear cell adenocarcinoma (Fig. 10-12A–C) is composed of a mixture of clear, hobnail, and flat cells, in combinations of one or more of four architectural patterns: solid, glandular, papillary, or cystic.[17] The neoplastic cells contain abundant glycogen in cytoplasm that is either clear or eosinophilic. Nuclear atypia and mitoses are prominent features. Since the architectural patterns have limited variability, nuclear grading is more reliably employed.[7] Clear cell carcinoma may occur in combination with other patterns of endometrial carcinoma.

Clear cell carcinoma should be distinguished from secretory and mucinous carcinomas, because clear cell carcinoma carries a significantly worse prognosis.[17] As mentioned previously, the cytoplasm of the cells of mucinous carcinoma contains abundant mucopolysaccharides, while those of a clear cell carcinoma do not. Secretory carcinoma, while containing glycogen, is architecturally distinguishable from a clear cell adenocarcinoma in most cases, and shows significantly less mitotic activity and nuclear atypia. The Arias–Stella reaction may be confused with a clear cell carcinoma, but may be distinguished by its occurrence in a younger pregnant woman, and by the fact that it lacks mitotic activity. Buckley and Fox[14] note that the distinction between a papillary pattern of clear cell carcinoma and a uterine papillary serous carcinoma may be difficult, particularly on curettings, but as both have a notably poor prognosis, this distinction is of no clinical significance.

Uterine Papillary Serous Carcinoma (UPSC)

This neoplasm resembles papillary serous cystadenocarcinoma of the ovary histologically (Fig. 10-8), and its pattern of spread over peritoneal surfaces and poor prognosis mimic that tumor as well. Unlike usual endometrioid adenocarcinoma of the endometrium, UPSC is a markedly aggressive tumor, usually diagnosed in an advanced stage in older women, with a poor prognosis. Histologically, the tumor is composed of fibrovascular cores lined by neoplastic epithelium exhibiting marked nuclear pleomorphism, sometimes with prominent nucleoli, nuclear stratification, and mitotic activity. Psammoma bodies may be present. The adjacent endometrium is usually atrophic.[18] The tumor tends to invade myometrium and myometrial lymphatics, with early spread. The nonsolid architecture of the tumor may erroneously lead to assignment of a FIGO grade of I, even with significant nuclear atypia, suggesting a better prognosis than there actually is. In one series,[18] there were poor outcomes even with only superficial myometrial invasion or tumor confined to an endometrial polyp, as well as when UPSC was admixed with other tumor types.

Differential diagnosis includes the villoglandular pattern of endometrioid adenocarcinoma, and papillary syncytial metaplasia. In the villoglandular

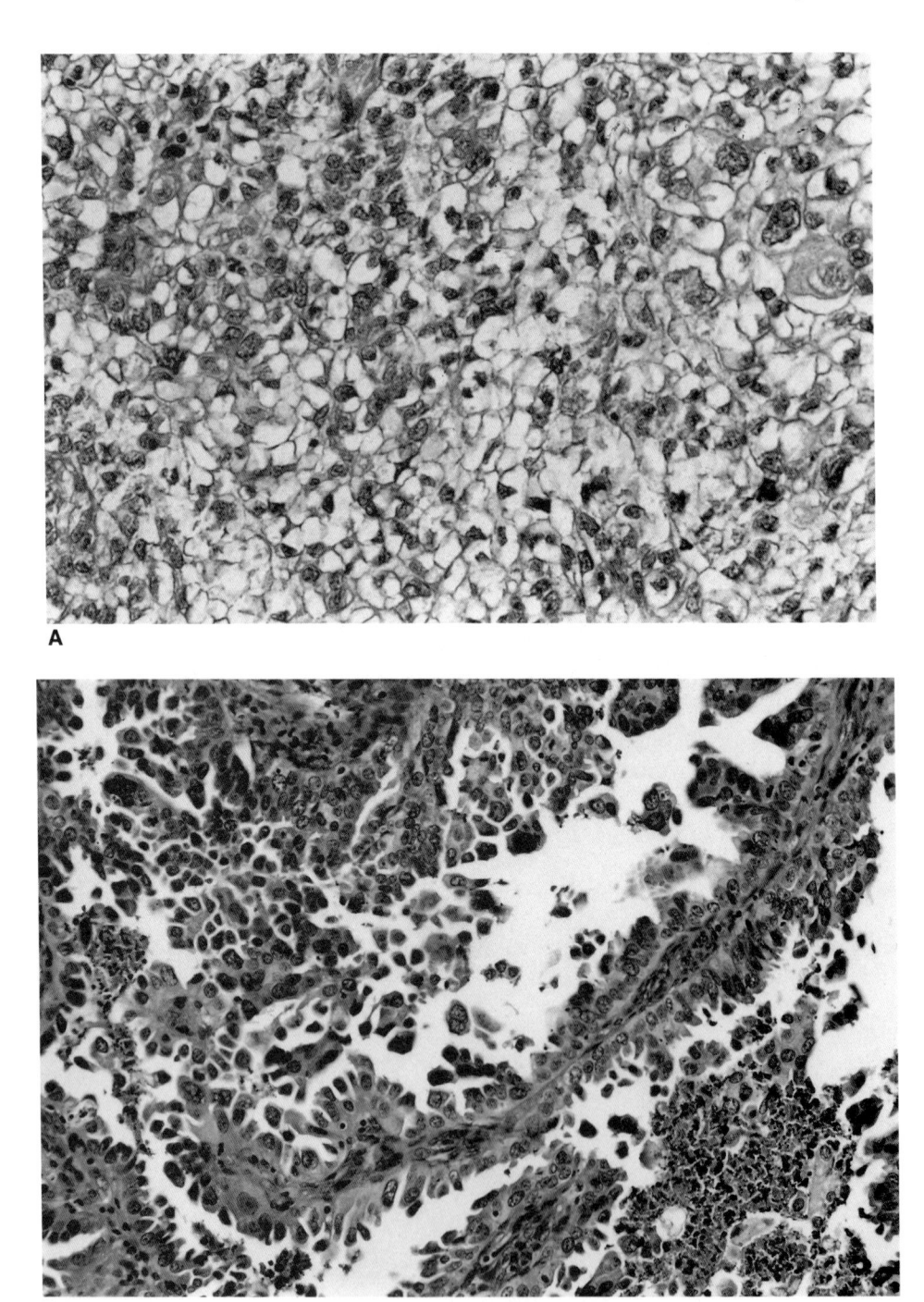

Figure 10-12. (A) Clear cell pattern of clear cell adenocarcinoma of the endometrium. (B) Hobnail cell pattern of clear cell adenocarcinoma of the endometrium.

Histologic Types of Endometrial Carcinoma 151

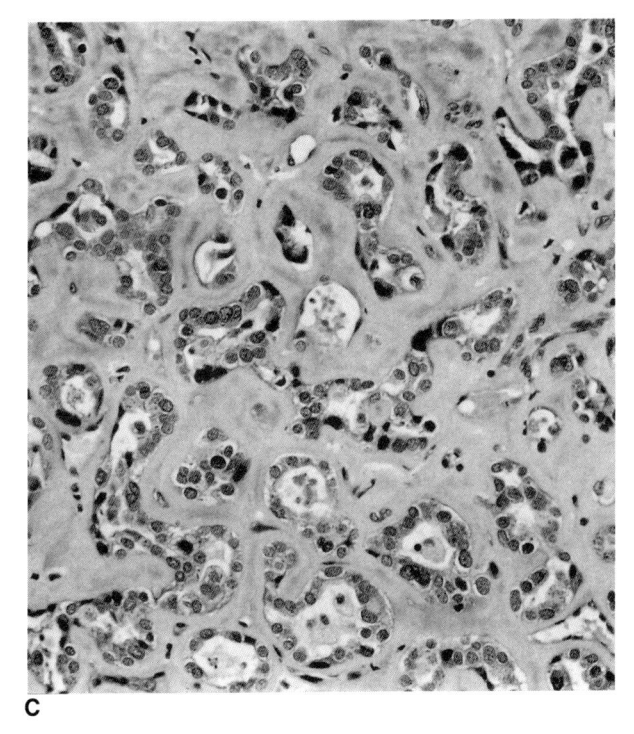

Figure 10-12. (C) Clear cell adenocarcinoma of the endometrium often shows areas of densely collagenized stroma.

pattern of endometrioid carcinoma, the papillary projections are more delicate, with less cytologic atypia of the epithelium. Villoglandular areas usually blend into areas with the more typical pattern of endometrioid adenocarcinoma.[18] Papillary syncytial metaplasia contains rare mitoses and bland nuclei, and lacks fibrovascular stalks. It is confined to the superficial endometrium, particularly the surface epithelium.[18]

Undifferentiated Carcinoma

Undifferentiated carcinoma of the endometrium lacks evidence of glandular, squamous, or sarcomatous differentiation (Fig. 10-13). Distinction from lymphomas can be made with immunohistochemical stains, since carcinomas won't stain with lymphoid markers such as leukocyte common antigen. There is some overlap of the staining patterns of carcinomas and sarcomas, and immunohistochemistry is not always helpful in these cases. Some undifferentiated carcinomas of the endometrium resemble small cell carcinoma of the lung, and contain neurosecretory granules. Others show a spindle cell or giant cell pattern.[14]

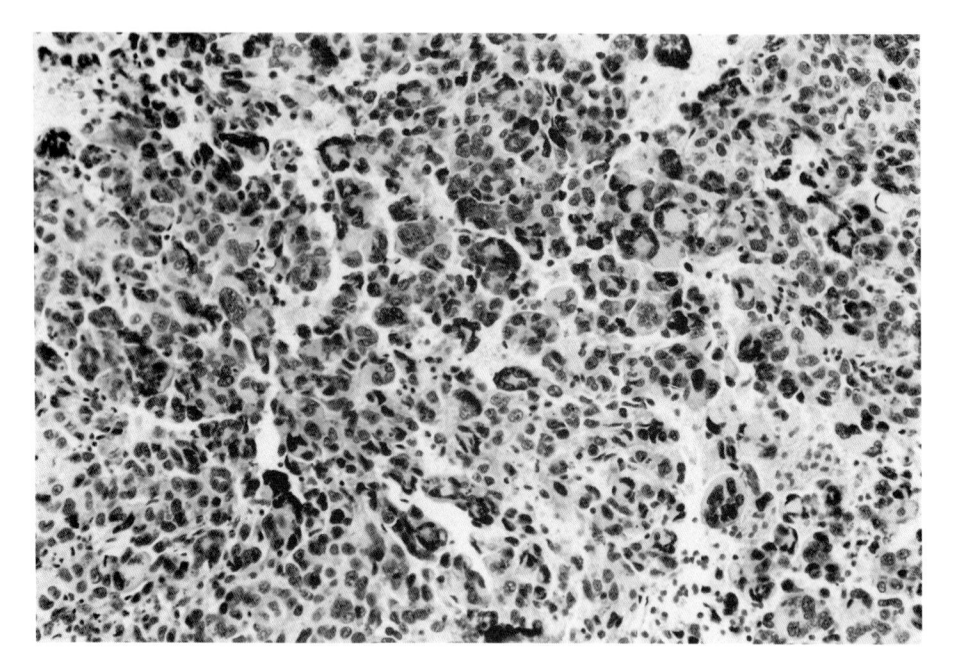

Figure 10-13. Undifferentiated carcinoma of the endometrium shows no obvious squamous or glandular differentiation.

Squamous Cell Carcinoma

Primary squamous cell carcinoma of the endometrium is exceedingly rare, with few reported cases.[19] The three diagnostic criteria of Fluhmann are stringent:[20] (1) there must be no coexisting glandular carcinoma, (2) there must be no connection between the tumor and the cervical squamous epithelium, and (3) there must be no primary cervical squamous cell carcinoma.

Of 26 reported cases of primary squamous cell carcinoma of the endometrium, 31% were associated with pyometra,[19] which may represent an antecedent or subsequent event. The cases occurred in a slightly older population than endometrial adenocarcinoma, with 70% of the patients over the age of 55. Prognosis was poor; in most cases invasive and/or metastatic disease was present at initial surgery.

Secondary squamous cell carcinoma of the endometrium can result from spread of a cervical lesion, either carcinoma in situ,[1] or from an invasive squamous cell carcinoma of the cervix.[21] This pattern is often associated with cervical stenosis, which may act as a mechanical block, preventing the more common downward vaginal spread of cervical carcinoma, and encouraging upward spread over the endometrial surface.[21] The spread over the surface of the endometrium does not change the staging of a cervical carcinoma, nor alter its prognosis,[21] although Perez[22] has noted a worse outcome in cervical squamous cell carcinoma invading the endometrial stroma.

Mixed-Cell-Type Endometrial Adenocarcinoma

It should be noted that endometrial carcinoma may occur as a mixture of histologic patterns. Tumors containing uterine papillary serous carcinoma (UPSC) as a component of a mixed epithelial tumor behave as aggressively as pure UPSC.[18]

Carcinoma Metastatic to the Endometrium

While the myometrium and ovaries are more common sites of metastases from extragenital malignancies, disease metastatic to the endometrium will occasionally be encountered. The most common extragenital malignancy to metastasize to the endometrium is carcinoma of the breast (Fig. 10-14), followed by colon carcinoma.[23]

Ovarian carcinoma can metastasize to the endometrium, but the reverse is more often the case.[24] With similar histologies, the possibility of synchronous primary tumors arises, most often if both tumors are of the endometrioid pattern of adenocarcinoma. Eifel et al[25] felt that the better than expected prognosis seen in cases of concomitant endometrioid adenocarcinoma of the endometrium and ovary speaks for lower-staged synchronous primaries, rather than for higher-staged metastatic disease from one organ to the other. They found a poorer prognosis in tumors of nonendometrioid or mixed endometrioid and nonendometrioid patterns, and postulated that in these cases the findings were more compatible with metastatic disease.

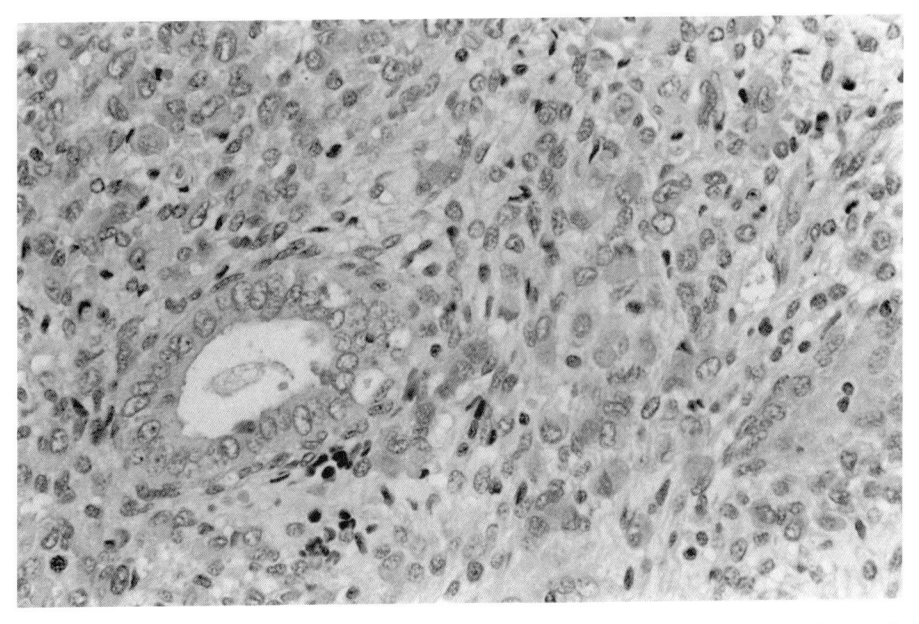

Figure 10-14. Metastatic carcinoma of the breast replacing endometrial stroma. Note the trapped benign endometrial gland.

Criteria for classifying a tumor as an endometrial primary with ovarian metastases include a multinodular ovarian pattern, small ovaries, bilateral ovarian involvement, deep myometrial invasion, vascular invasion, and tubal lumen involvement.[24] Scully calls a lesion "metastatic" when it is large in one organ and small in the other, and when direct extension is seen, and further states that a typical endometrial carcinoma with surface ovarian implants, or intraluminal tubal spread of tumor also speak for an endometrial primary.[26]

DISTINCTION BETWEEN ENDOMETRIAL ADENOCARCINOMA AND ENDOCERVICAL ADENOCARCINOMA

The similar histologic appearance of mucinous adenocarcinomas of the endometrium and endocervix may make their separation difficult, but it is important to try to make the distinction because therapy differs. Czernobilsky et al[27] noted that in most primary endometrial adenocarcinomas, the endocervical-type pattern is focal, and distinction can be made by assessing the endometrioid component elsewhere. They commented on certain factors that favor an endometrial primary: a transition between the endocervical-type carcinoma and more typical endometrioid carcinoma, areas of tufting, pseudostratification and atypia within the endocervix-like carcinoma, and endometrial stroma within the endocervical-type fragments. The presence of concomitant adenomatous hyperplasia favors an endometrial primary.[1] The presence of concomitant cervical intraepithelial neoplasia (CIN), or endocervical adenocarcinoma in situ (ACIS), favors an endocervical primary.[1] Fractional curettage and imaging studies may be of assistance in making the distinction. Special stains are not usually helpful. In general, normal endocervical mucosa, neoplastic endocervical mucosa, and mucinous endocervical-type patterns of endometrial carcinoma have similar staining characteristics for mucin, and similar immunohistochemical staining patterns as well. The presence of strong positive staining for carcinoembryonic antigen favors an endocervical primary over an endometrial, although there are positives and negatives in both types of neoplasia.[28,29]

ENDOMETRIAL CARCINOMA IN ADENOMYOSIS

Endometrial carcinoma can be seen in adenomyosis, and this should be distinguished from myometrial invasion (Fig. 10-15). Evidence suggests that the presence of endometrial adenocarcinoma in adenomyosis, even if deeper than the depth of myometrial invasion of that tumor, does not worsen the prognosis beyond that of the myometrial invasion.[30] Identification of carcinoma in a focus of adenomyosis rests on finding endometrial stroma, which is absent in true myometrial invasion. Residual nonneoplastic glands may also still exist in the focus of adenomyosis.

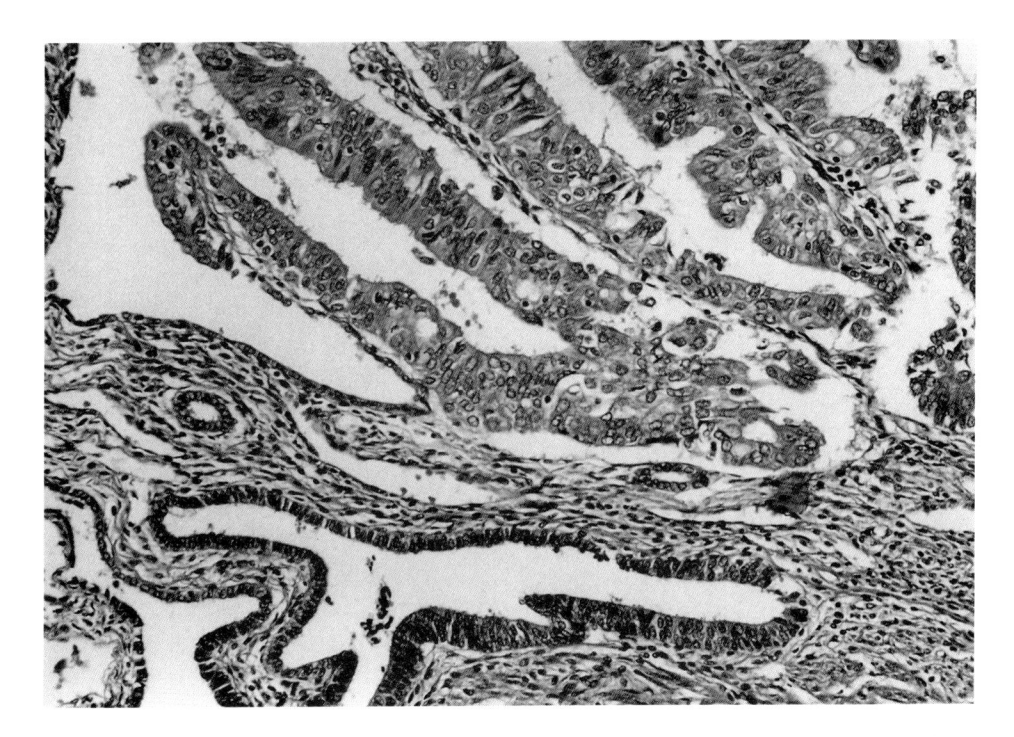

Figure 10-15. Endometrial carcinoma in adenomyosis. Note the benign glandular and stromal elements at the bottom of the photomicrograph.

PYOMETRA

The finding of pyometra (Fig. 10-16) in a postmenopausal woman is a red flag to search for an endometrial carcinoma, although this will not be proved true in all cases.

RADIATION EFFECT ON ENDOMETRIAL CARCINOMA

With the new surgical staging, preoperative radiation prior to hysterectomy is less common than previously; however, radiation change is more prevalent in archival material, so a brief discussion is in order. Silverberg et al[31] found no morphologic difference between tumor in preradiation curettages and residual carcinoma in the radiated hysterectomy specimen. They noted that the radiation had induced bizarre cytologic changes in residual benign glands (Fig. 10-17). Kurman and Norris[1] state that there may be minimal changes, or severe cytologic atypia in both benign and malignant glands, and grading in this case rests on the architecture.

The effect of radiation on cells is one of enlarged pleomorphic nuclei with hyperchromasia and chromatin clumping. Cytoplasm is increased in amount, and may be vacuolated, as may nuclei.[1]

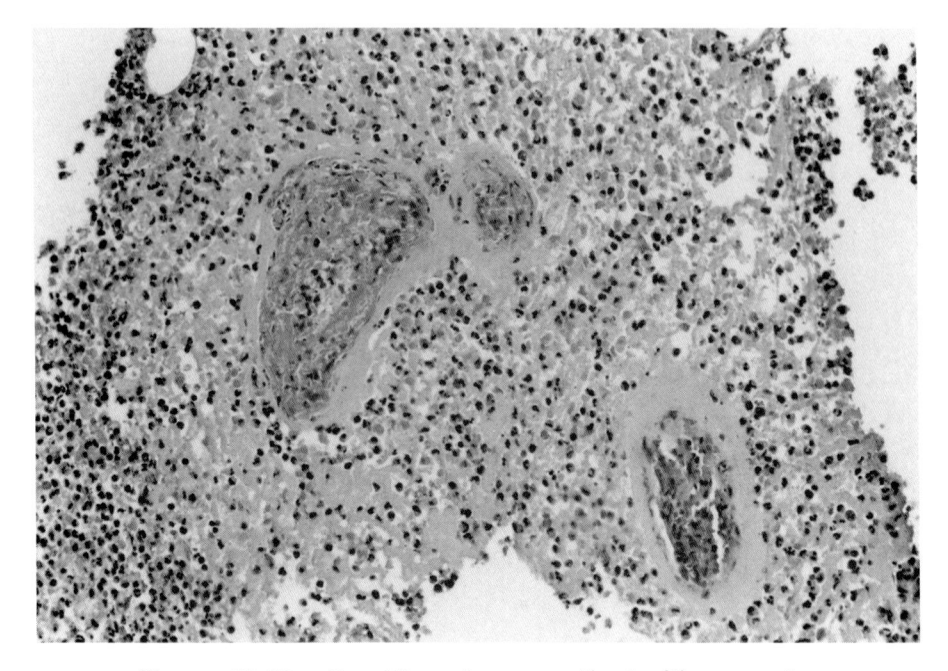

Figure 10-16. Curettings from a patient with pyometra.

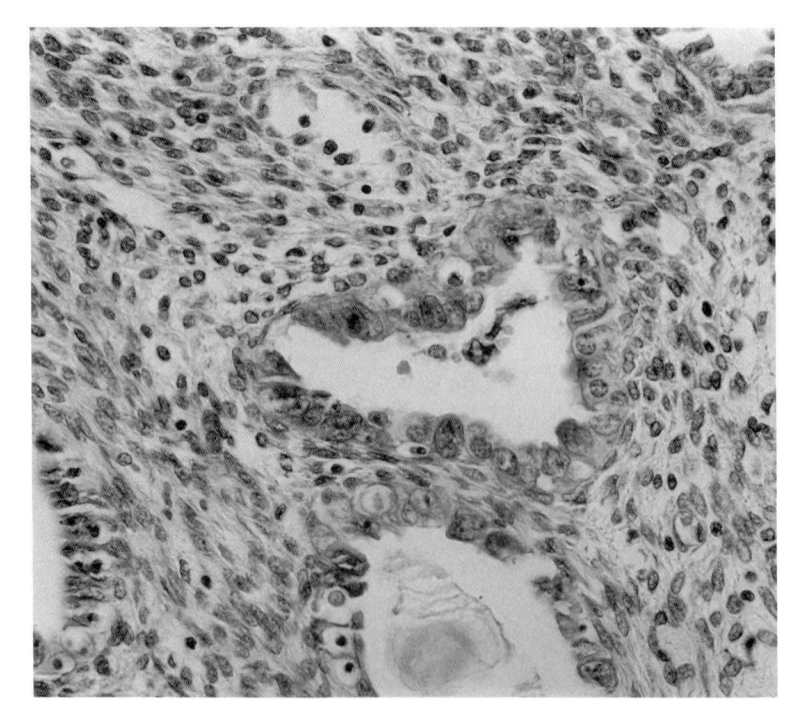

Figure 10-17. Radiation atypia in benign glands after radiotherapy for endometrial carcinoma.

TABLE 10-2. Mesenchymal Neoplasms Involving the Endometrium

Pure mesenchymal neoplasms—homologous
  Stromal neoplasms
    Stromal nodule
    Low-grade endometrial stromal sarcoma
    High-grade endometrial stromal sarcoma and/or undifferentiated sarcoma
  Smooth muscle neoplasms (when submucosal)
    Leiomyoma
    Leiomyosarcoma
    Smooth muscle tumors of uncertain malignant potential

Pure mesenchymal neoplasms—heterologous
  Rhabdomyosarcoma
  Chondrosarcoma
  Osteosarcoma

Mixed epithelial–mesenchymal neoplasms
  Adenofibroma
  Adenosarcoma
  Malignant mixed Müllerian tumors
    Homologous
    Heterologous

MESENCHYMAL NEOPLASMS INVOLVING THE ENDOMETRIUM

Müllerian-derived stem cells are multipotential, and may give rise to purely epithelial, purely mesenchymal, or mixed neoplasms. Mesenchymal elements may be homologous, that is native to the uterus, or heterologous, consisting of tissue types not found in the normal uterus (Table 10-2).[32]

PURE MESENCHYMAL NEOPLASMS—HOMOLOGOUS

Endometrial Stromal Lesions

The endometrial stroma can occasionally give rise to a benign neoplasm, the stromal nodule, and more often to endometrial stromal sarcomas, both low- and high-grade.

Stromal nodules usually present with abnormal bleeding. The median age is 47 years, with a wide range of occurrence. There may be pelvic pain and/or uterine enlargement, but stromal nodules may be incidental findings, and range in size from 0.8 to 15 cm.[33] Stromal nodules are well-circumscribed lesions, which is important in distinguishing them from low-grade endometrial stromal sarcoma. The cells resemble proliferative phase endometrial stromal cells, with a prominent vasculature. There is no cytologic atypia, and mitotic activity is usually minimal. Epithelial differentiation can occasionally be seen. The main feature that distinguishes a stromal nodule from low-grade endometrial stromal sarcoma is its lack of infiltration. This distinction cannot be made when fragments of a stromal proliferation are picked up on a curettage specimen.

Low-grade endometrial stromal sarcoma (Fig. 10-18A,B) histologically resembles stromal nodule, except that the neoplasm is infiltrative. Its former name, endolymphatic stromal myosis relates to its propensity to invade vascular and lymphatic myometrial spaces. These tumors generally behave as low-grade malignancies, with indolent behavior.[34] The endometrial component of the lesion is usually polypoid, while the myometrium may be diffusely thickened, may contain a discrete mass, or may contain a poorly circumscribed mass infiltrating in wormlike cords.[33] Mitotic activity can be up to 9 mitoses per 10 high-power fields, but is usually less than 3 per 10 high-power fields.[33] Nuclear atypia is less than in high-grade endometrial stromal sarcoma.

High-grade endometrial sarcoma behaves as an aggressive malignancy. Atypia is usually more pronounced than in low-grade stromal sarcoma, but the differential diagnosis is classically made on the mitotic count, which is 10 or more mitoses per 10 high-power fields in the high-grade lesion.[33]

It should be noted that in one study, the degree of mitotic activity and atypia failed to predict recurrences in stage I patients.[35] Some authors now divide these lesions into low-grade endometrial sarcoma for tumors with minimally atypical endometrial stroma-like cells and up to 15 mitoses per 10 high-power fields, and undifferentiated uterine sarcomas for high-grade tumors not resembling endometrial stroma (Fig. 10-19).[36]

Smooth Muscle Neoplasms Involving the Endometrium

While smooth muscle neoplasms generally occur in the myometrium rather than in the endometrium, occasionally fragments of a submucous smooth muscle tumor are encountered in uterine curettings. Smooth muscle neoplasms are divided into benign, malignant, or of uncertain malignant potential on the basis of their mitotic counts and cytologic atypia. This distinction may be difficult on a small biopsy specimen, as mitoses are counted per 10 high-power fields.

PURE MESENCHYMAL NEOPLASMS— HETEROLOGOUS

Pure rhabdomyosarcoma, chondrosarcoma, and osteosarcoma are rare in the uterus. If obtained in endometrial biopsy specimens, they are more likely

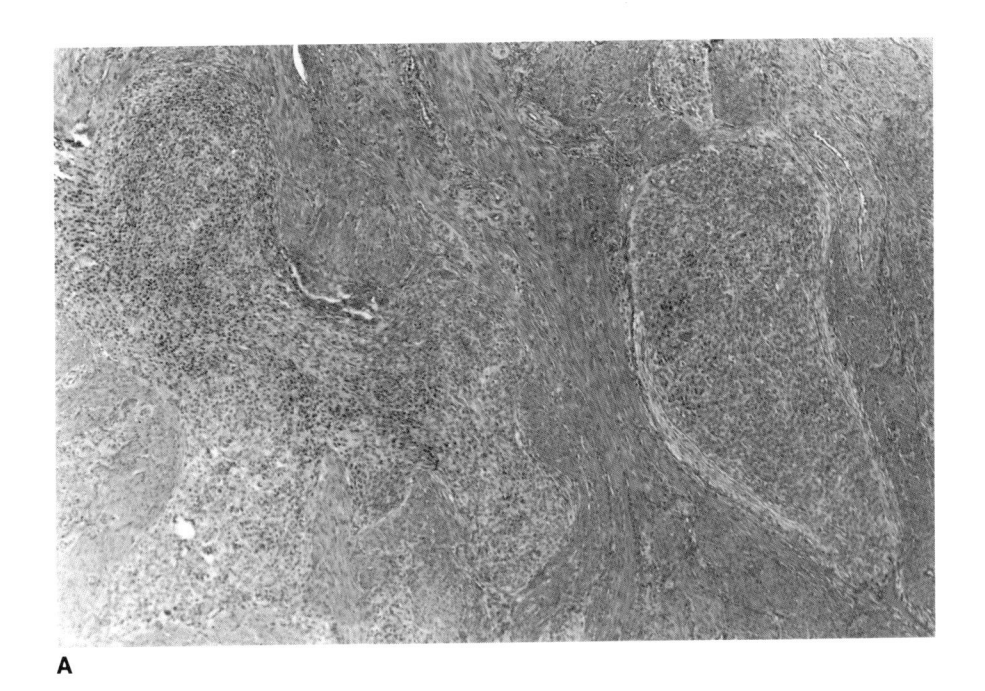

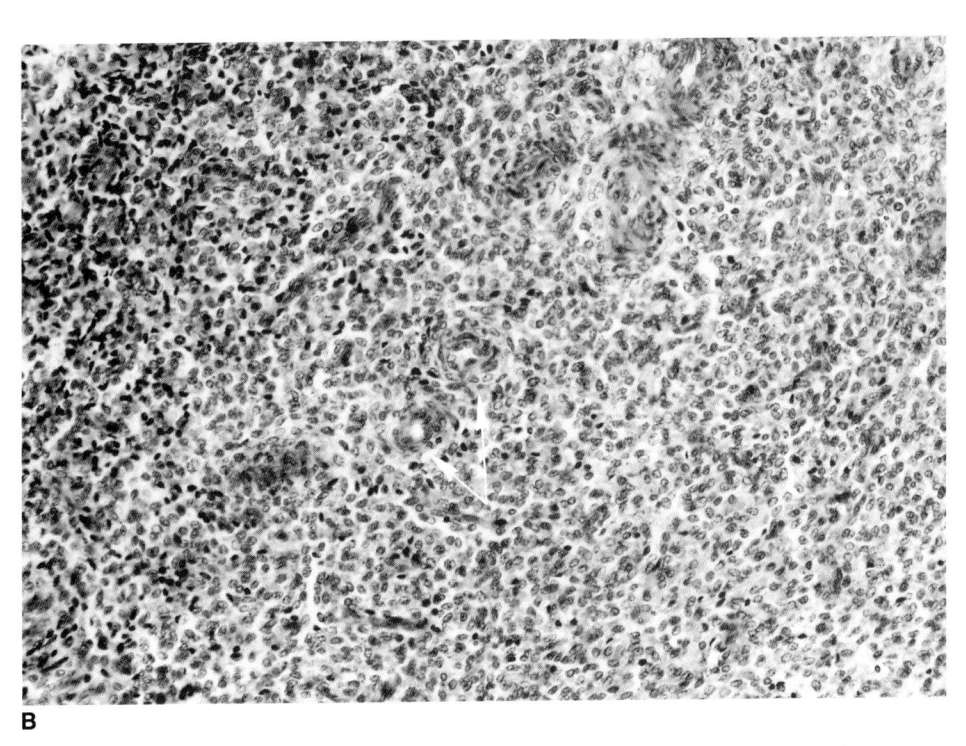

Figure 10-18. (A) Low-grade endometrial stromal sarcoma infiltrating myometrium. (B) At higher power, low-grade endometrial stromal sarcoma is seen to resemble cellular endometrial stroma. Mitotic activity is variable. Prominent vessels are often present (arrow).

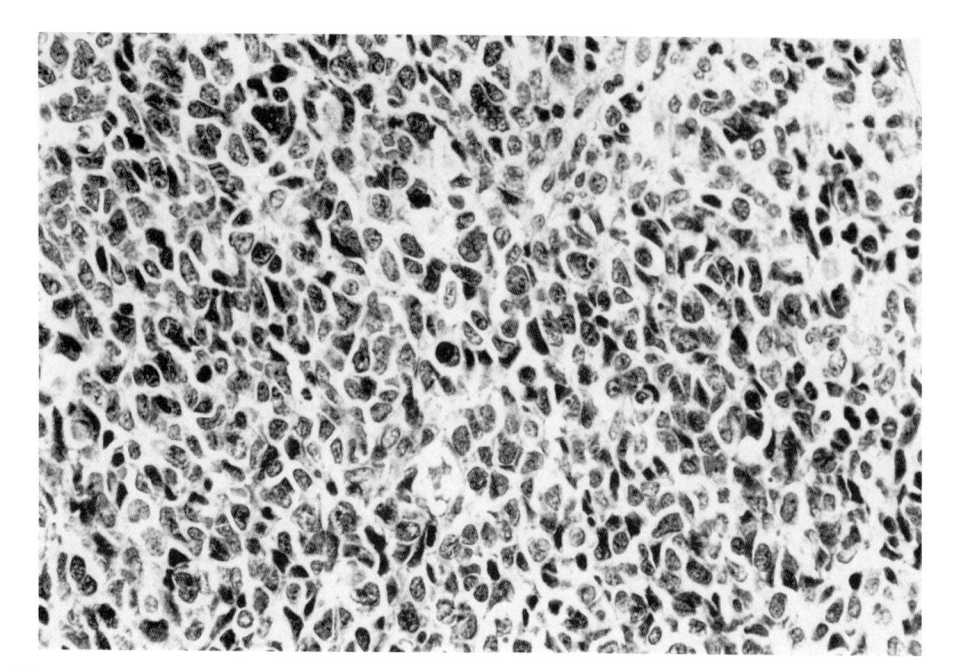

Figure 10-19. High-grade stromal sarcoma (undifferentiated sarcoma) of the endometrium.

to represent the mesenchymal component of a malignant mixed Müllerian tumor (MMMT).

MIXED EPITHELIAL–MESENCHYMAL TUMORS

Adenofibroma and Adenosarcoma

Adenofibromas are uncommon benign tumors, usually occurring in postmenopausal women who present with bleeding, pain, or uterine enlargement.[37] They are polypoid or papillary epithelium-lined neoplasms resembling papillary serous cystadenofibroma of the ovary. There is no cytologic atypia and minimal mitotic activity in the stroma.[37] The diagnosis of adenofibroma as opposed to adenosarcoma of the endometrium should be made with caution.

Adenosarcomas contain a benign glandular epithelial component and a malignant stromal component. They occur over a wide age range, with a median age of 57 years.[37] The most common symptom is abnormal bleeding. Like adenofibromas, they are fleshy polypoid lesions, but tend to be larger, with areas of necrosis. Stromal mitotic counts are generally greater than or equal to 4 mitoses per 10 high-power fields, and the degree of atypia varies.[37] The stroma usually resembles endometrial stroma or fibroblasts, but heterologous elements may occur. A characteristic feature is the condensation of stromal cells around the benign glandular elements (Fig. 10-20A,B). Mitotic activity may only be present in these areas, and the stroma may appear

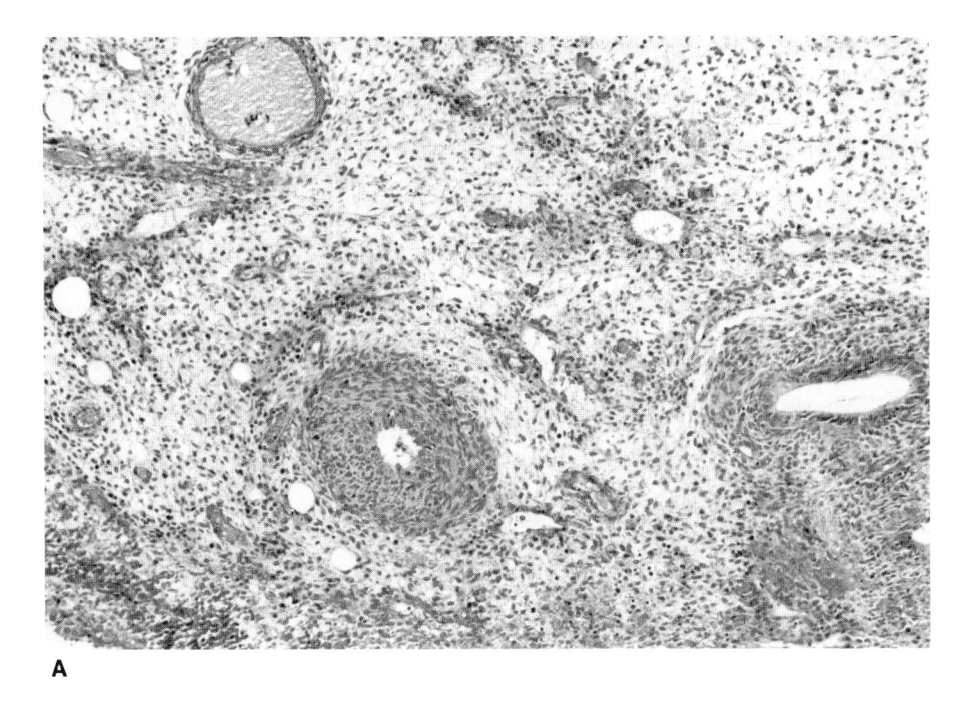

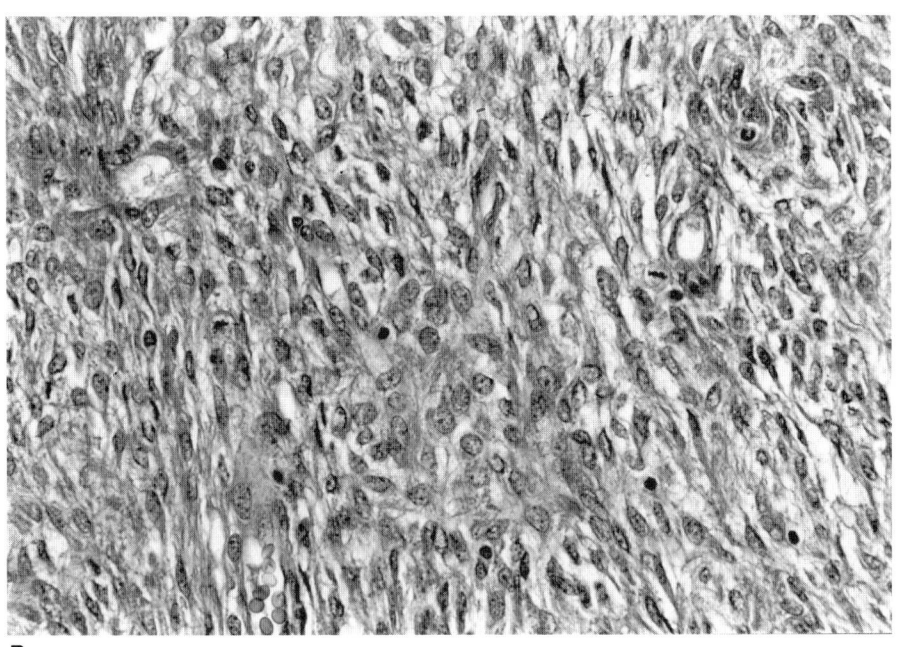

Figure 10-20. (A) Adenosarcoma. The sarcomatous element often condenses around the benign glands. (B) Higher-power view of the sarcomatous portion of the adenosarcoma shows a spindle cell tumor with mitotic activity.

deceptively benign. Although malignant, they are less aggressive in behavior than MMMTs, from which they must be distinguished.[38]

Malignant Mixed Müllerian Tumors

These aggressive tumors contain malignant epithelial and mesenchymal elements, and thus have been called "carcinosarcomas" by some. They occur as fleshy polypoid masses protruding into the endometrial cavity, and present most often with postmenopausal bleeding. The malignant carcinomatous element usually resembles endometrioid adenocarcinoma, although patterns such as UPSC, clear cell adenocarcinoma, squamous cell, and undifferentiated carcinomas do occur.[39] The sarcomatous portion of the tumor may be composed of a homologous tissue type, such as endometrial stromal sarcoma or leiomyosarcoma (Fig. 10-21), or may contain heterologous elements, such as rhabdomyosarcoma, osteosarcoma, or chondrosarcoma (Fig. 10-22). Frequently there are large undifferentiated areas, where it is unclear whether there is carcinomatous or sarcomatous differentiation. Unfortunately, in cases where the differential diagnosis is between MMMT and undifferentiated carcinoma, immunohistochemistry is often of limited help, because of the overlapping reactivities of the carcinomatous and sarcomatous areas. It is this overlapping of features, as well as the relative rarity of purely sarcomatous metastases, that has given rise to a newer theory of origin, metaplastic carcinoma, over the older stem cell theory.[40,41]

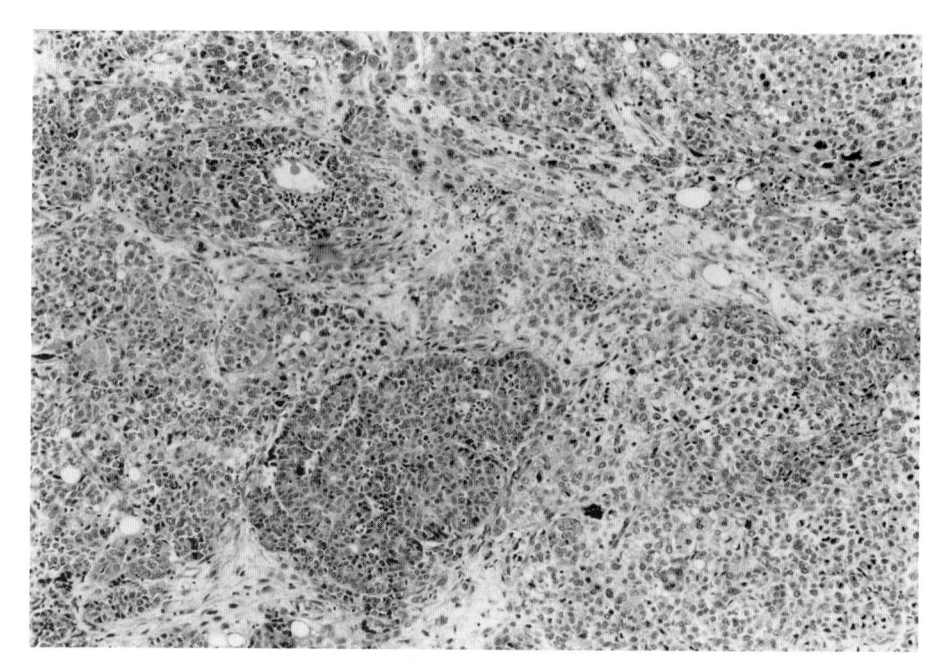

Figure 10-21. Homologous malignant mixed Müllerian tumor showing adenocarcinomatous areas in a nonspecific sarcomatous background.

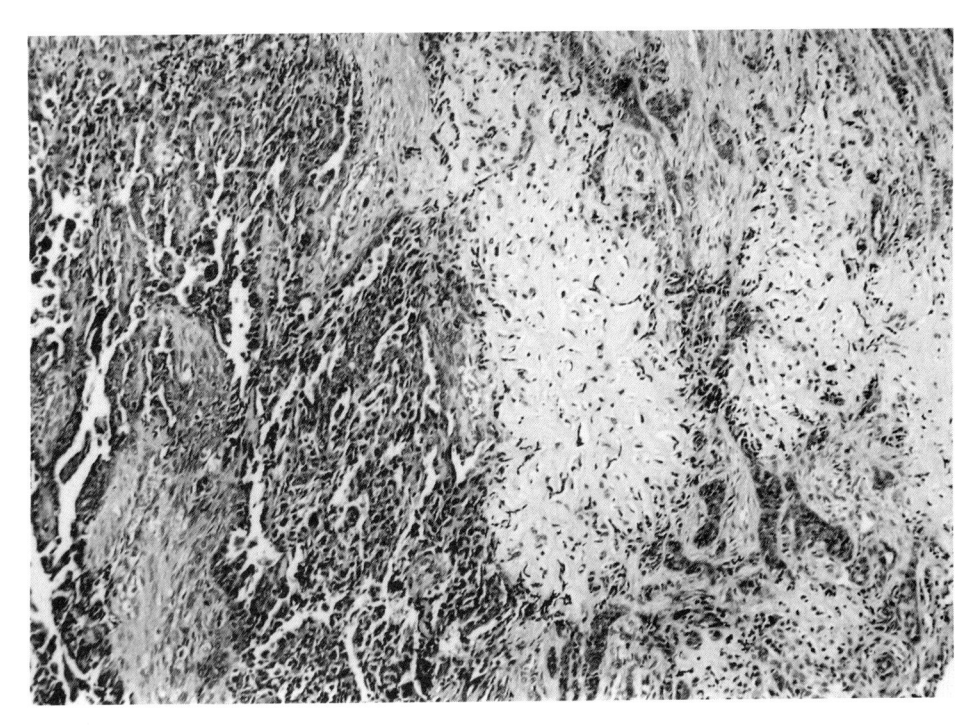

Figure 10-22. Heterologous malignant mixed Müllerian tumor showing chondroid differentiation.

REFERENCES

1. Kurman RJ (ed): *Blaustein's pathology of the female genital tract,* 3rd ed. Springer-Verlag, New York, 1987, pp 338–372.
2. Norris HJ, Tavassoli FA, Kurman RJ: Endometrial hyperplasia and carcinoma—diagnostic considerations. *Am J Surg Pathol* 7:839–847, 1983.
3. Kurman RJ, Norris HJ: Evaluation of criteria for distinguishing atypical endometrial hyperplasia from well-differentiated carcinoma. *Cancer* 49:2547–2559, 1982.
4. Silverberg SG: Hyperplasia and carcinoma of the endometrium. *Semin Diagn Pathol* 5:135–153, 1988.
5. Hendrickson MR, Ross JC, Kempson RL: Toward the development of morphologic criteria for well differentiated adenocarcinoma of the endometrium. *Am J Surg Pathol* 7:819–838, 1983.
6. Kurman RJ: The identification of stromal invasion in the distinction of atypical endometrial hyperplasia from well differentiated adenocarcinoma. *Verh Dtsch Ges Path* 75:371–372, 1991.
7. Creasman WT: New gynecologic cancer staging. *Obstet Gynecol* 75:287–288, 1990.
8. Hendrickson M, Ross J, Eifel P, et al: Uterine papillary serous carcinoma—a highly malignant form of endometrial adenocarcinoma. *Am J Surg Pathol* 6:93–108, 1982.
9. Bokhman JV: Two pathogenetic types of endometrial carcinoma. *Gynecol Oncol* 15:10–17, 1983.
10. Zaino RJ, Kurman R, Herbold D, et al: The significance of squamous differentia-

tion in endometrial carcinoma-data from a gynecologic oncology group study. *Cancer* 68:2293–2302, 1991.
11. Zaino RJ, Kurman RJ: Squamous differentiation in carcinoma of the endometrium: a critical appraisal of adenoacanthoma and adenosquamous carcinoma. *Semin Diagn Pathol* 5:154–171, 1988.
12. Christopherson WM, Alberhasky RC, Connelly PJ: Carcinoma of the endometrium: I—a clinicopathologic study of clear cell carcinoma and secretory carcinoma. *Cancer* 49:1511–1523, 1982.
13. Tobon H, Watkins GJ: Secretory adenocarcinoma of the endometrium. *Int J Gynecol Pathol* 4:328–335, 1985.
14. Buckley CH, Fox H: *Biopsy pathology of the endometrium*. Raven Press, New York, 1989, pp 166–194.
15. Hendrickson MR, Kempson RL: Ciliated carcinoma—a variant of endometrial adenocarcinoma: a report of 10 cases. *Int J Gynecol Pathol* 2:1–12, 1983.
16. Tiltman AJ: Mucinous carcinoma of the endometrium. *Obstet Gynecol* 55:244–247, 1980.
17. Kurman RJ, Scully RE: Clear cell carcinoma of the endometrium—an analysis of 21 cases. *Cancer* 37:872–882, 1976.
18. Sherman ME, Bitterman P, Rosenshein NB, et al: Uterine serous carcinoma. A morphologically diverse neoplasm with unifying clinicopathologic features. *Am J Surg Pathol* 16:600–610, 1992.
19. Simon A, Kopolovic J, Beyth Y: Primary squamous cell carcinoma of the endometrium. *Gynecol Oncol* 31:454–461, 1988.
20. Fluhmann C: Squamous epithelium in the endometrium in benign and malignant conditions. *Surg Gynecol Obstet* 46:309–316, 1928.
21. Kanbour A, Stock J: Squamous cell carcinoma in situ of the endometrium and fallopian tube as superficial extension of invasive cervical carcinoma. *Cancer* 42:570–580, 1978.
22. Perez C, Zivnuska F, Askin F, et al: Prognostic significance of endometrial extension from primary carcinoma of the uterine cervix. *Cancer* 35:1493–1504, 1975.
23. Kumar NB, Hart WR: Metastases to the uterine corpus from extragenital cancers—a clinicopathologic report of 63 cases. *Cancer* 50:2163–2169, 1982.
24. Ulbright TM, Roth LM: Metastatic and independent cancers of the endometrium and ovary. A clinicopathologic study of 34 cases. *Hum Pathol* 16:28–34, 1985.
25. Eifel P, Hendrickson M, Ross J, et al: Simultaneous presentation of carcinoma involving the ovary and the uterine corpus. *Cancer* 50:163–170, 1982.
26. Scully RE: Tumors of the ovaries and maldeveloped gonads. In *AFIP atlas of tumor pathology,* 2nd series, fascicle 16, Washington DC, 1979, pp 325–326.
27. Czernobilsky B, Katz Z, Lancet M, et al: Endocervical-type epithelium in endometrial carcinoma—a report of 10 cases with emphasis on histochemical methods for differential diagnosis. *Am J Surg Pathol* 4:481–489, 1980.
28. Wahlström T, Lindgren J, Korhonen M, et al: Distinction between endocervical and endometrial adenocarcinoma with immunoperoxidase staining of carcinoembryonic antigen in routine histological tissue specimens. *Lancet* 2:1159–1160, 1979.
29. Cohen C, Shulman G, Budgeon LR: Endocervical and endometrial adenocarcinoma—an immunoperoxidase and histochemical study. *Am J Surg Pathol* 6:151–157, 1982.
30. Hall JB, Young RH, Nelson JH: The prognostic significance of adenomyosis in endometrial carcinoma. *Gynecol Oncol* 17:32–40, 1984.
31. Silverberg SG, DeGiorgi LS: Histopathologic analysis of preoperative radiation therapy in endometrial carcinoma. *Am J Obstet Gynecol* 119:698–704, 1974.

References

32. Buckley CH, Fox H: *Biopsy pathology of the endometrium*. Raven Press, New York, 1989, pp 195–219.
33. Zaloudek C, Norris HJ: Mesenchymal tumors of the uterus. In Kurman R (ed): *Blaustein's pathology of the female genital tract,* 3rd ed. Springer-Verlag, New York, 1987, pp 373–408.
34. Fekete PS, Vellios F: The clinical and histologic spectrum of endometrial stromal neoplasms. A report of 41 cases. *Int J Gynecol Pathol* 3:198–212, 1984.
35. Chang KL, Crabtree GS, Lim-Tan SK, et al: Primary uterine endometrial stromal neoplasms—a clinicopathologic study of 117 cases. *Am J Surg Pathol* 14:415–438, 1990.
36. Hendrickson MR, Kempson RL: The uterine corpus. In Sternberg S (ed): *Diagnostic surgical pathology*. Raven Press, New York, 1989, pp 1591–1564.
37. Zaloudek CJ, Norris HJ: Adenofibroma and adenosarcoma of the uterus—a clinicopathologic study of 35 cases. *Cancer* 48:354–366, 1981.
38. Clement PB, Scully RE: Müllerian adenosarcoma of the uterus. A clinicopathologic analysis of ten cases of a distinctive type of Müllerian mixed tumor. *Cancer* 34:1138–1149, 1974.
39. Mixed epithelial and mesenchymal neoplasms: mixed Müllerian neoplasia. In Hendrickson MR, Kempson RL: *Surgical pathology of the uterine corpus*. Saunders, Philadelphia, 1980, pp 418–438.
40. Silverberg SG, Major FJ, Blessing JA, et al: Carcinosarcoma (malignant mixed mesodermal tumor) of the uterus—a gynecologic oncology group pathologic study of 203 cases. *Int J Gynecol Pathol* 9:1–19, 1990.
41. DeBrito PA, Silverberg SG, Orenstein JM: Carcinosarcoma (malignant mixed Müllerian [mesodermal] tumor) of the female genital tract: immunohistochemical and ultrastructural analysis of 28 cases. *Hum Pathol* 24:132–142, 1993.

11

Pregnancy and Related Conditions

Debra S. Heller, M.D.

A common organic cause of abnormal uterine bleeding in the reproductive age group is loss of a first-trimester pregnancy. Other pregnancy-related conditions can present with abnormal bleeding, and are often investigated and sometimes treated with endometrial curettage. In order to better recognize these entities, an understanding of the findings in normal gestation is necessary, and an overview follows.

NORMAL INTRAUTERINE PREGNANCY

Syncytiotrophoblasts and cytotrophoblasts have long been recognized histologically in specimens submitted as products of conception. Recently the presence of a third type of trophoblastic tissue, the intermediate trophoblast, has been described.[1] Cytotrophoblasts are small cells with distinct intercellular borders, and are hormonally inactive. They give rise to the intermediate and syncytiotrophoblasts. Syncytiotrophoblasts are multinucleated large cells with indistinct cell borders, and produce predominantly human chorionic gonadotropin (HCG). Intermediate trophoblastic cells have features between cyto- and syncytiotrophoblasts, with cells larger than cytotrophoblasts, with more distinct cell borders than syncytiotrophoblasts. Intermediate trophoblasts arising from chorionic villi have clear or amphophilic cytoplasm, and in general are mononuclear. At the implantation site they are more often multinucleated. Intermediate trophoblast produces predominantly human placental lactogen (HPL), and little HCG.[1]

Normal Intrauterine Pregnancy

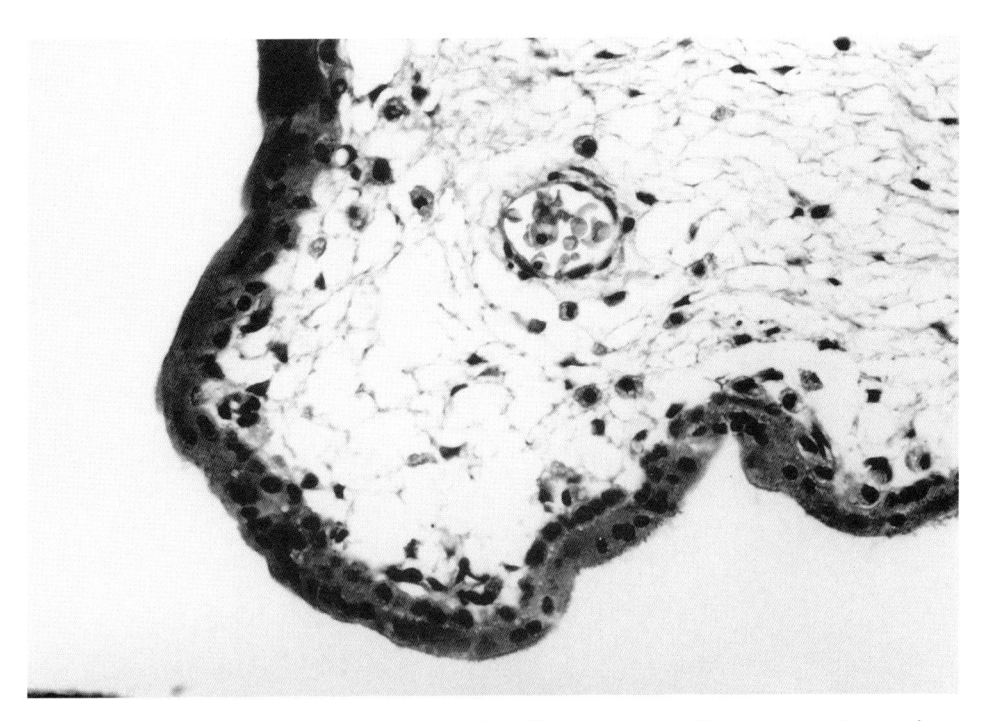

Figure 11-1. First-trimester chorionic villus showing the inner cytotrophoblast layer and the outer syncytiotrophoblast layer. Note the nucleated red blood cells in a fetal vessel.

During the first trimester, chorionic villi are covered by two layers, an inner cytotrophoblast, and an outer syncytiotrophoblast layer (Fig. 11-1). Anchoring villi show proliferation of trophoblast at one pole, where the spectrum of cyto-, intermediate, and syncytiotrophoblast may be seen (Fig. 11-2).[1] Intermediate trophoblasts are also seen at the implantation site infiltrating decidua and myometrium (Fig. 11-3), where they often become multinucleated, forming the placental-site giant cells. Prior to 6 weeks gestational age (dated from the last menstrual period), fetal vessels are not generally seen in the chorionic villi. By 8 weeks gestational age, abundant nucleated fetal red blood cells may be seen in fetal vessels, decreasing to about 10% of the red cell population in fetal vessels by about 10–12 weeks gestation[2] (Fig. 11-1). After 12 weeks, anucleate red blood cells are seen in fetal vessels. As pregnancy progresses, villous ramification increases, and the villi become smaller. Little cytotrophoblast is seen in the second trimester (Fig. 11-4), and by the third, only an attenuated layer of syncytiotrophoblast covers the chorionic villi. This attenuation leads to the juxtaposition of fetal vessels against the thinnest portion of the villous surface, forming the so-called "vasculosyncytial" membranes (Fig. 11-5), felt to be important for optimal exchange.

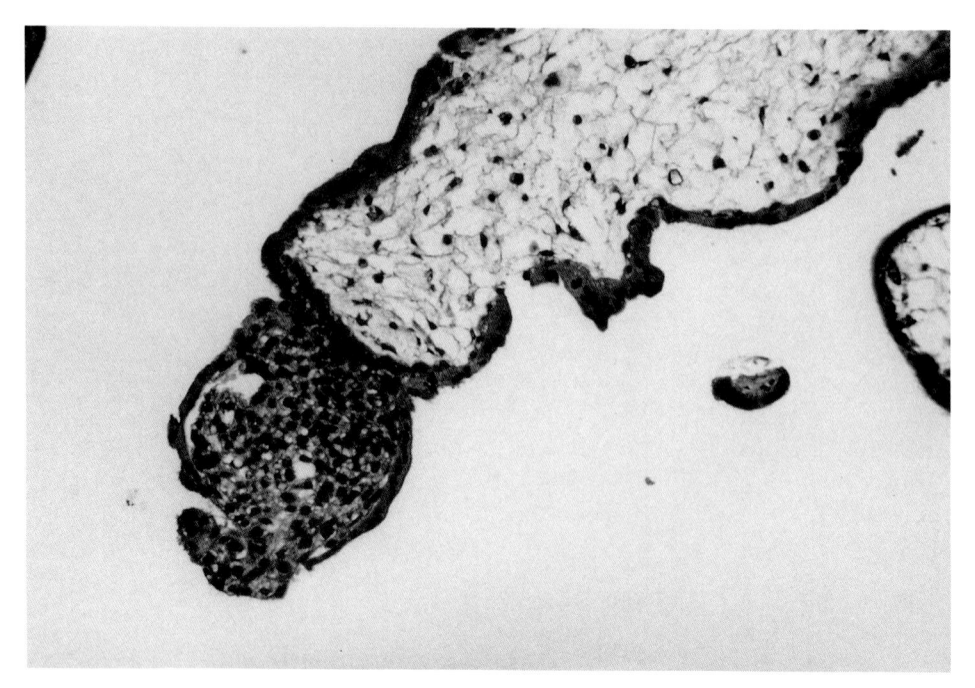

Figure 11-2. Anchoring first-trimester chorionic villus showing polar trophoblastic proliferation.

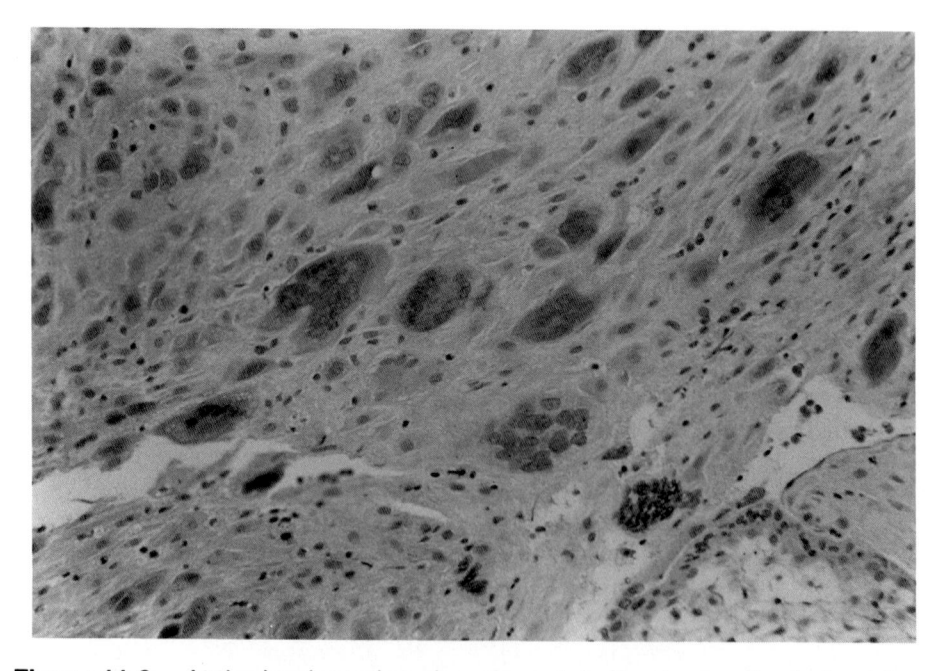

Figure 11-3. At the implantation site, placental-site giant cells, derived from intermediate trophoblast, are seen. A chorionic villus is present in the right lower corner. The presence of placental-site giant cells is diagnostic of a recent intrauterine gestation even in the absence of chorionic villi.

Normal Intrauterine Pregnancy

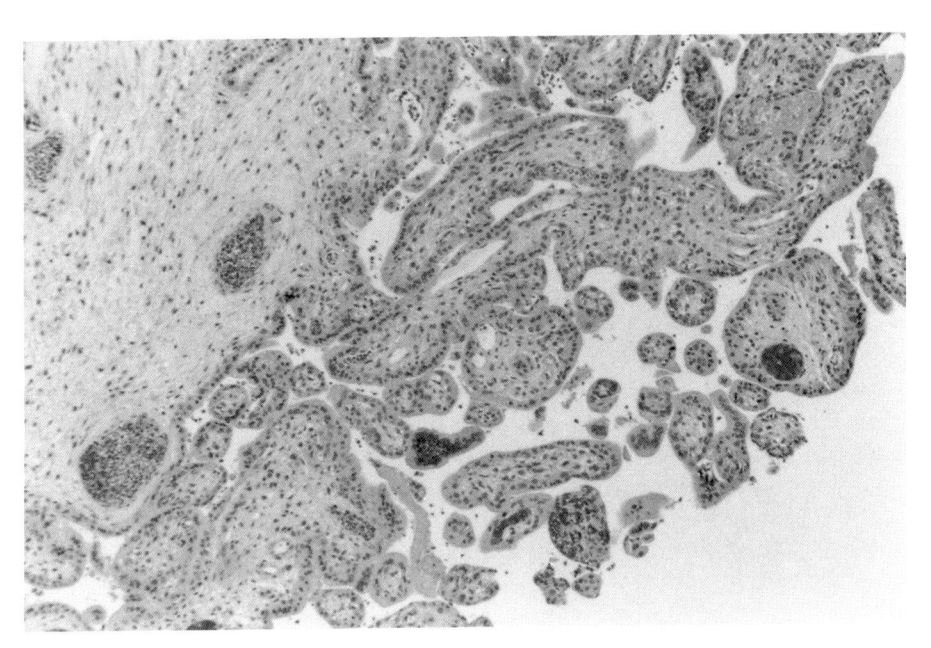

Figure 11-4. Second-trimester villi are smaller than in the first trimester, although larger than at term. The cytotrophoblast layer is less prominent, and is essentially gone by the third trimester.

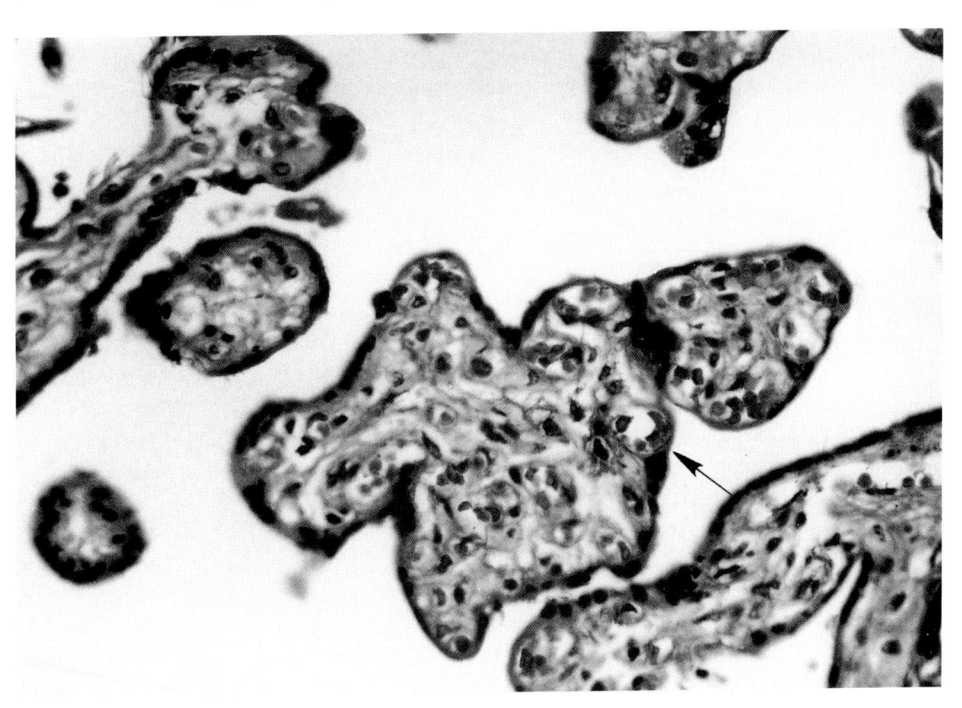

Figure 11-5. High-power view of third-trimester chorionic villi. Fetal vessels have proliferated, and abut the attenuated syncytiotrophoblast, forming the so-called vasculosyncytial membrane (arrow).

FIRST TRIMESTER PREGNANCY LOSS

Intrauterine first trimester pregnancy loss may be clinically divided into threatened, inevitable, incomplete, complete, and missed abortion, depending on the findings. Threatened abortion refers to bleeding, and inevitable abortion to cervical dilatation, usually with the products of conception at the cervical os. In threatened and inevitable abortions, the products of conception have not yet spontaneously passed. In incomplete and complete abortions, the products of conception have either partially or completely passed spontaneously. Missed abortion refers to the intrauterine death of the gestation, or a blighted ovum, without passage of tissue. In cases where the pregnancy cannot be maintained, therapeutic suction curettage is usually performed to remove tissue, and prevent hemorrhage and infection. Two major concerns may arise during pathologic evaluation of these pregnancy loss specimens. In cases of complete abortion, there are no chorionic villi present in curettings, and an ectopic pregnancy must always be considered. The other problem is that the degenerative changes seen in missed abortions must be distinguished from hydatidiform moles.

Specimens received by the pathology laboratory labeled "products of conception" may consist of tissue and/or blood clots passed per vagina or protruding from the cervical os, or may represent true intrauterine tissue. Gross recognition of fetal parts is always helpful, as is gross recognition of chorionic villi. Chorionic villi consist of fronds of tissue that float on water. Although this finding is useful in selecting suspected villous tissue for microscopic examination, the definitive diagnosis of chorionic villi rests on histologic confirmation.

If first-trimester villi are present, they may appear normal, fibrotic if there has been time for degeneration (Fig. 11-6), or hydropic (Fig. 11-7), particularly with a missed abortion. Hydropic avascular villi may raise the concern of molar disease, but the lack of trophoblast proliferation as well as lack of central cistern formation, both seen in molar disease, usually makes the distinction possible.

One of the most common specimens received by the gynecologic pathology laboratory is the curettage specimen from a young woman with a history of 6 weeks of amenorrhea, positive pregnancy test, and vaginal bleeding. The pathologist is often called on to distinguish between an incomplete or complete abortion, and a possible ectopic pregnancy. The absence of chorionic villi is not diagnostic of an ectopic pregnancy however, and the finding of placental-site giant cells, even without chorionic villi, confirms that an intrauterine gestation took place.[3] Except in the exceedingly rare instance of concomitant intrauterine and extrauterine gestations, the finding of placental-site giant cells in a curettage specimen effectively rules out an ectopic pregnancy. The implantation site is the most reliable evidence of an intrauterine gestation, because rarely, chorionic villi from a tubal or cornual pregnancy may be removed by suction curettage, and be observed to be loose among the curettings. While intrauterine pregnancy can be diagnosed by finding placental site giant cells, and in most cases chorionic villi, their ab-

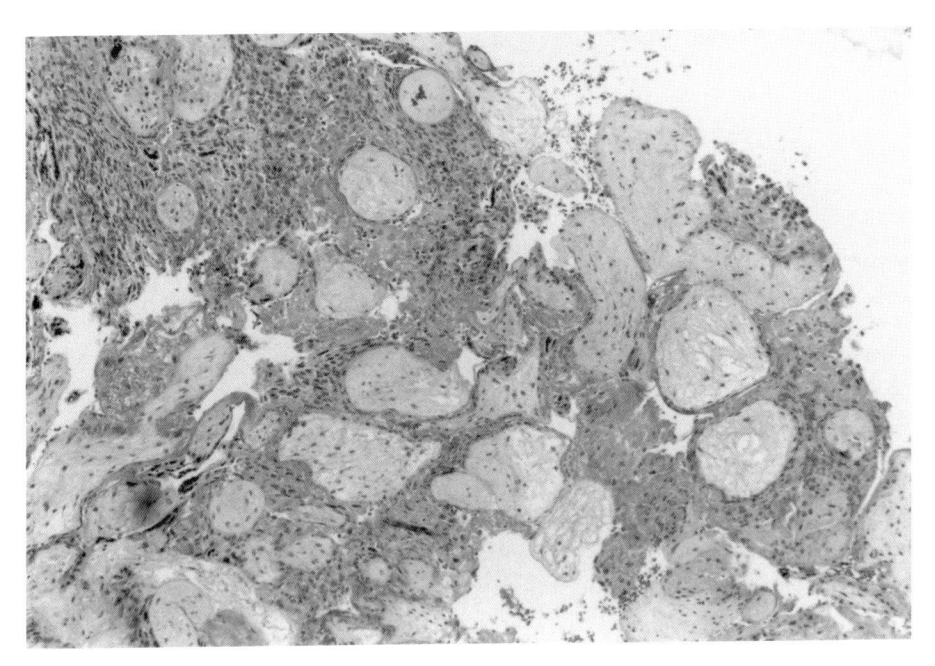

Figure 11-6. Fibrotic, nonviable chorionic villi.

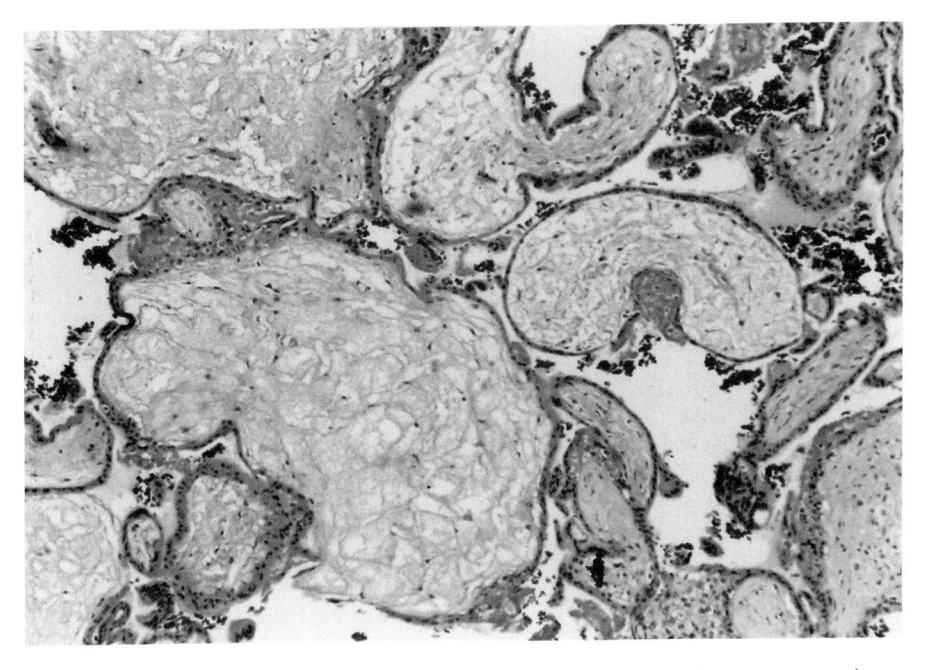

Figure 11-7. Missed (hydropic) abortion. The villi are edematous and avascular, but lack the trophoblastic proliferation seen with a hydatidiform mole.

sence does not confirm an ectopic pregnancy, and clinical evaluation is necessary. In this situation, in the absence of any chorionic derivatives, the clinician must be notified, and clinical evaluation by examination and serial HCG titers can be performed if concern exists.

EXAGGERATED IMPLANTATION SITE

As mentioned previously, intermediate trophoblast invades the decidua and myometrium at the site of implantation. At times this can be most exuberant, forming an exaggerated implantation site (Fig. 11-8). This was previously termed "syncytial endometritis," a misnomer, as it does not represent an inflammatory condition. Exaggerated implantation sites must be distinguished from gestational trophoblastic disease, particularly placental-site trophoblastic tumor (PSTT). This can be difficult on curettage. Focality of the lesion, rare or absent mitoses, hyalinization, and the presence of decidua and chorionic villi favor an exaggerated placental site.[4] Although not neoplastic in and of themselves, exaggerated placental sites are often seen in association with hydatidiform moles.[4]

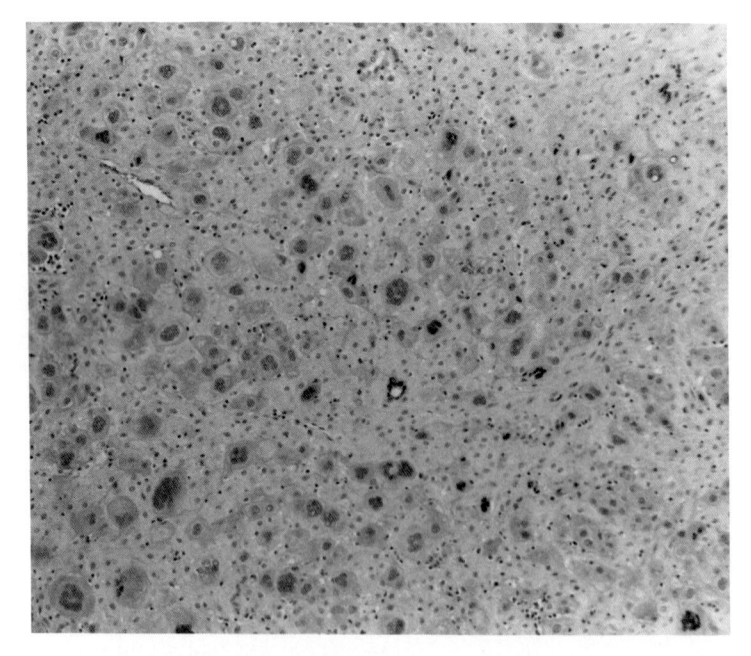

Figure 11-8. Exaggerated placental site. Intermediate trophoblast can be prominent at the implantation site, and this should not be mistaken for a placental-site trophoblastic tumor.

PLACENTAL-SITE NODULES AND PLAQUES

Endometrial or superficial myometrial nodules or plaques consisting of intermediate trophoblast surrounded by extensive hyalinization may on occasion be detected on curettage for abnormal bleeding. These lesions may also be incidental findings[4,5] (Fig. 11-9A,B). Placental-site nodules and plaques appear to be incompletely absorbed placental sites, and may be detected many years from a known pregnancy.[4] Unlike PSTT, with which they may be confused, placental-site plaques and nodules are discrete focal lesions, with abundant hyalinization, and unlike PSTT, there is usually no thought of the patient being pregnant at the time of diagnosis.[4]

THE ENDOMETRIUM IN ECTOPIC PREGNANCY

The endometrium in extrauterine gestations can have a variety of appearances. Most commonly, with continued viability of the gestation and continued HCG production, the endometrium is hypersecretory, and is seen intermingling with sheets of decidua, where the stromal elements predominate. This is much as is seen with an intrauterine pregnancy (Fig. 11-10), without the chorionic derivatives. The Arias–Stella reaction, characterized by clear or hobnail cells showing nuclear atypia without mitotic activity in hypersecretory glands (Fig. 11-11), may be seen in some ectopic pregnancies, but can occur in intrauterine gestations as well, and is not diagnostic of an ectopic pregnancy. If the ectopic gestation has died, the endometrium may slough, and the breakdown of the hypersecretory endometrium is similar in histologic appearance to the endometrium seen after a complete abortion. If the decidua has been shed, proliferative endometrial changes may be seen.

SECOND- AND THIRD-TRIMESTER BLEEDING

Bleeding later in pregnancy may be due to placental abnormalities such as placental abruption or placenta previa. These topics are discussed in standard obstetric texts.

POSTPARTUM HEMORRHAGE

Curettage is often performed after postpartum hemorrhage. The differential diagnosis includes subinvolution of the uterus, retained placenta, and placenta accreta.

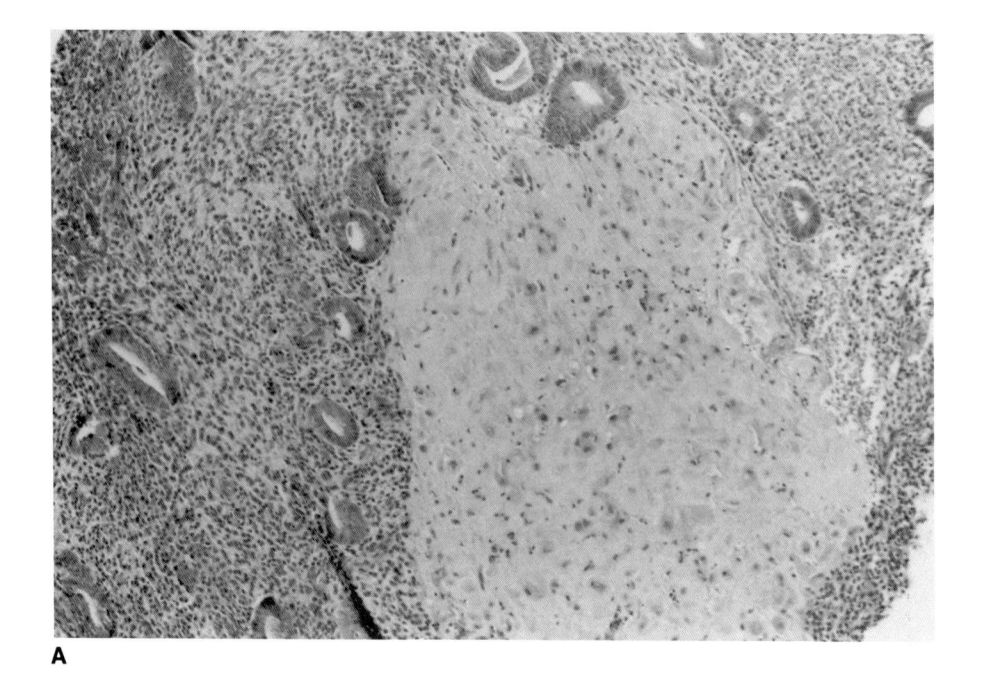

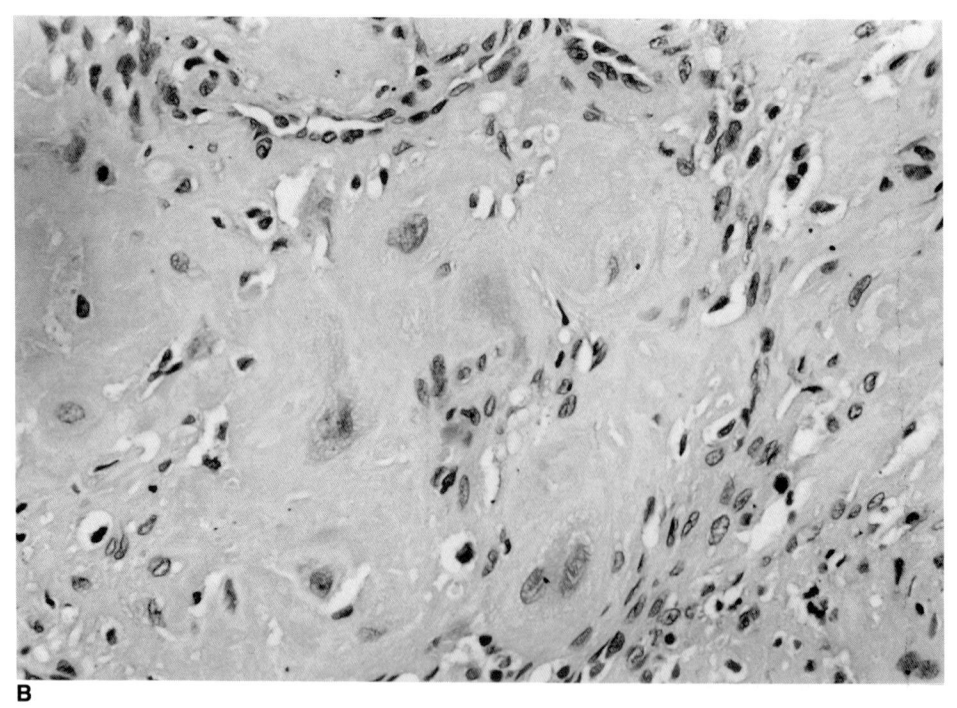

Figure 11-9. (A) Placental-site nodule in curettings. (B) Placental-site nodule contains intermediate trophoblast in a markedly hyalinized background.

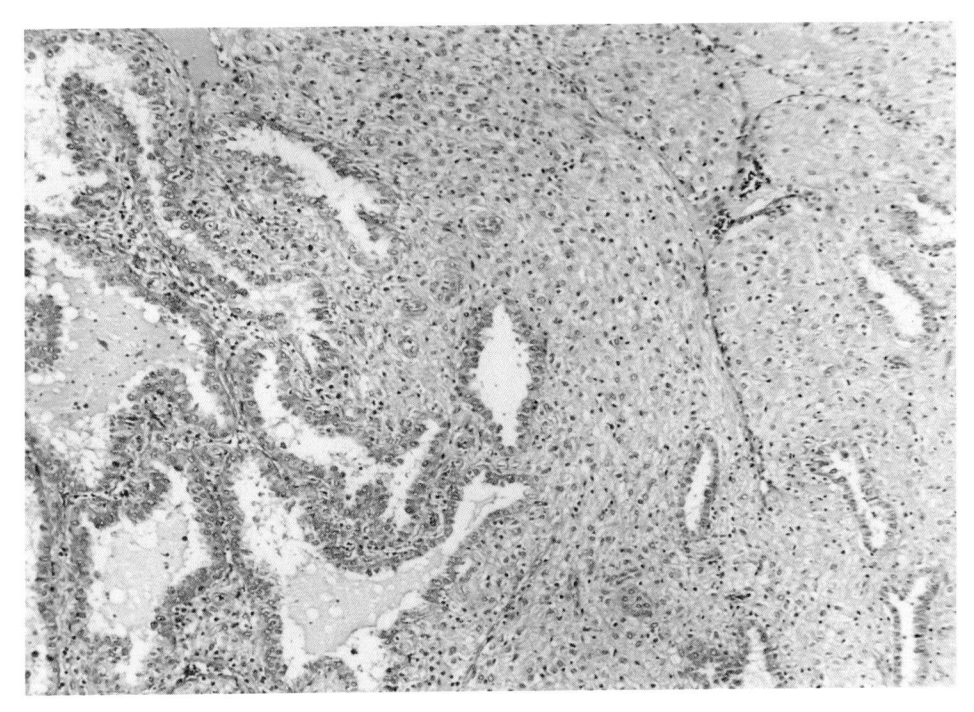

Figure 11-10. Curettings from an ectopic pregnancy may show sheets of decidua and hypersecretory endometrium.

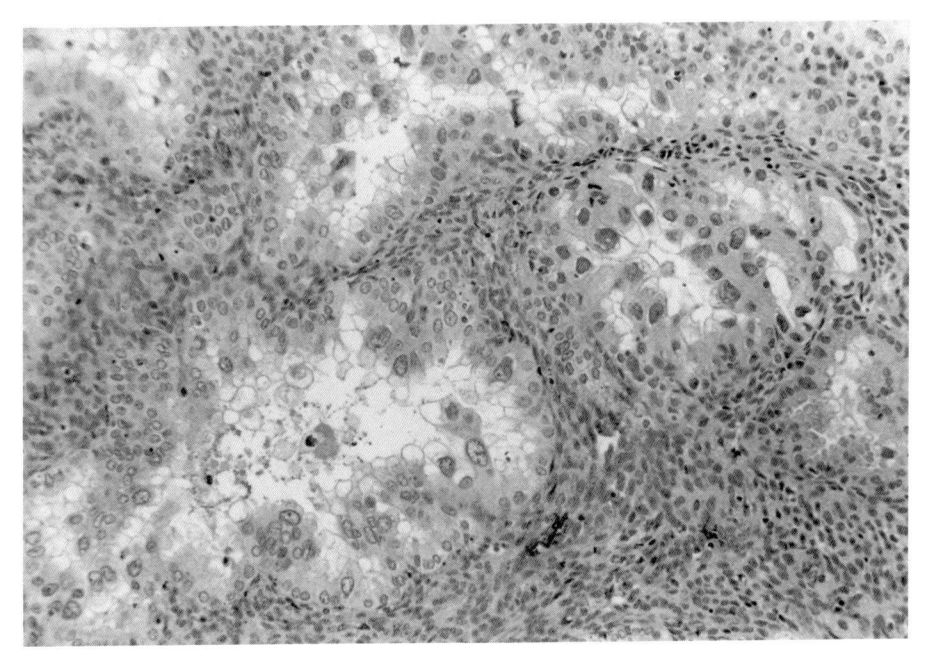

Figure 11-11. Arias–Stella reaction showing hypersecretory glands with nuclear atypia.

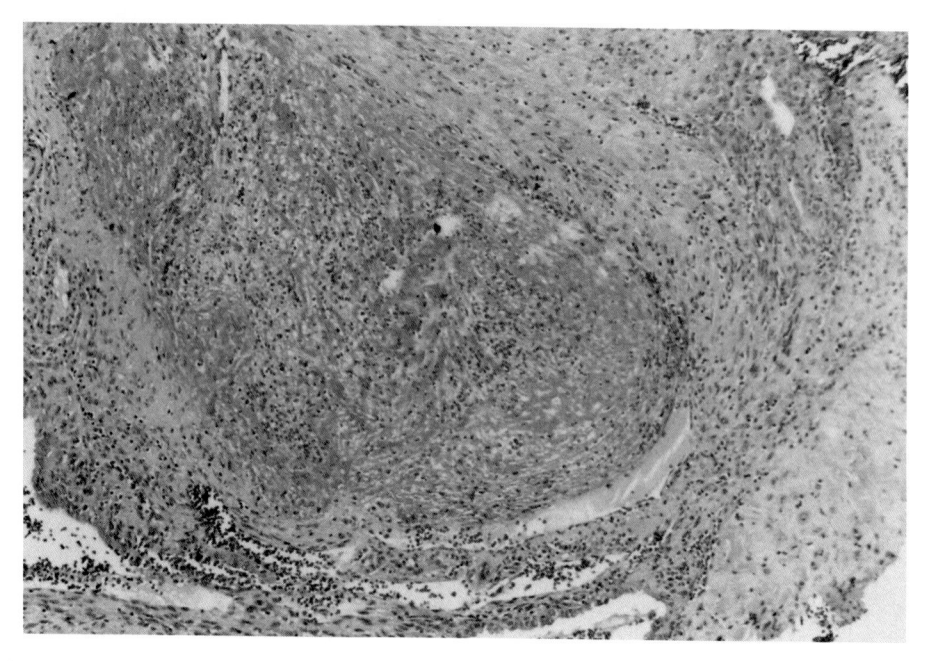

Figure 11-12. In subinvolution, distended thrombosed vessels are seen in the decidua.

Subinvolution of the Uterus

Normally the decidual vessels of the placental bed involute by spasm and thrombosis. In subinvolution, partially hyalinized decidual vessels are distended and incompletely occluded by fresh and old thrombi (Fig. 11-12).

Retained Placenta

Retained third-trimester placenta may be hyalinized or necrotic, depending on the time from delivery (Fig. 11-13).

Placenta Accreta

In the absence of the usually intervening decidua basalis, the placenta becomes abnormally adherent to the myometrium. When the placenta adheres directly to the myometrial surface, the condition is termed *placenta accreta* (Fig. 11-14). Nitabuch's fibrinoid layer is present and may be defective. When the chorionic villi invade the myometrium, this is termed *placenta increta,* and if the villi penetrate the entire uterine wall, *placenta percreta* is the diagnosis.

The diagnosis of placenta accreta on histology is challenging, even in hysterectomy specimens, due to the normally irregular interface between villi, decidua, and myometrium, as well as because of the abundant hyaliniza-

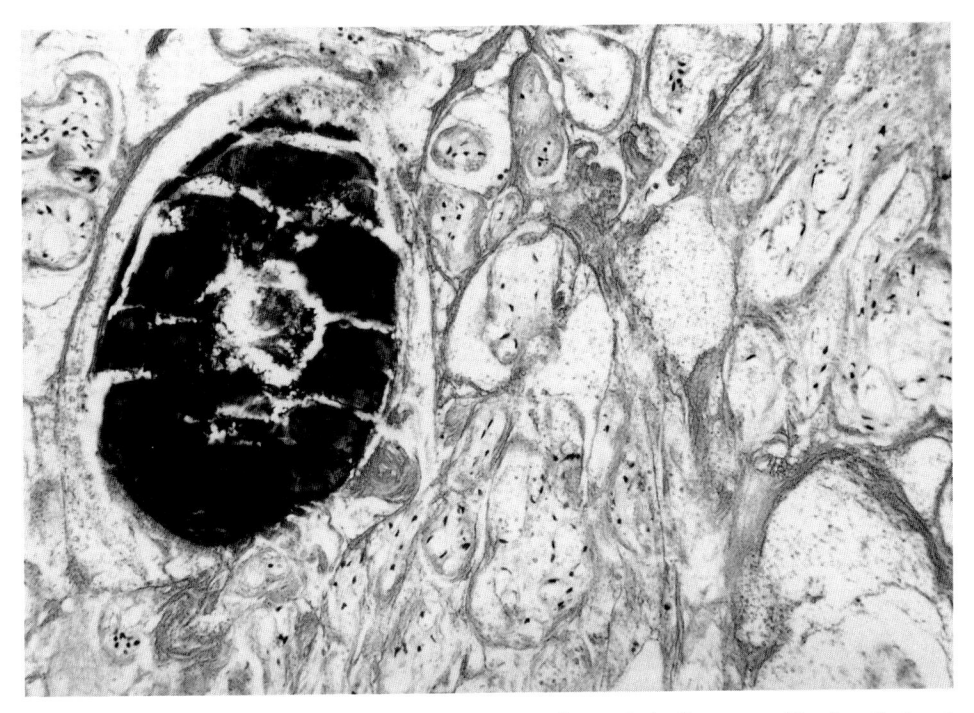

Figure 11-13. Retained third-trimester placental tissue with hyalinized "ghost" villi and calcification.

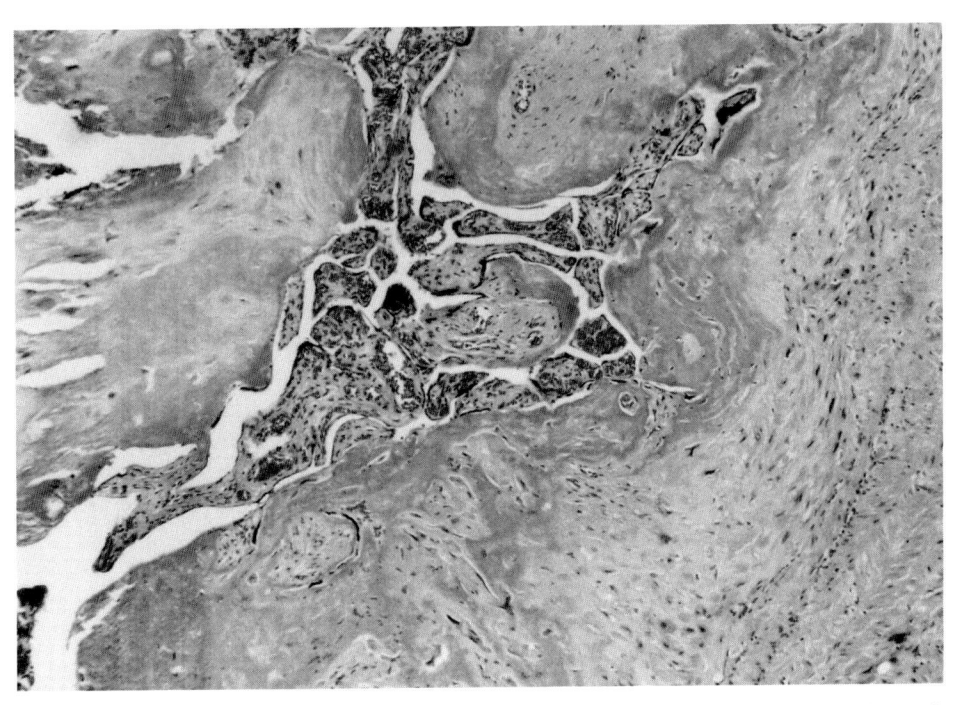

Figure 11-14. Placenta accreta showing chorionic villi directly implanted on the myometrium. A layer of fibrinoid (Nitabuch's layer) is present, but no decidua intervenes between the villi and myometrium.

tion that occurs in this region at term. Attempts at removal of the placenta prior to hysterectomy make the surface more irregular and difficult to interpret histologically. In curettings, placenta accreta can only be diagnosed if myometrial tissue with the abnormally implanted placental tissue is present in the specimen.

GESTATIONAL TROPHOBLASTIC DISEASE

Gestational trophoblastic disease is divided by the World Health Organization (WHO) into hydatidiform mole, complete or partial; invasive mole; choriocarcinoma; placental site trophoblastic tumor; miscellaneous trophoblastic lesions, including exaggerated placental sites, placental nodules and plaques; and unclassified trophoblastic lesions.[4] Exaggerated placental sites and placental nodules and plaques do not have metastatic potential and are frequently incidental findings. In many cases of persistently elevated HCG titers after evacuation of a molar pregnancy, subsequent histologic diagnosis is not obtained, and if recurettage is performed, it is often difficult to interpret. Management in many of these cases is based on the clinical parameters of what is classified simply as gestational trophoblastic disease.

Complete Hydatidiform Mole

The majority of complete hydatidiform moles are 46*xx*, although 46*xy*, triploid, and tetraploid moles do occur. All genetic material is of paternal origin.[4] Clinically, complete moles most often present in the second trimester. Uterine size is often greater than that of gestational age, there may be bleeding, passage of "grapes" (markedly hydropic villi), and possibly hyperemesis, pregnancy-induced hypertension, or even rarely, hyperthyroidism. Serum HCG titers are usually markedly elevated, and ultrasound examination of the uterus typically shows a "snowstorm" pattern, with no evidence of a fetus.

Histologically, in complete hydatidiform moles, there is generally no evidence of fetal tissue. All the chorionic villi are involved, and are markedly edematous, often with central cistern formation. Fetal vessels are absent, or only vestiges remain. Trophoblast proliferation of all three cell types occurs, and is circumferential or multifocal around villi, rather than polar as in a normal gestation (Fig. 11-15A,B). Approximately 10–30% of complete hydatidiform moles progress to persistent trophoblastic disease.[4]

Partial Hydatidiform Mole

Usually triploid, the majority of partial hydatidiform moles are 69*xxy*, with the occasional 69*xxx* or 69*xyy*.[4] Clinically, partial moles often present as second-trimester missed abortions. The uterus may be smaller than expected for gestational age, and HCG titers are seldom as elevated as in complete

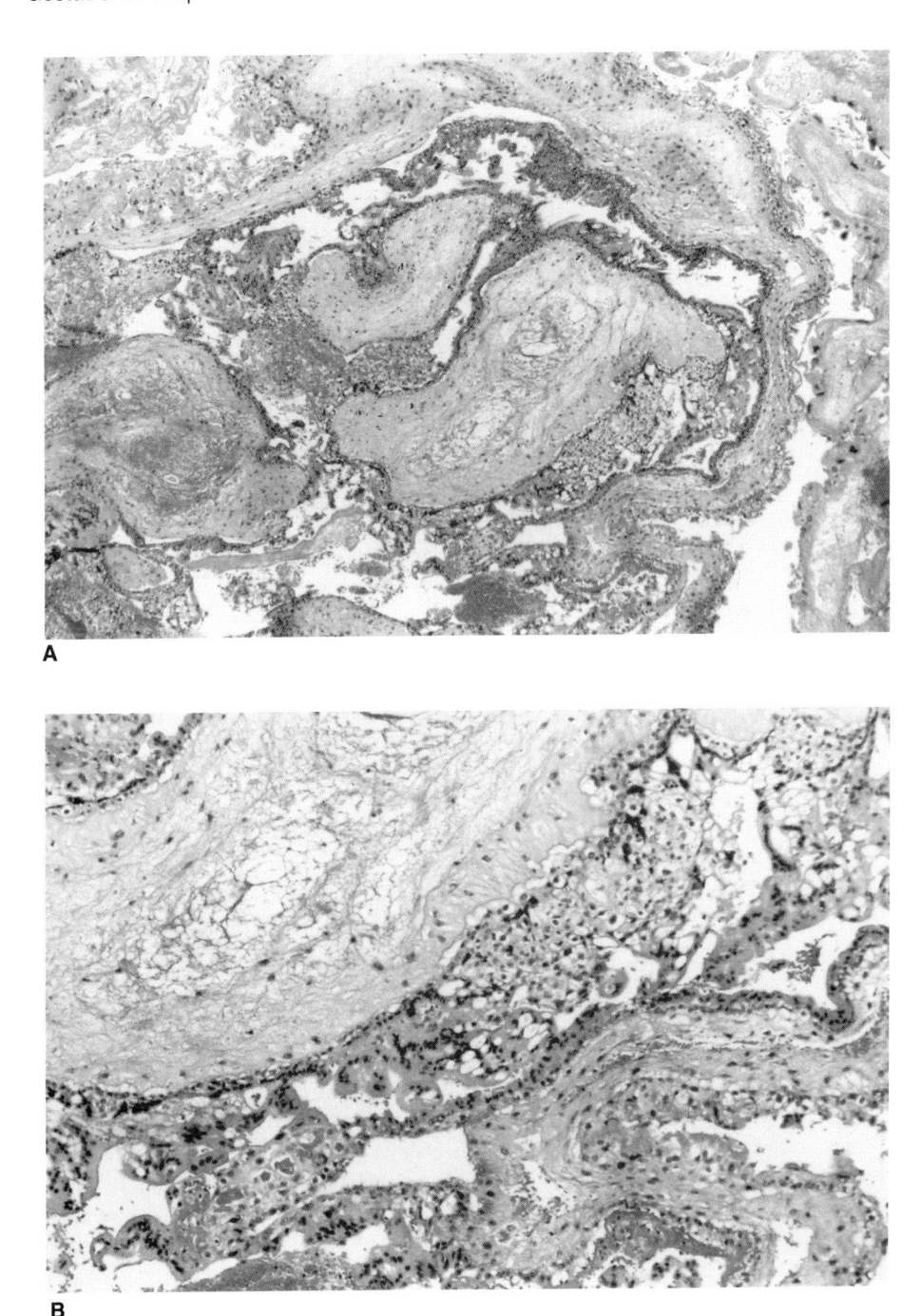

Figure 11-15. (A,B) Complete hydatidiform mole showing hydropic avascular chorionic villi with trophoblast proliferation.

moles. A fetus is usually present at some point, and when identified grossly is often malformed.

Histologically, partial moles are composed of a mixture of normal-sized chorionic villi admixed with larger hydropic ones (Fig. 11-16A). Fetal tissue or evidence of a fetus such as nucleated red blood cells in fetal vessels must be searched for. In general, villi are less edematous in a partial mole than in a complete mole, with less cistern formation. Trophoblastic proliferation is not as exuberant, and the villous outline is frequently "scalloped." Trophoblastic inclusions are often seen (Fig. 11-16B). Fibrotic villi are common. Proliferating intermediate trophoblast is uncommon.[4] Most persistent gestational trophoblastic disease (GTD) after a partial mole is confined to the uterus, with choriocarcinoma exceedingly rare,[4] and the development of persistent GTD is less than in a complete mole, with only a 4–11% risk.[4] Although it is preferable to separate complete from partial moles for prognostic purposes, clinical follow-up is the same. More important clinically is the separation of a hydropic abortion from a partial hydatidiform mole. Diagnosis of a partial hydatidiform mole is often an area of diagnostic difficulty for the pathologist.[6] When the diagnosis could not be made on morphologic grounds, flow cytometry has been utilized by some to demonstrate polyploidy in partial moles.[7]

Invasive Mole

Molar villi invade the myometrium in this condition. This is a difficult diagnosis to make on curettage, requiring the presence of myometrial tissue invaded by molar villi.

Choriocarcinoma

Fifty percent of gestational choriocarcinoma arises after a complete hydatidiform mole (4), the rest occuring after a normal term pregnancy, spontaneous abortion, or ectopic gestation. The tumor is very hemorrhagic and necrotic, and biopsy specimens may contain necrotic material only. The tumor is generally biphasic, consisting of cytotrophoblast or intermediate trophoblast, with syncytiotrophoblast (Fig. 11-17). Choriocarcinoma contains no chorionic villi (except in the extremely rare case arising in a normal placenta). Biopsy diagnosis is difficult, because in the absence of demonstrable myometrial invasion, one can only diagnose suspicious nonvillous trophoblast. If the finding of proliferating trophoblastic tissue, whether villous or nonvillous, occurs after evacuation of a known molar pregnancy, the diagnosis of persistent GTD is confirmed. After a normal pregnancy, villous trophoblast in a curettage represents retained products of conception, but the finding of proliferating nonvillous trophoblast, particularly if excessive and/or atypical, is highly suspicious of choriocarcinoma.

Gestational Trophoblastic Disease

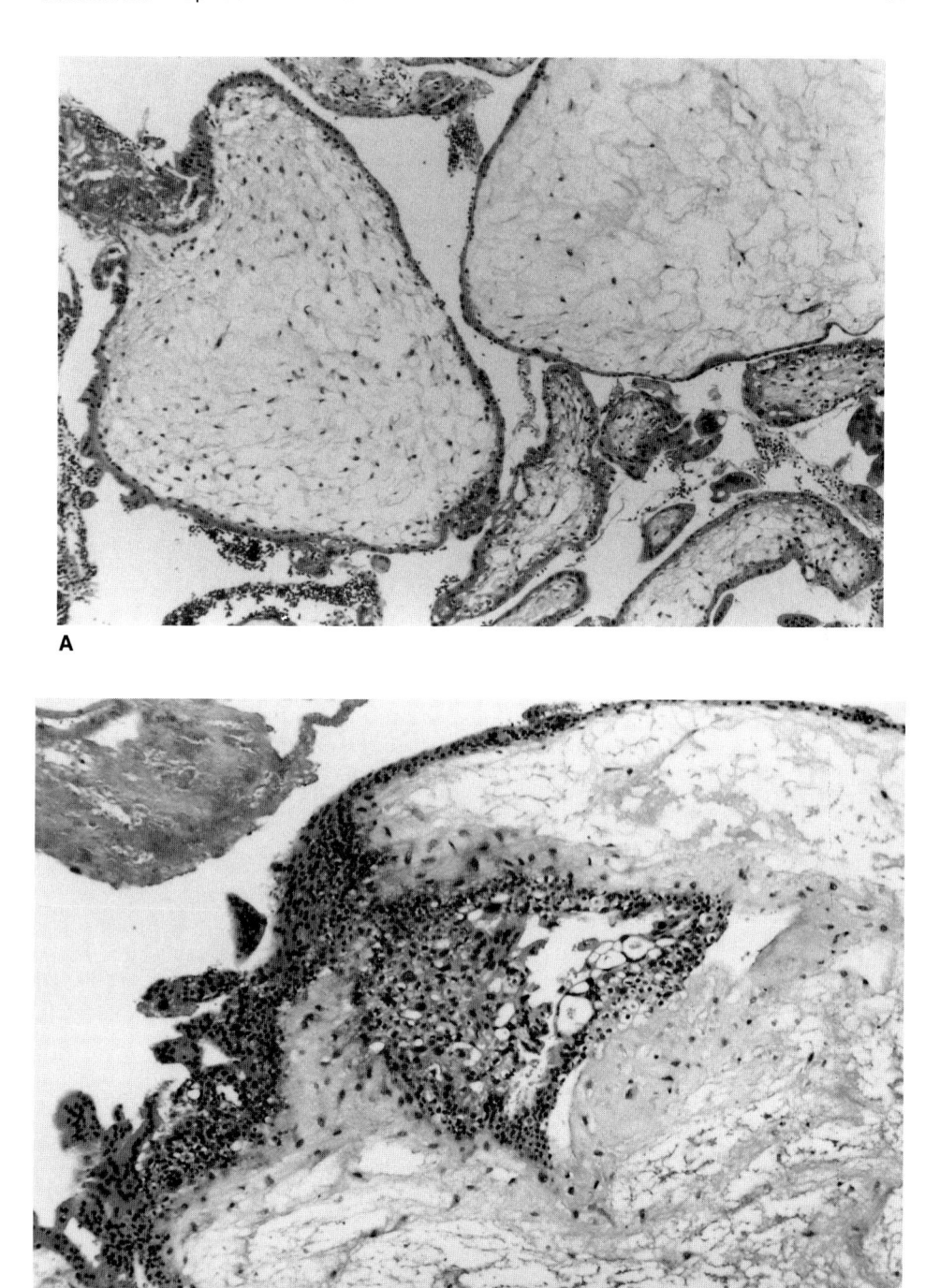

Figure 11-16. (A) Partial hydatidiform mole showing a mixture of normal-sized and hydropic villi. (B) Partial mole showing trophoblastic inclusion.

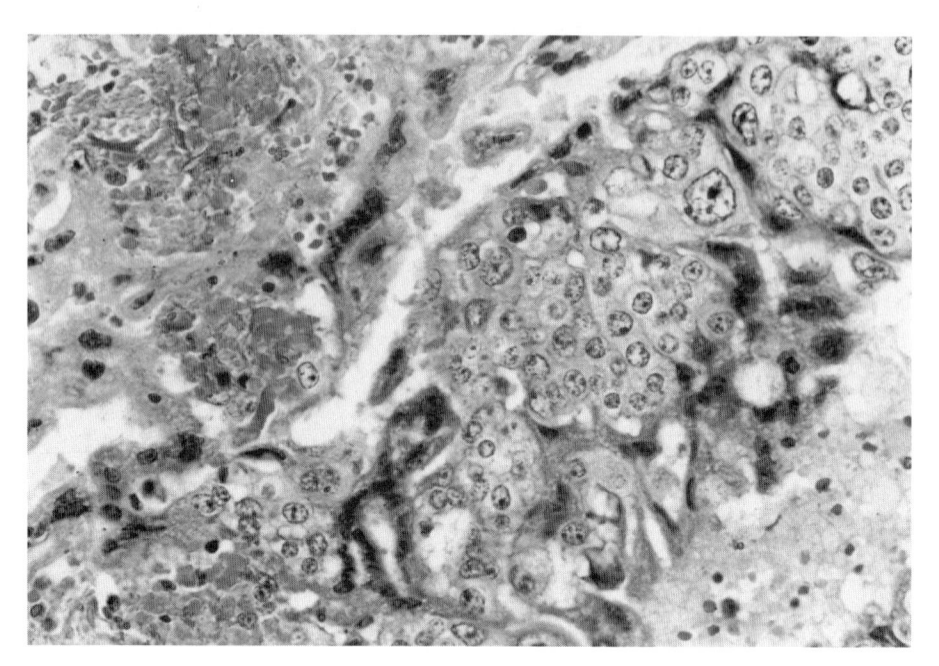

Figure 11-17. Choriocarcinoma showing biphasic cell proliferation and hemorrhage. No chorionic villi are present.

Placental-Site Trophoblastic Tumor

An uncommon tumor, most placental-site trophoblastic tumors (PSTT), occur in the reproductive age group, and the majority present with amenorrhea or menorrhagia.[8] While most of these tumors are associated with some form of pregnancy, the type of gestation (hydatidiform mole, term pregnancy, spontaneous abortion), as well as the time elapsed from the pregnancy, can vary considerably. The uterus may grow for a time then stop, with HCG titers elevated but not substantially so, suggesting a missed abortion.[4] Histologically, the tumor is composed predominantly of intermediate trophoblasts, which infiltrate between bundles of myometrium (Fig. 11-18A,B). Staining for HPL is strong, while HCG staining is weaker. Most behave in a benign fashion, although approximately 10–15% of reported cases have been malignant.[4] Curettage of the tumor or the presence of the tumor itself may lead to uterine perforation, and although curettage is occasionally therapeutic, to date hysterectomy has been the treatment of choice in most cases.[8] PSTT must be distinguished from exaggerated placental site, and from choriocarcinoma. The second distinction can be made histologically from the different immunohistochemical staining patterns, with strong HPL in PSTT, and strong HCG in choriocarcinoma, as well as by the monophasic nature of PSTT as opposed to the biphasic choriocarcinoma. Exaggerated placental sites are discrete lesions with hyalinization and general lack of mitotic activity, and are more likely to occur temporally closer to a known gestation.

Gestational Trophoblastic Disease

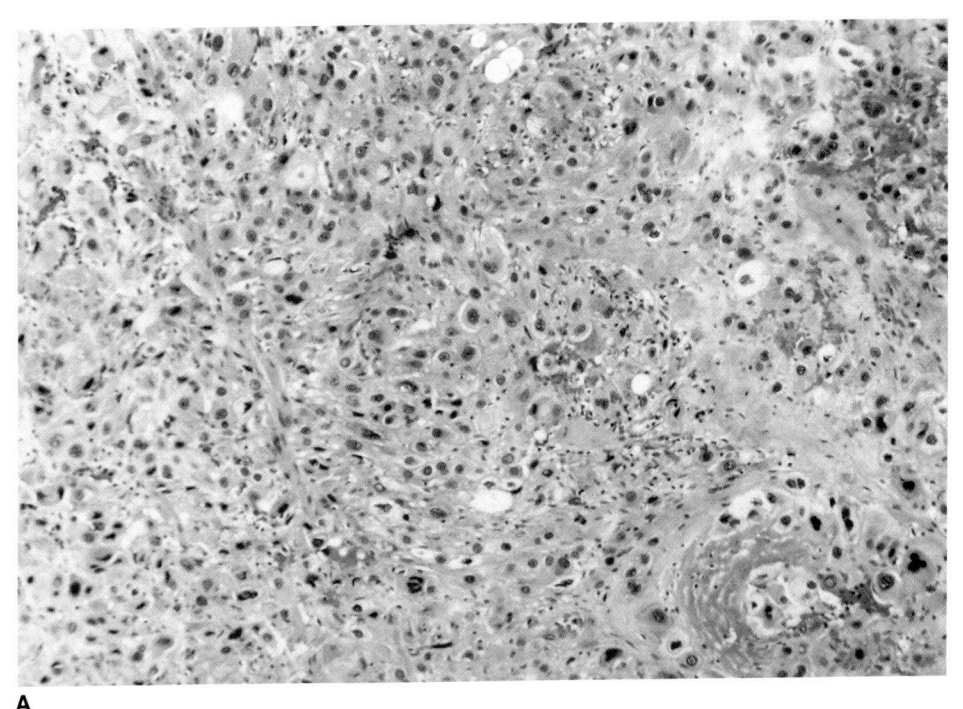

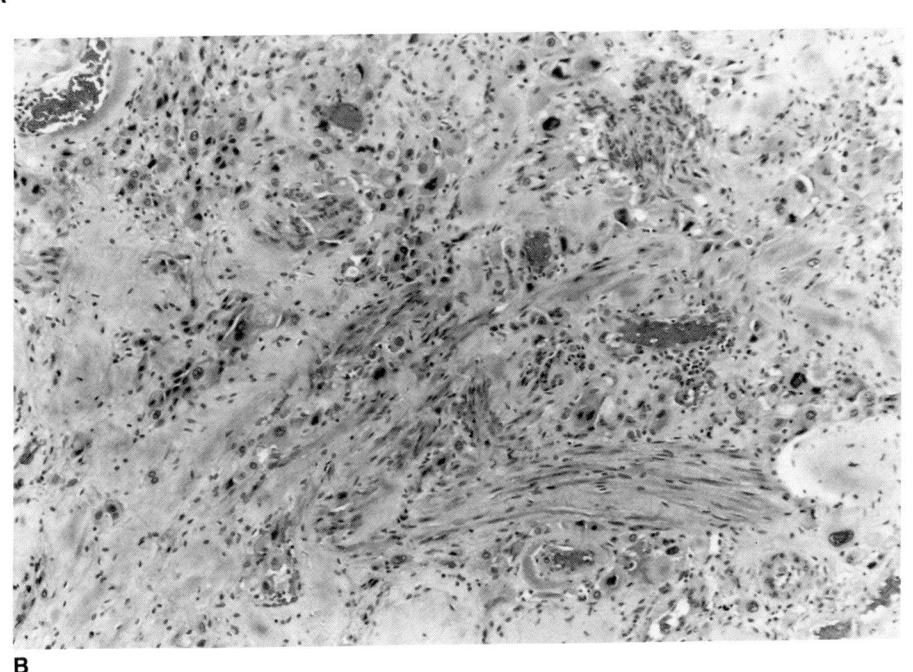

Figure 11-18. (A) Placental-site trophoblastic tumor is composed predominantly of intermediate trophoblast. (B) Placental-site trophoblastic tumor tends to dissect between smooth muscle bundles in the myometrium.

If chorionic villi and decidua are present, an exaggerated placental site is favored.[4]

THE ROLE OF IMMUNOHISTOCHEMISTRY IN PREGNANCY-RELATED CONDITIONS

Immunocytochemical studies utilizing antibodies to human chorionic gonadotropin (HCG) and human placental lactogen (HPL) have been helpful in characterizing the histogenesis of both normal and neoplastic trophoblastic tissue.[9] The patterns of distribution of staining for HCG, HPL, and placental alkaline phosphatase have been found to differ in complete and partial hydatidiform moles.[8] While immunohistochemistry is not necessary in most cases, these staining patterns may be of some use in the differential diagnosis of pregnancy-related lesions.

REFERENCES

1. Kurman RJ: The morphology, biology, and pathology of intermediate trophoblast: a look to the present. *Hum Pathol* 22:847–855, 1991.
2. Sternberg SS (ed): *Histology for pathologists.* Raven Press, New York, 1992, pp 835–863.
3. O'Connor DM, Kurman RJ: Intermediate trophoblast in uterine curettings in the diagnosis of ectopic pregnancy. *Obstet Gynecol* 72:665–670, 1988.
4. Silverberg SG, Kurman RJ: Tumors of the uterine corpus and gestational trophoblastic disease. In *Atlas of tumor pathology,* 3rd series, Fascicle 3. AFIP, Washington, DC, 1992.
5. Young RH, Kurman RJ, Scully RE: Placental site nodules and plaques. A clinicopathologic analysis of 20 cases. *Am J Surg Pathol* 14:1001–1009, 1990.
6. Messereli ML, Parmley T, Woodruff JD, et al: Inter- and intra-pathologist variability in the diagnosis of gestational trophoblastic neoplasia. *Obstet Gynecol* 69:622–626, 1987.
7. Van Oven MW, Schouts JF, Oosterhuis JW, et al: The use of DNA flow cytometry in the diagnosis of triploidy in human abortions. *Hum Pathol* 20:238–242, 1989.
8. Young RH, Scully RE: Placental-site trophoblastic tumor—current status. *Clin Obstet Gynecol* 27:248–258, 1984.
9. Kurman RJ, Young RH, Norris HJ, et al: Immunocytochemical localization of placental lactogen and chorionic gonadotropin in the normal placenta and trophoblastic tumors, with emphasis on intermediate trophoblast and the placental site trophoblastic tumor. *Int J Gynecol Pathol* 3:101–121, 1984.
10. Brescia RJ, Kurman RJ, Main CS, et al: Immunocytochemical localization of chorionic gonadotropin, placental lactogen, and placental alkaline phosphatase in the diagnosis of complete and partial hydatidiform moles. *Int J Gynecol Pathol* 6:213–229, 1987.

12

Endometrial Cytology on Cervicovaginal Smears

Ruth Kreitzer, M.D.

The conventional Pap (Papanicolaou) smear is a widely accepted screening modality for cervical carcinoma and its precursors. Its usefulness in the detection of endometrial carcinoma has been largely disputed. Using the cervical Pap smear, the diagnostic accuracy rate for endometrial carcinoma is 25–60%,[1-4] and the false-negative rate averages 50–80%.[5] Detecting endometrial carcinoma by this method is almost fortuitous. In fact, one is more likely to discover endometrial cells in a vaginal pool specimen than a cervical smear.[6] Even when these cells are present, they are often difficult to interpret because of marked degeneration and obscuring fresh blood.

Efforts to improve on these disappointing data resulted in a number of studies designed to evaluate the various endometrial sampling devices (EndoPap sampler, Isaacs sampler, Mi-Mark sampler, sponges, brushes, cannulas, etc.). The ideal device should be inexpensive, easy to use, cause minimal discomfort, have few complications, and yield adequate diagnostic material that can easily be interpreted.[4,7-9] Many of the sampling devices showed high sensitivities and specificities for detecting endometrial carcinoma in both the asymptomatic and symptomatic population.[2,6-10] Some reported marked patient discomfort; however, the most limiting factor was the difficulty in diagnosing endometrial hyperplasia.[2,6-9,11,12] To help overcome this

---

The author thanks everyone at Kyto Diagnostics for their help in collecting the case material, especially to Saru Naini, Maria Susco, Kris Johnson, and Beth Phillips, and also Dr. Ellen Greenebaum for her contributions.

drawback, Meisels et al addressed this issue in a study of 1465 women using the Endopap sampler. They determined that the following five criteria were "useful" in diagnosing endometrial hyperplasia: cellular overlap, nucleoli, anisokaryosis, granular chromatin, and sheets of stromal cells. Their diagnostic accuracy rate depended on how many of these criteria were present together.[11] The adoption of general screening for endometrial carcinoma using these methods is unlikely, but it may have a promising role in evaluating patients over 45 and in the high-risk population (e.g., unopposed estrogen use, obesity, infertility, diabetes, abnormal uterine bleeding, hypertension, late menopause, failure to ovulate, tamoxifen administration).[1,4,5,10,13]

BENIGN ENDOMETRIAL CELLS ON PAP SMEARS AND THEIR SIGNIFICANCE

In premenopausal women there is a normal physiologic disintegration of the endometrial lining on day 28, and a subsequent exfoliation of endometrial cells up through and including day 12 of the menstrual cycle. A Pap smear taken at this time may show benign endometrial glandular cells, benign endometrial stromal cells, and/or both in a background of blood, inflammatory cells, and histiocytes (exodus).

The endometrial glandular cells may be seen isolated, in clusters or in compact uniform sheets. The latter can be differentiated from endocervical cell sheets by their smaller cell size (approximately equal to the size of an intermediate cell nucleus) and decreased amount of cytoplasm (Figs. 12-1, 12-2). They may also be seen in ball-like arrangements encircling a tight inner core of stromal cells (Figs. 12-3, 12-4). Generally, the nuclear size does not vary, the chromatin is evenly distributed, and the nucleoli are relatively inconspicuous. Deep endometrial stromal cells approximate the size of a red blood cell. They are more easily recognized by their coarse chromatin pattern, indistinct cytoplasm, and nuclear molding and spindling (Figs. 12-5, 12-6). They appear on low-power view as tight aggregates of small darkly staining cells (Fig. 12-7). The superficial stromal cells are often difficult to discern from the accompanying histiocytes (Fig. 12-8).

Benign endometrial cells are sometimes found in premenopausal women after day 12 of the menstrual cycle (out-of-phase). The significance of this finding depends on the clinical situation; however, the etiology is usually benign in this age group. Most can be explained by the presence of an IUD, a concomitant biopsy procedure, endometritis, polyps, hormonal therapy, submucosal leiomyomas, impending or recent abortions, pregnancy, or anovulatory bleeding.[1,14,15,16] There may be additional findings on the Pap smear to suggest one of these etiologies. For instance, in the case of a submucosal leiomyoma, the bulging mass can cause an ulceration of the endometrium and subsequently shed endometrial cells and possibly benign smooth muscle cells derived from the leiomyoma as well (Fig. 12-9). In the situation of a pregnant patient, it is possible to find additional pregnancy-related cells such

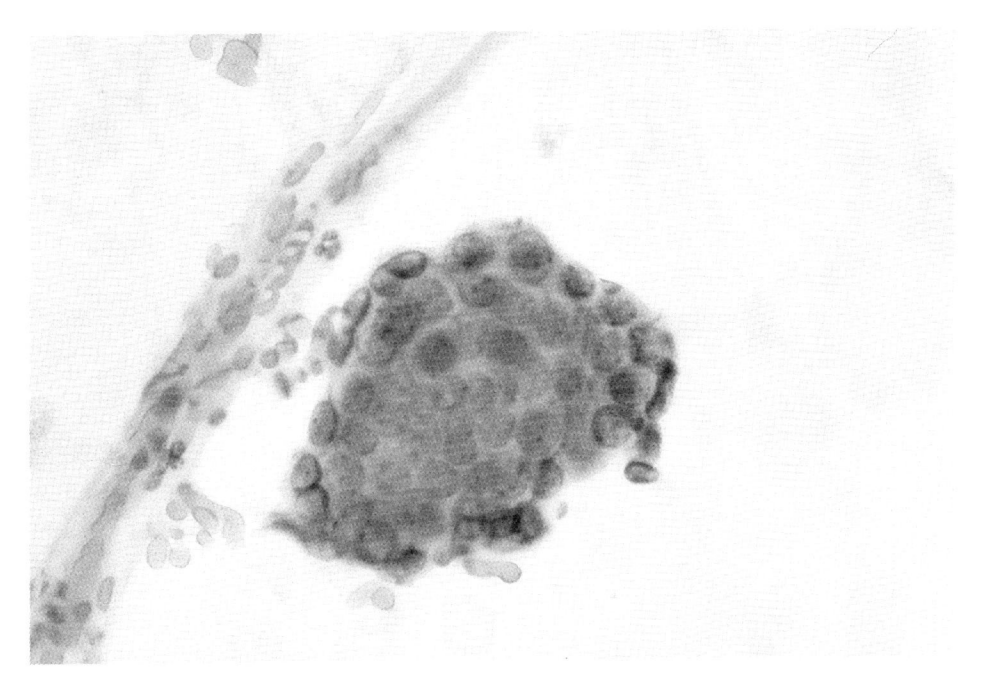

Figure 12-1. Benign endometrial glandular cells seen in a tight cluster. Note the uniform nuclei, even chromatin distribution and inconspicuous nucleoli. Compare with the endocervical glandular cells in Fig. 12-2. (40×).

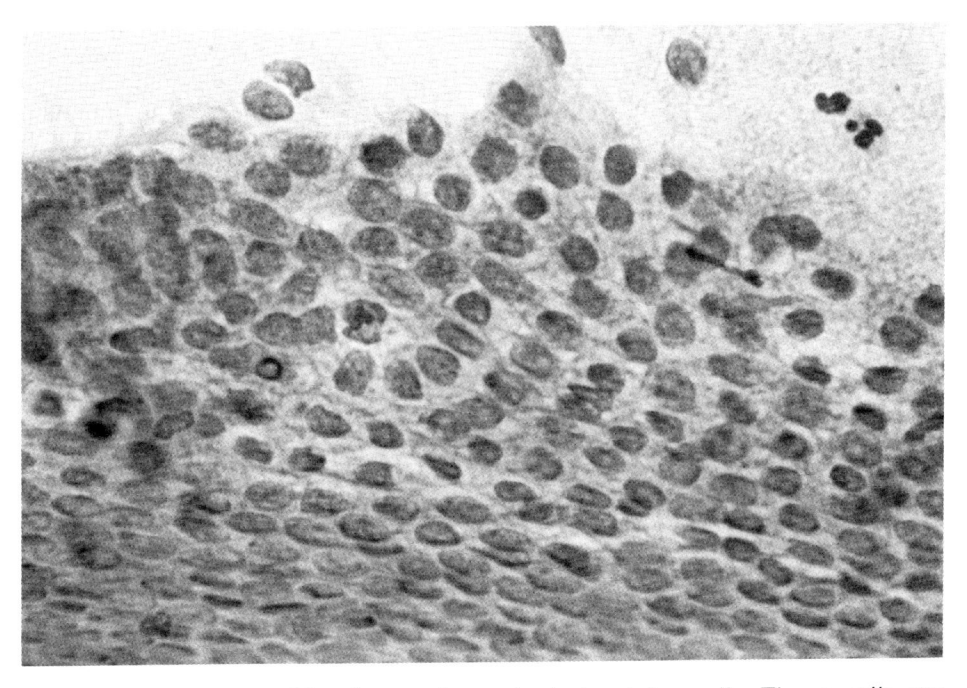

Figure 12-2. Sheet of benign endocervical glandular cells. These cells are more widely spaced than endometrial glandular cells because of an increased amount of cytoplasm. Note the typical honeycomb pattern between cells created by the adjacent cell membranes. (40×).

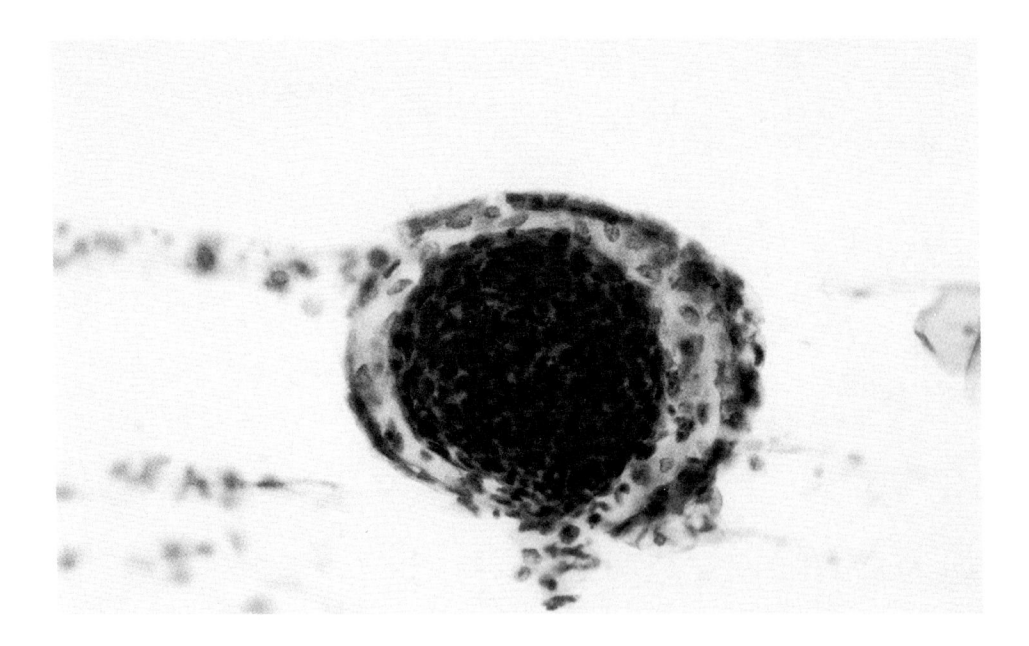

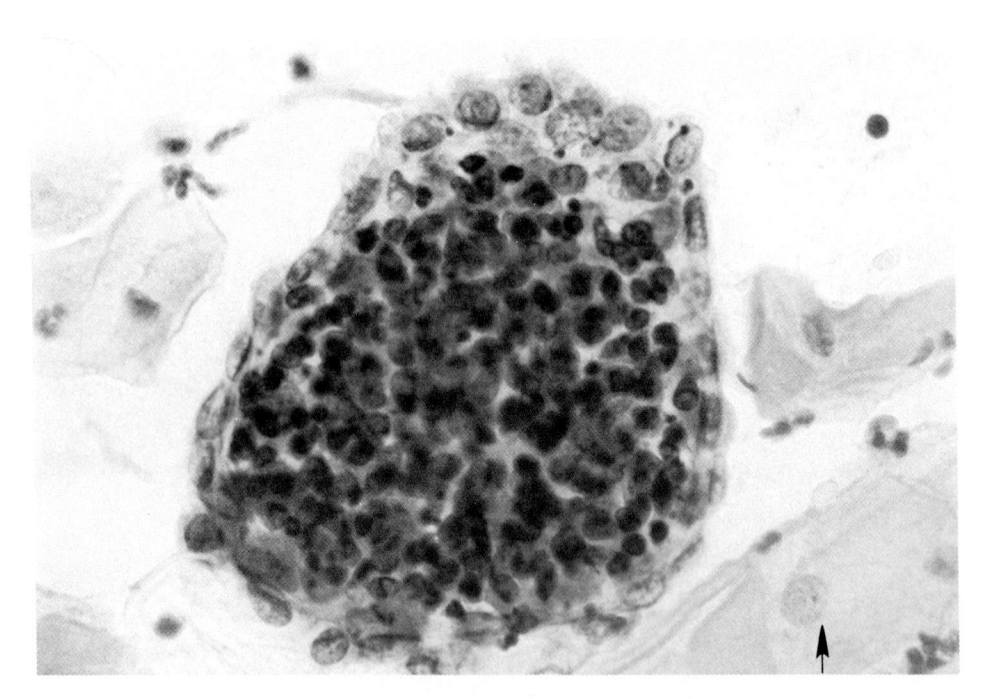

Figures 12-3, 12-4. Menstrual endometrium. The ball-like clusters here are composed of a tight inner core of endometrial stromal cells enveloped by a rim of endometrial glandular cells. The latter cell size is often compared to an intermediate squamous cell nucleus (arrow). (20×, 40×).

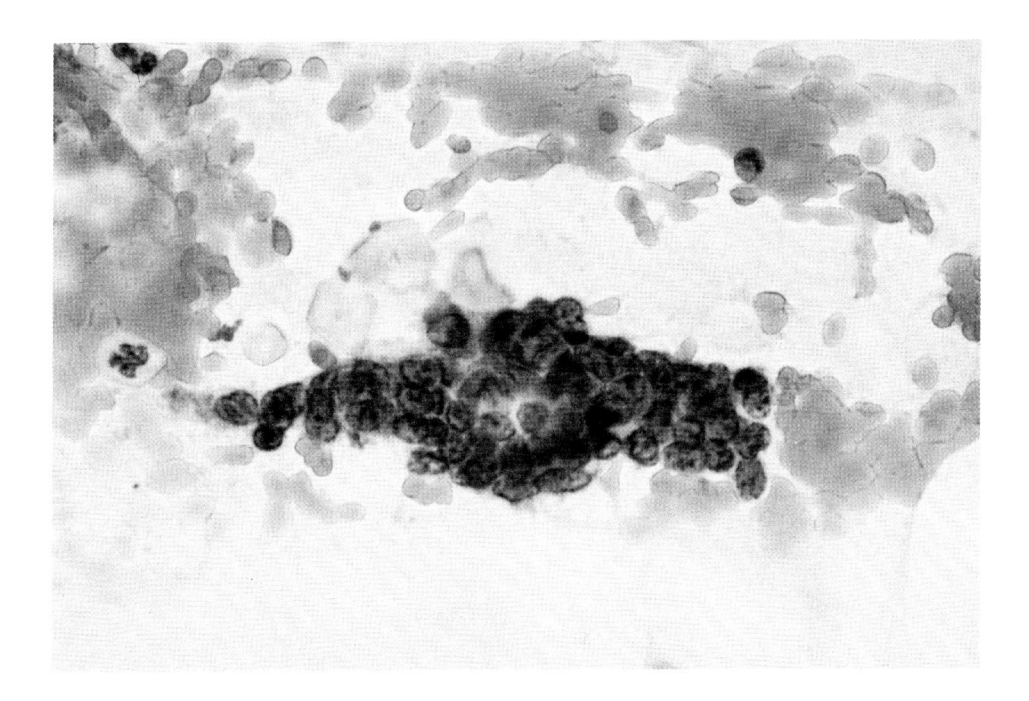

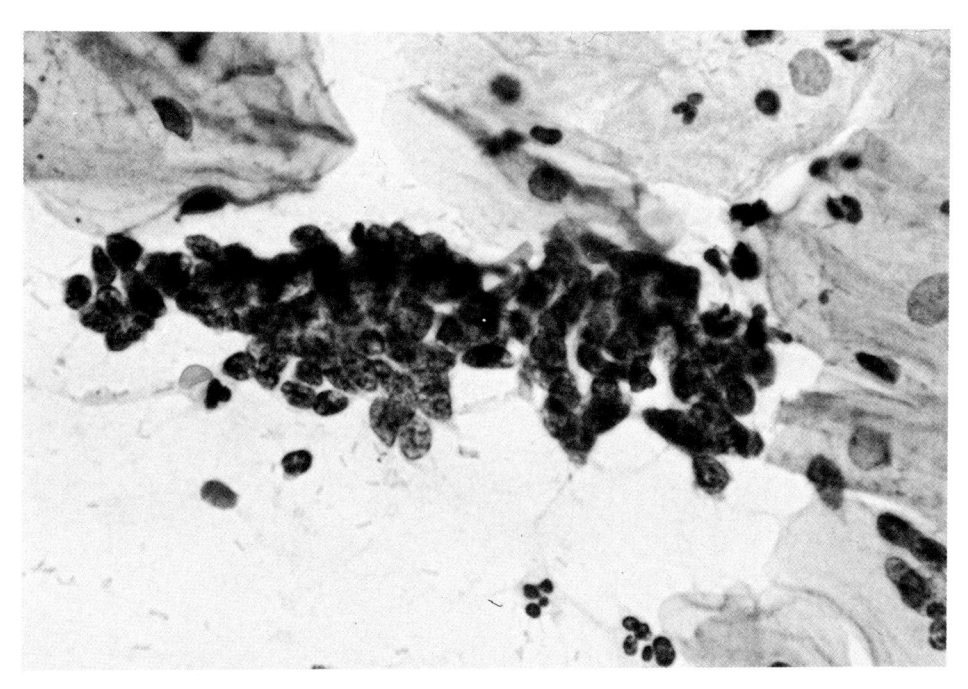

Figures 12-5, 12-6. Deep stromal cells. Note the coarse chromatin, indistinct cytoplasm and nuclear molding. Compare cell size to red blood cells in the background. (20×, 40×).

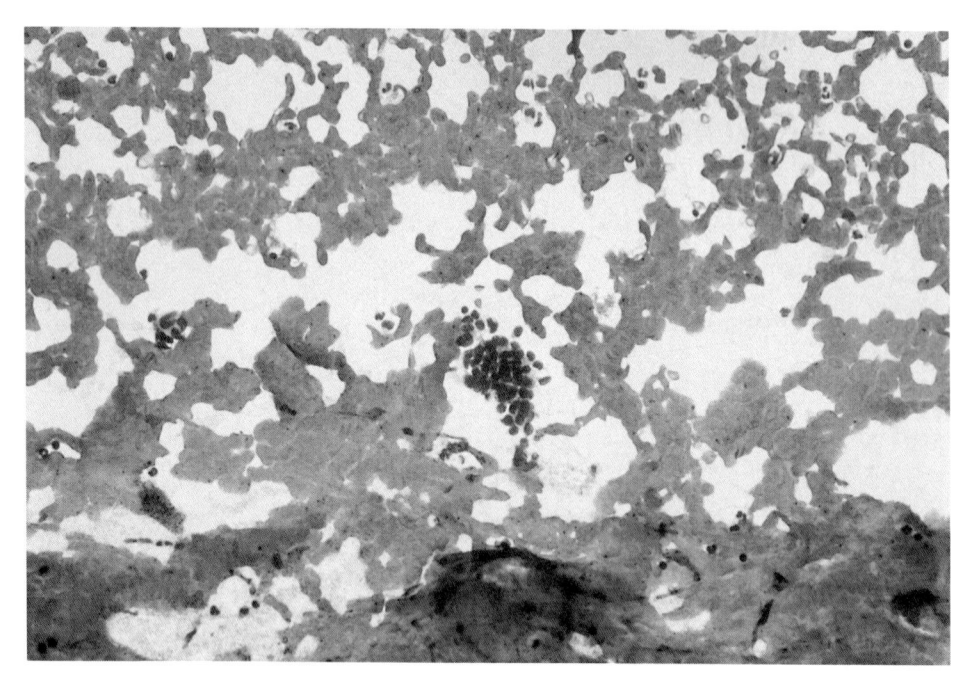

Figure 12-7. On lower power the deep stromal cells appear as darkly staining small cells. (10×).

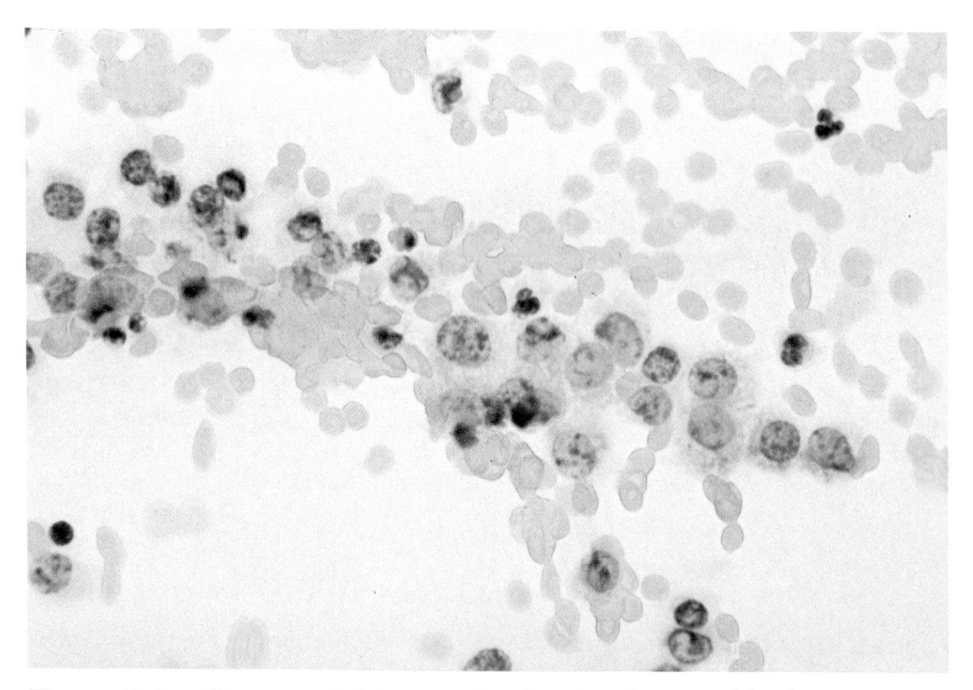

Figure 12-8. The superficial stromal cells closely resemble the accompanying histiocytes. Their cytoplasm is less distinct and chromatin more variable than that of the histiocytes. (40×).

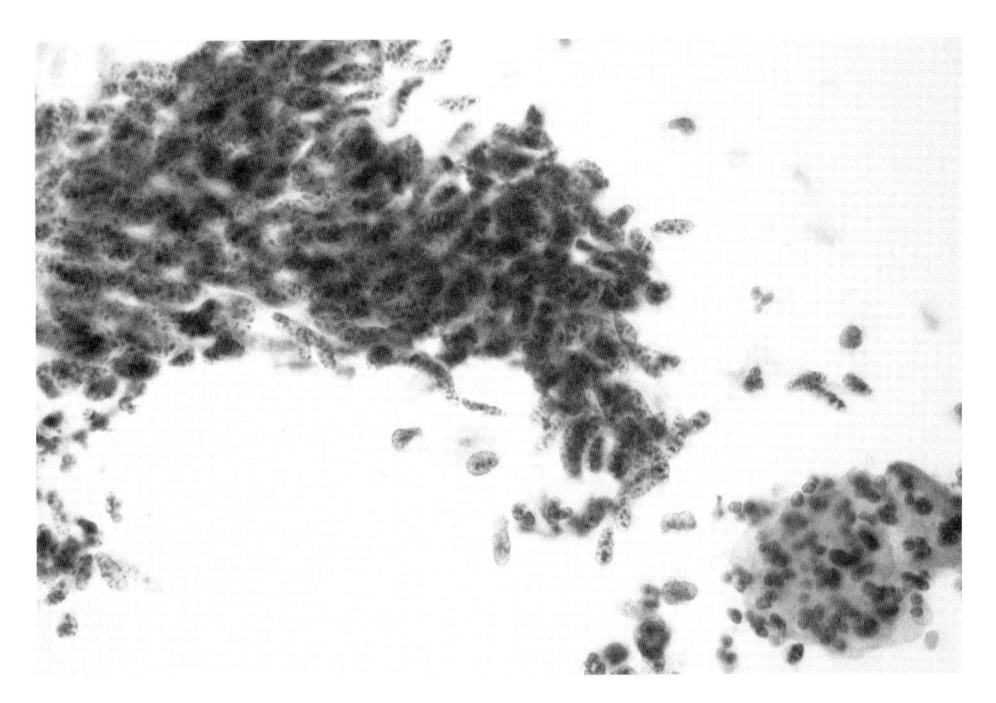

Figure 12-9. Smooth muscle cells derived from a submucosal leiomyoma. (40×).

as syncytiotrophoblast cells, Arias–Stella cells and decidualized stromal cells (Figs. 12-10 through 12-12). Arias–Stella changes include hypersecretory glandular cells which appear hyperchromatic, hobnail-like, and vacuolated. Historically, these cells were mistaken for malignancy. Hence, it is essential that the cytopathologist be provided with the complete clinical history including hormonal therapy, pregnancy status, past history, bleeding, instrumentation, LMP (last menstrual period), age, and presence of IUD (intrauterine device) in order to determine the significance of the Pap smear findings.

In the event that benign endometrial cells are discovered in a postmenopausal or perimenopausal patient, further investigation is necessitated. Reports indicate that 12–20% of patients with normal appearing endometrial cells on Pap smear had significant endometrial pathology when biopsied.[1,3,14–16] This may be the only indication of an endometrial lesion (hyperplasia or carcinoma) in the asymptomatic patient!

INFLAMMATION-RELATED CONDITIONS

Endometrial cells having degenerative changes, reactive changes, and even some nuclear atypia may be seen in association with inflammatory processes. Endometritis may be seen in the postpartum period, with IUD use, in PID (pelvic inflammatory disease), and rarely with tuberculosis and vi-

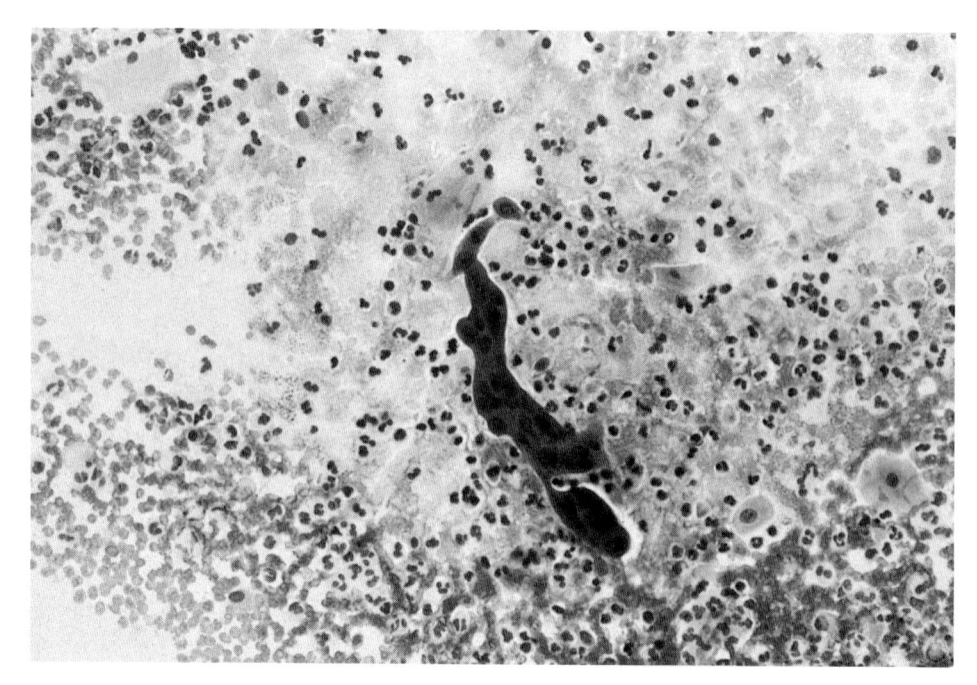

Figure 12-10. Syncytiotrophoblastic cell from a pregnant patient. These are large, irregular multinucleated cells with dense cytoplasm. (10×).

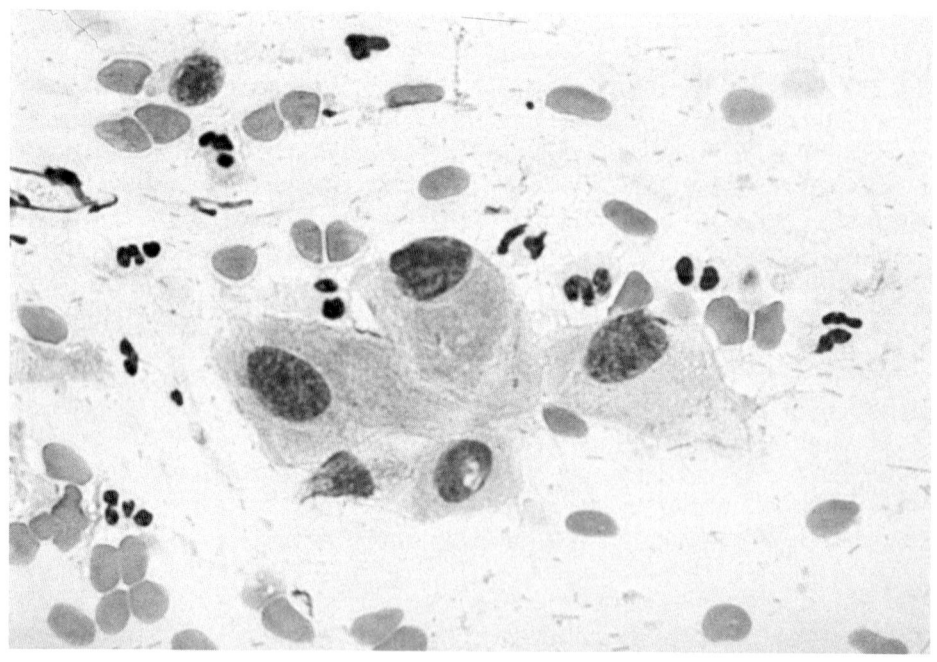

Figure 12-11. Decidualized stromal cells may be seen on occasion either singly or in flat sheets as seen here. The nucleus may be large and fairly central and may have a prominent nucleolus. The cytoplasm is basophilic and wispy or smudgy. These polygonal cells may be mistaken for dysplastic squamous cells. (40×).

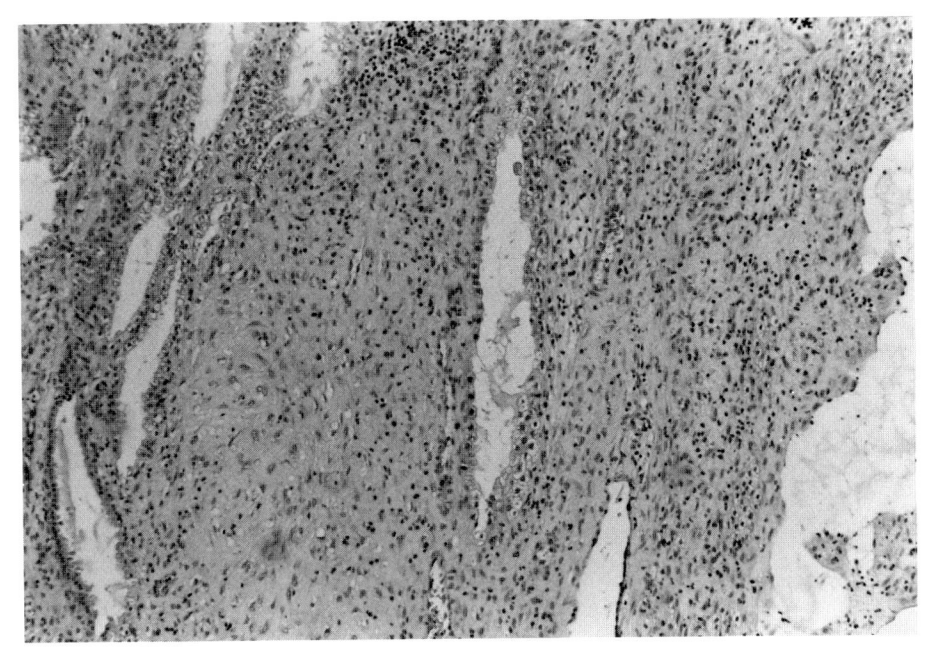

Figure 12-12. A decidualized polyp was the origin of the decidual cells discussed in Fig. 12-11. (10×).

ruses.[4] The Pap smear in acute endometritis secondary to an IUD may also show a dense inflammatory exudate and organisms such as *Actinomyces* may be present (Figs. 12-13, 12-14). The presence of plasma cells on Pap smear suggests the diagnosis of chronic endometritis (Fig. 12-15). Endometritis secondary to tuberculosis is now uncommon in the United States. The Pap smear may contain highly atypical endometrial cell clusters and possibly a granulomatous reaction. The finding of specific viral inclusions is diagnostic for viral endometritis, however this is an exceedingly rare finding.

ATYPICAL AND SUSPICIOUS ENDOMETRIAL CELLS ON PAP SMEAR

The finding of atypical endometrial cells on a Pap smear warrants further investigation. It is possible to find either benign-appearing and/or atypical endometrial clusters in patients who have endometrial polyps, inflammatory conditions, exogenous hormone administration, regenerating endometrium, IUDs, and hyperplasias.[17] These benign etiologies must be considered in a young asymptomatic patient with atypical appearing endometrial cells on Pap smear. Moreover, care must be taken not to overdiagnose menstrual endometrial clusters that may at times show cytoplasmic vacuolization due to late secretory changes and associated neutrophils that are typically found during this phase.

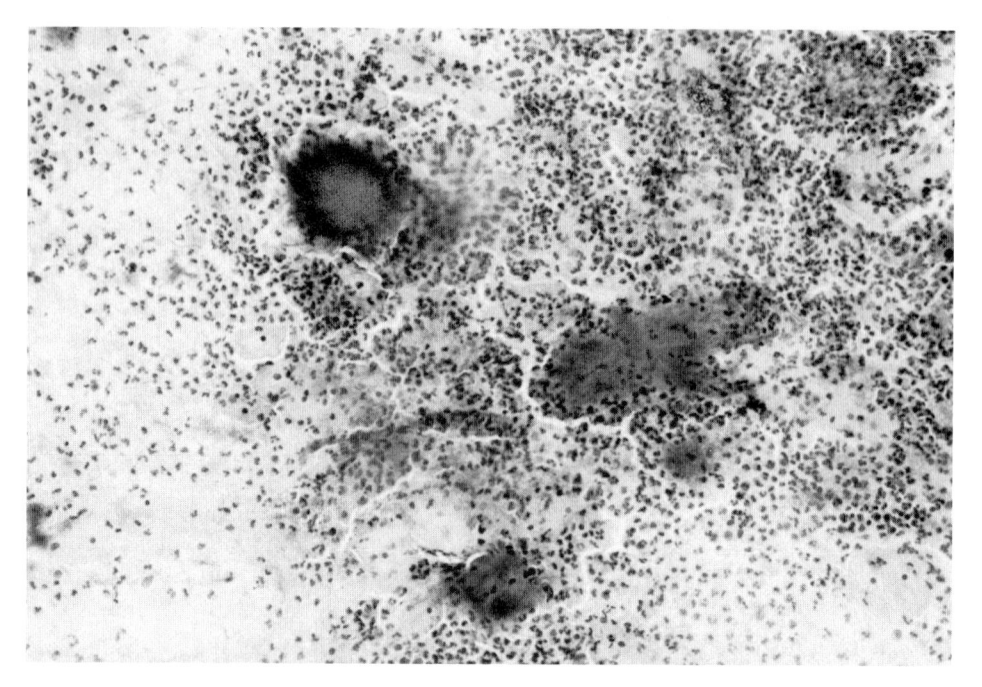

Figure 12-13. Actinomycosis in a Pap smear. Note the characteristic radiating filaments. The background shows marked acute inflammation. (10×).

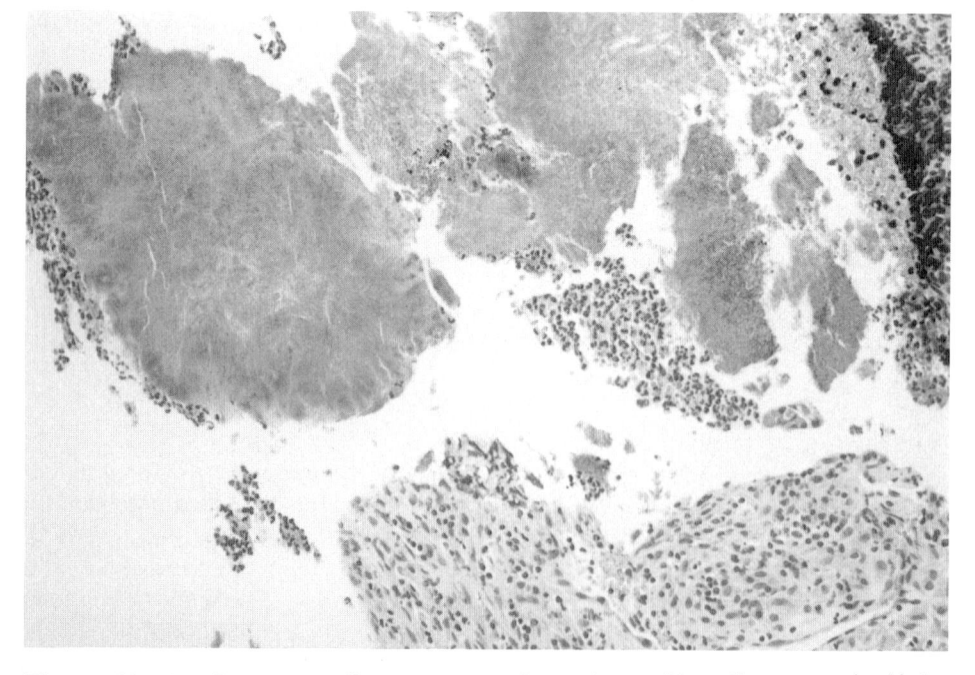

Figure 12-14. Corresponding curettage in patient with actinomycosis. Note the dense inflammatory infiltrates and classic sulfur granule. (10×).

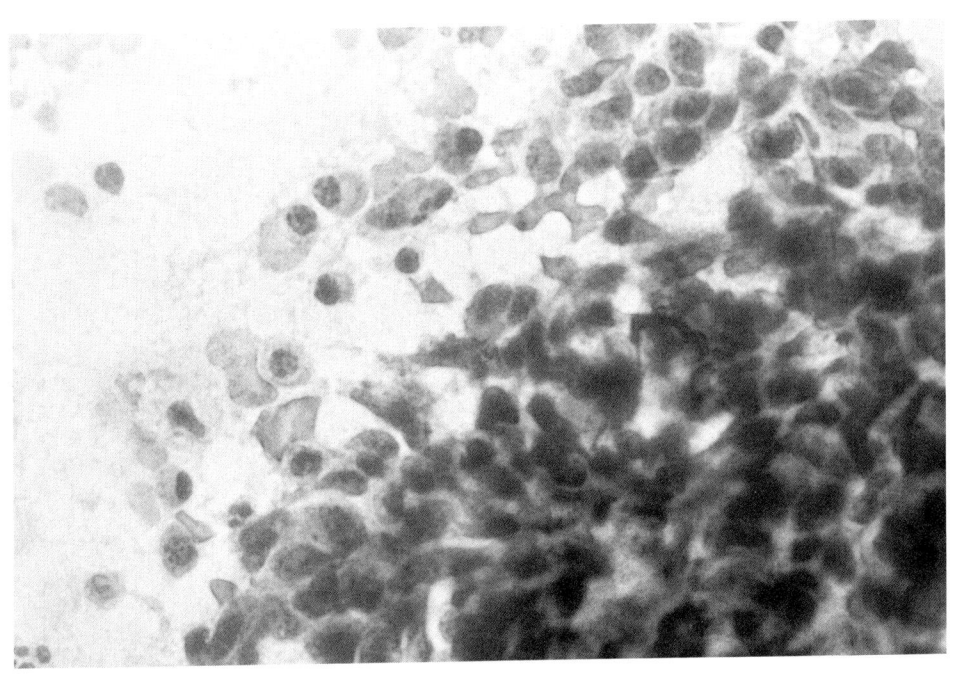

Figure 12-15. Pap smear showing endometrial cluster, blood, and plasma cells, suggestive of chronic endometritis. (40×).

Endometrial Polyps

Endometrial polyps (Figs. 12-16 through 12-18) account for 20–25% of the cases in which endometrial cells are abnormally present in a Pap smear.[4] Histologically, these polypoid lesions are composed of either functioning or inactive endometrial glands found in a dense stroma containing a rather prominent vasculature. Endometrial polyps are usually covered by a proliferative-type endometrium. Most polyps are nonfunctional and remain asymptomatic. Functional polyps, because they respond cyclicly, may enlarge rapidly and outgrow their blood supplies. This will result in necrosis and subsequent bleeding and shedding of endometrial cells.[1,4,18] The endometrial clusters frequently appear totally benign; however, nuclear enlargement, cytoplasmic vacuolization, and nucleoli can also be seen. The endometrial glands within polyps can undergo hyperplasia, and rarely malignant transformation as well. There are no findings diagnostic of an endometrial polyp on Pap smear; therefore, its presence may only be suggested.[4,18]

IUD

The endometrium undergoes a reactive process secondary to the presence of the intrauterine device. The resultant Pap smear may show an inflammatory infiltrate, macrophages, organisms, repair, and possibly endometrial cell

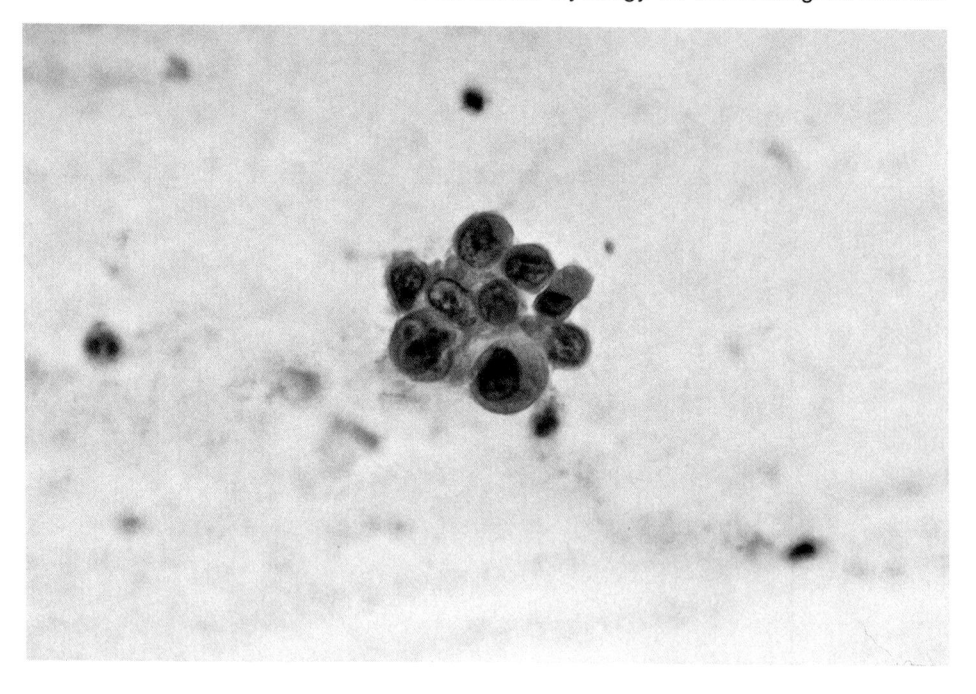

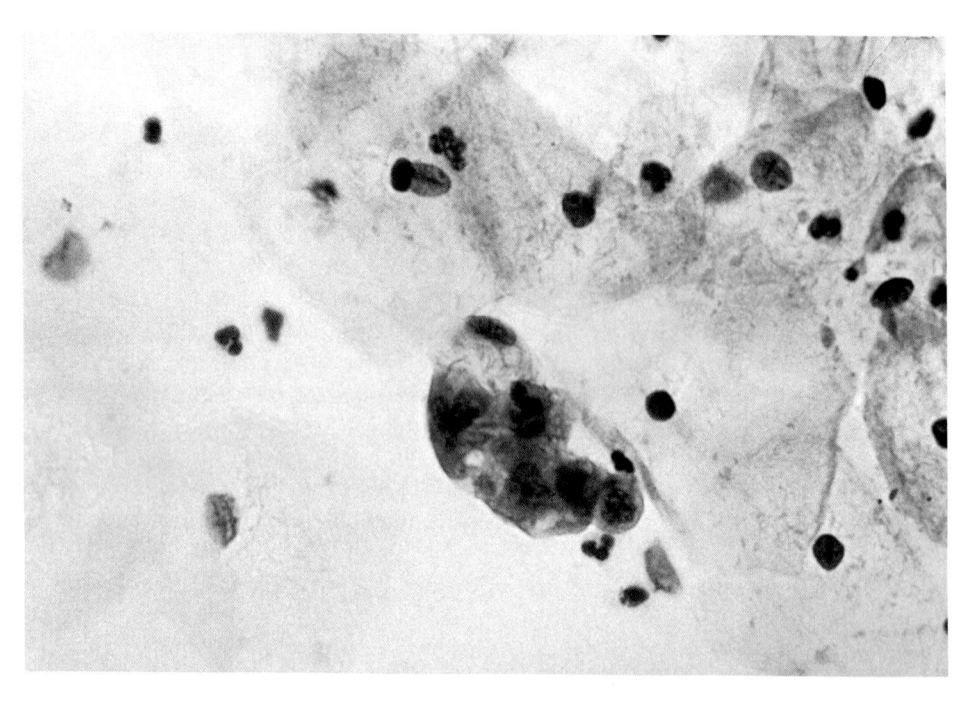

Figures 12-16, 12-17. Clusters of endometrial glandular cells found in a Pap smear of a 68-year-old postmenopausal woman. Patient has a history of atypical hyperplasia. Note the minimal nuclear atypia and nucleoli. (40×, 40×).

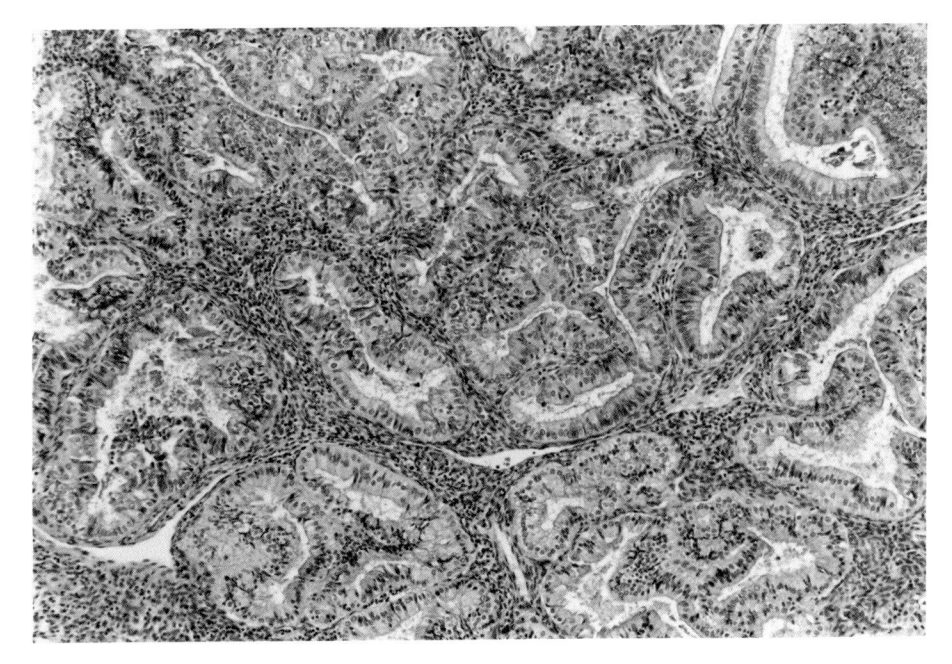

Figure 12-18. Recent biopsy on patient in Figs. 12-16 and 12-17 showed an endometrial polyp with complex hyperplasia. (4×).

clusters. Both endometrial and endocervical cell clusters can exhibit marked cytoplasmic vacuolization and nuclear eccentricity, features also shared with adenocarcinoma. A clinical history of an IUD can help eliminate any false-positive diagnoses in such cases. Koss reported associated psammoma bodies and metaplastic squamous foci seen in IUD users.[18]

Regenerative Endometrium

Regenerating tissue can be mistaken for malignant change due to its bizarre appearance and high mitotic activity. One must be careful not to overdiagnose endometrial cells that are detected following a recent operative procedure or pregnancy.

Endometrial Hyperplasia

The range of endometrial hyperplasias includes simple (with mild glandular crowding and/or cystic dilatation), complex (in which the glands are complex, branching, and closely packed), and atypical (with marked nuclear enlargement, chromatin alterations, and nucleoli). Cytologically, it is extremely difficult to diagnose endometrial hyperplasia without direct endometrial sampling. Even then it requires a cytopathologist who is experienced in this area.

A small proportion of patients with endometrial hyperplasia are totally asymptomatic. The presence of out of cycle endometrial cells in the Pap may be the only clue to their underlying pathology. However, the majority of the patients with endometrial hyperplasia will have abnormal bleeding. Most of these women will be over 40 years old and generally post- or perimenopausal.

Endometrial hyperplasia is not easily diagnosed by Pap smear because of the erratic shedding of the lesion and the advanced state of cellular degeneration. Furthermore, the range of appearances of the endometrial clusters varies considerably depending on the severity of the hyperplasia. In general, the more atypical the histology, the more likely it is to find atypical features in the endometrial cellular clusters on Pap smear.[1,4,14,18,19] Therefore, in cases of simple hyperplasia one may see perfectly benign or minimally enlarged and hyperchromatic endometrial cells singly or in small clusters (Figs. 12-19 through 12-21). Whereas, in cases of atypical hyperplasia, the endometrial clusters present may be more complex, exhibit increased cellular variation, coarse chromatin, and macronucleoli. In severe cases it may not be possible to differentiate atypical hyperplasia from endometrial adenocarcinoma (Figs. 12-22 through 12-28).

In general, when endometrial cells are discovered on a Pap smear in a postmenopausal patient there is a higher incidence of endometrial disease than in premenopausal patients. In addition, the more atypical the endometrial cells appear, the more likely one will find significant endometrial pathology.[3,14,16,19]

MALIGNANT CRITERIA ON PAP SMEARS

The most common malignancy of the endometrium is adenocarcinoma. Malignant endometrial glandular cells are usually round, with enlarged slightly eccentric nuclei, having a variable chromatin distribution and prominent eosinophilic irregular nucleoli. The cytoplasm is basophilic and typically scant; however, finely vacuolated cytoplasm and large degenerative vacuoles showing polymorphonuclear leukocyte infiltration may be seen as well (Figs. 12-29 through 12-31). Single malignant cells are more difficult to detect than malignant clusters; however, if one meticulously searches, they are usually present as well. In malignant cell clusters the cells have all the same features mentioned above, but now the cells are arranged three-dimensionally. The groupings may show cellular overlap, indistinct cell borders, loss of polarity, and variation in nuclear size (Figs. 12-32, 12-33). Clusters can vary in configuration, including smooth ball-like arrangements, papillary clusters, files, and rosette formations (Figs. 12-34 through 12-36). The nuclei may be polarized and protrude out of the cluster imparting a knobby surface to the cluster (Fig. 12-34). Vacuoles can displace and indent the nuclei creating a signet ring appearance (Figs. 12-37, 12-38). In general, the better differentiated the

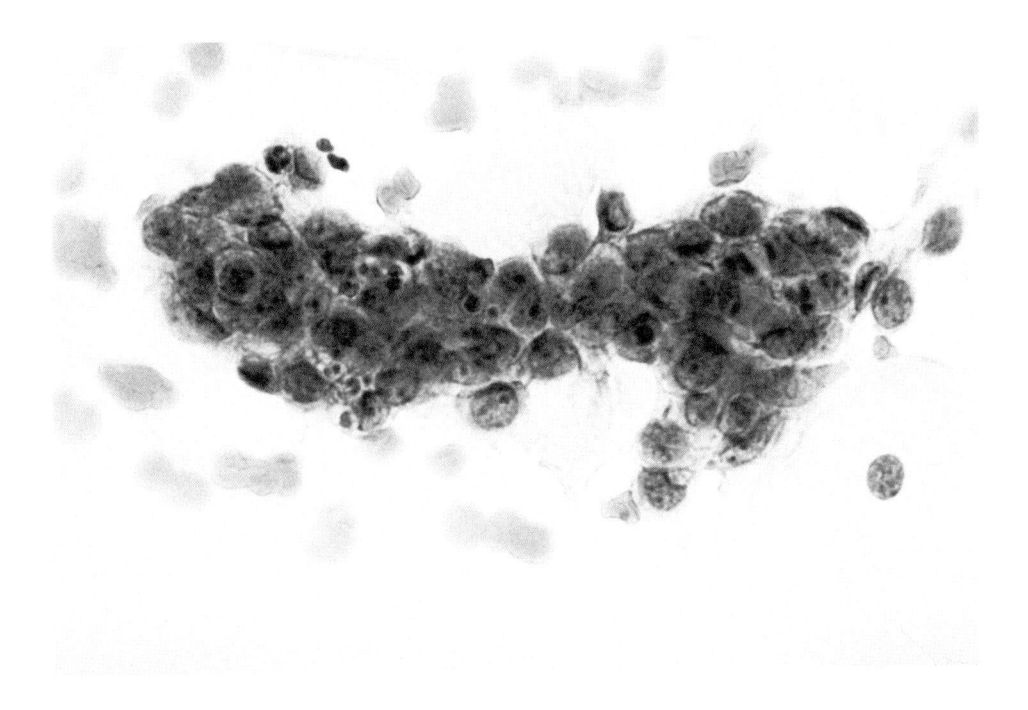

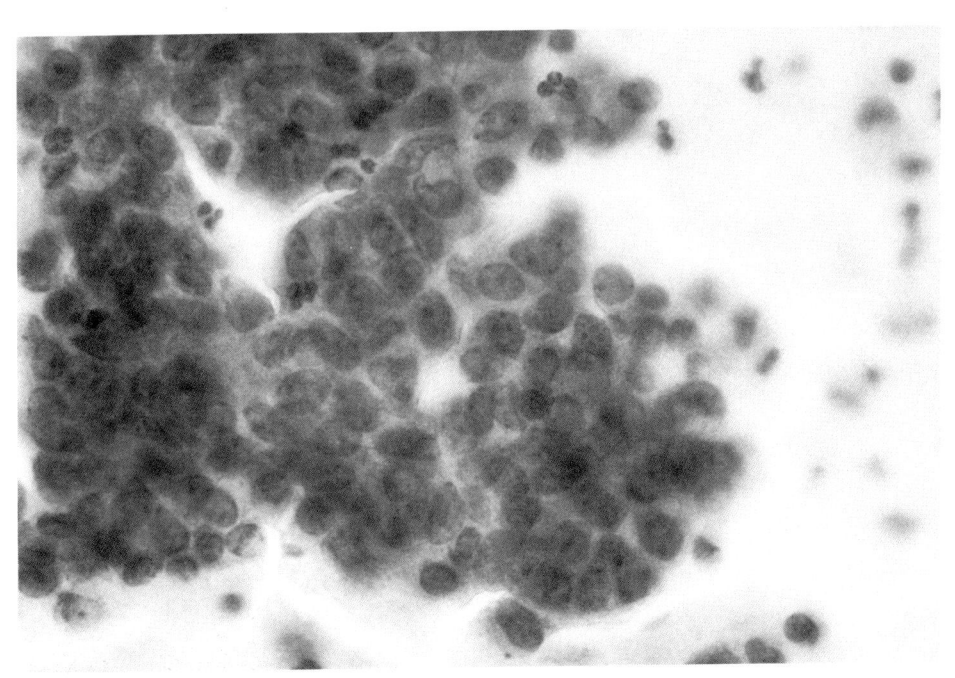

Figures 12-19, 12-20. 56-year-old postmenopausal patient with "abnormal bleeding." Rare endometrial glandular clusters were found on Pap smear. Note the branching cluster and mild atypia. (40×, 40×).

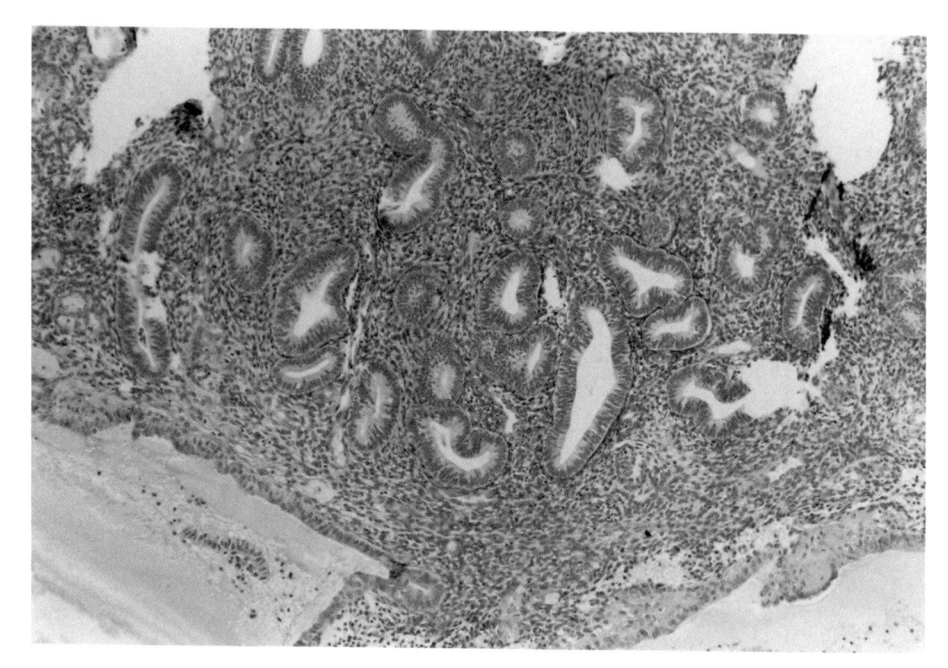

Figure 12-21. Biopsy on patient in Figs. 12-19 and 12-20 revealed simple hyperplasia. (4×).

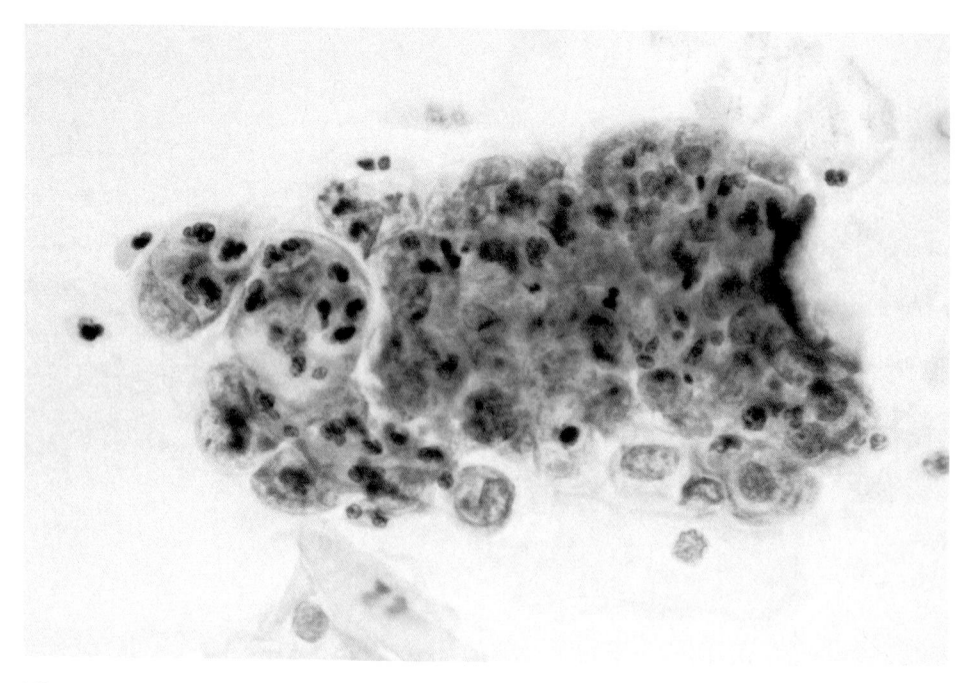

Figure 12-22. Markedly atypical endometrial gland in a 54-year-old postmenopausal patient with history of bleeding. Note the cytoplasmic vacuoles scalloping the nuclei, prominent PMN (polymorphonuclear) infiltration, and cellular overlap. (40×).

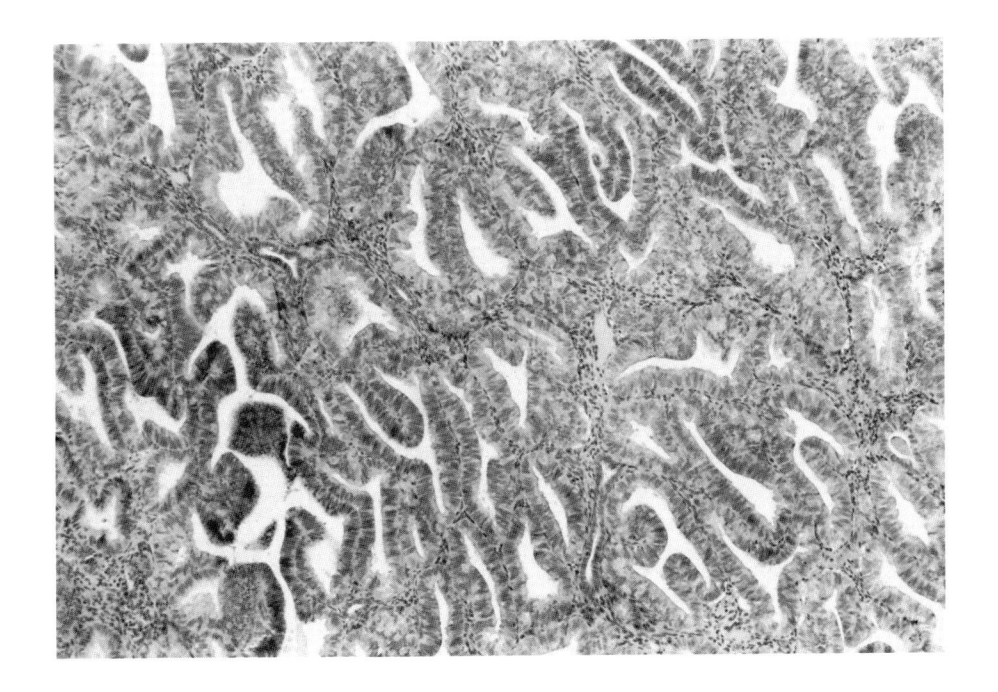

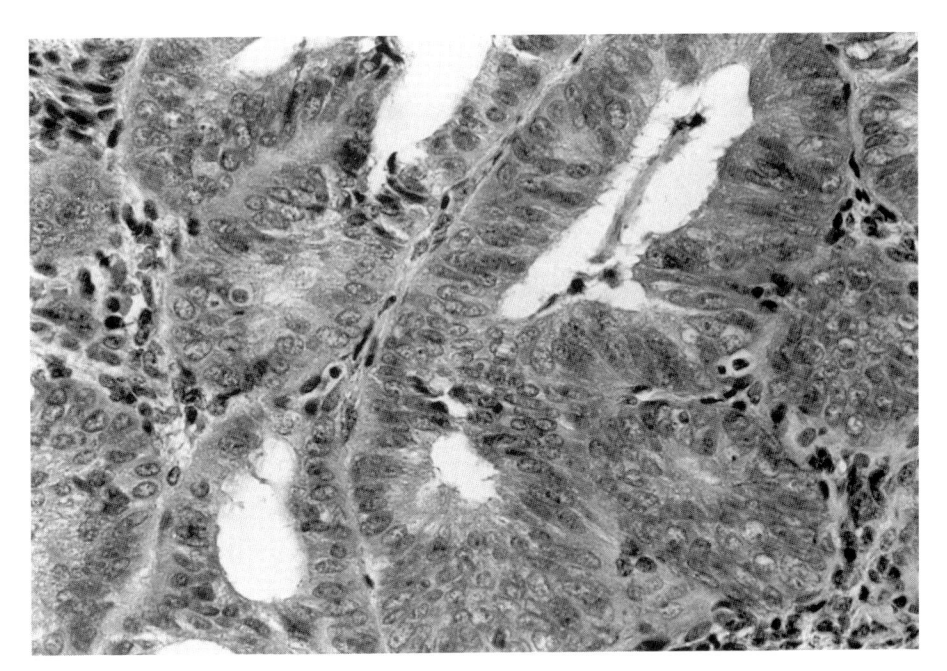

Figures 12-23, 12-24. Endometrial biopsy on patient in Fig. 12-22 showing atypical adenomatous hyperplasia, r/o adenocarcinoma. (4×, 40×).

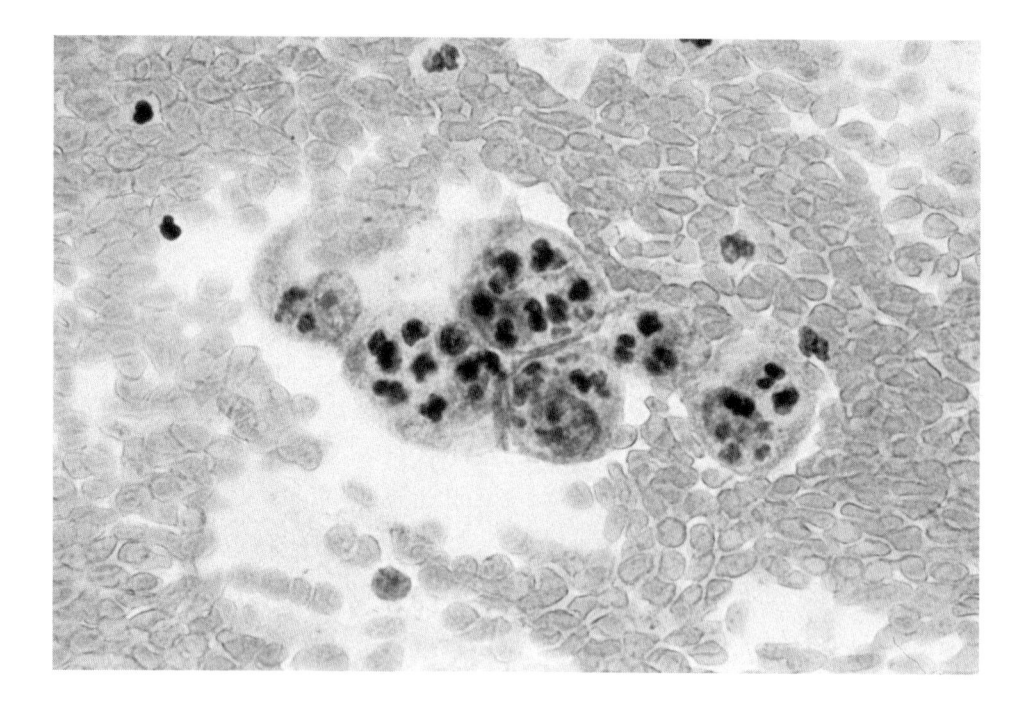

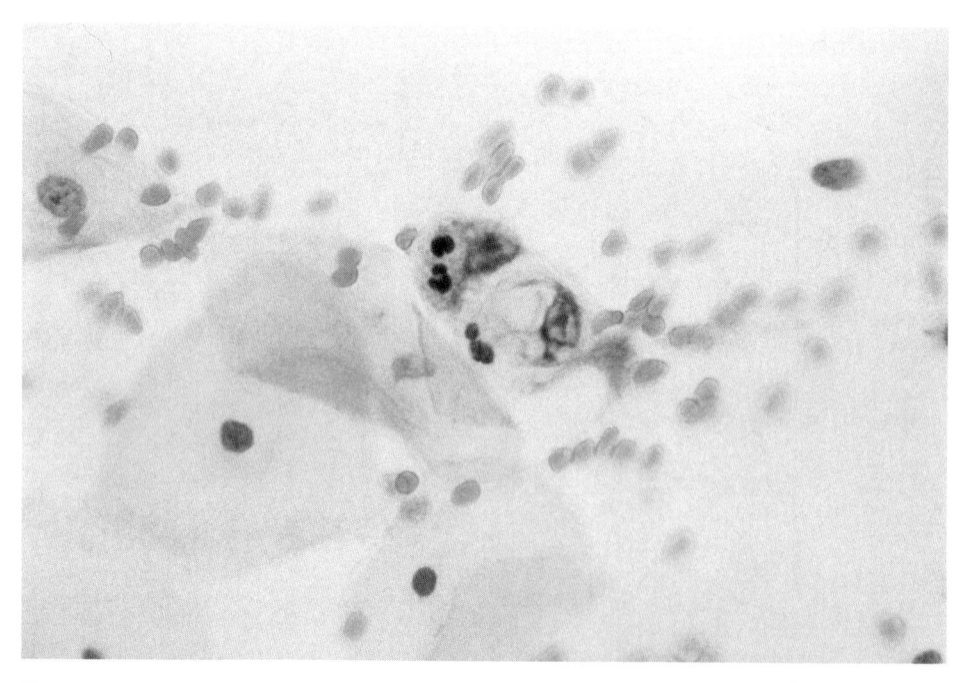

Figures 12-25, 12-26. 77-year-old patient with highly atypical endometrial glandular cell clusters on Pap smear. Note the blood in the background. Similar suspicious cytologic features as in previous case. Also note the increased nuclear size compared to the intermediate cell nucleus. (40×, 40×).

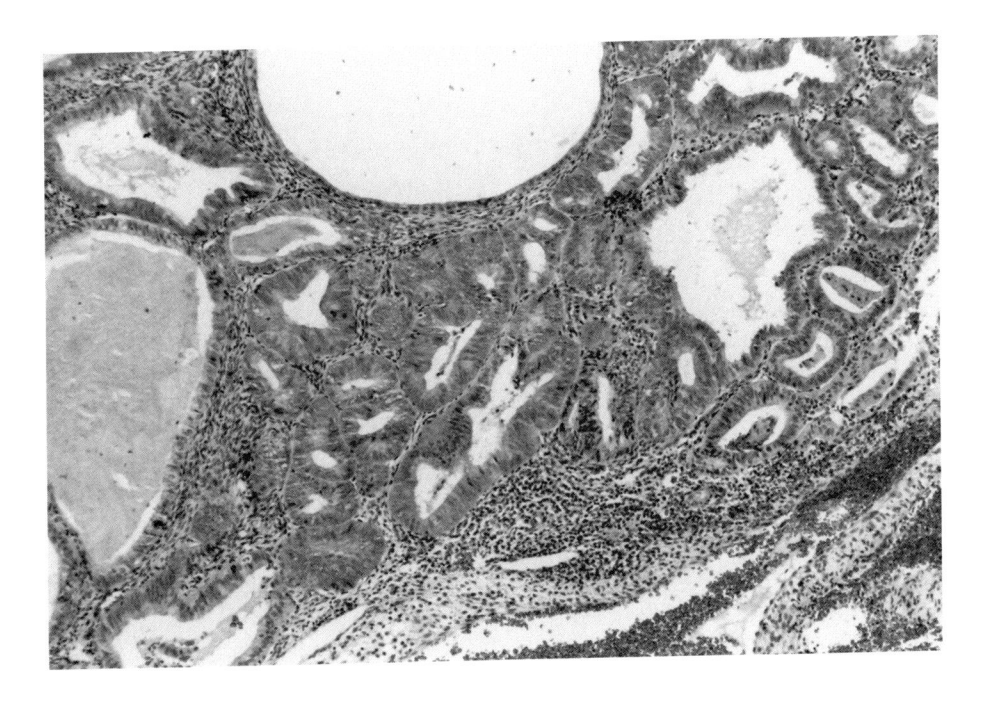

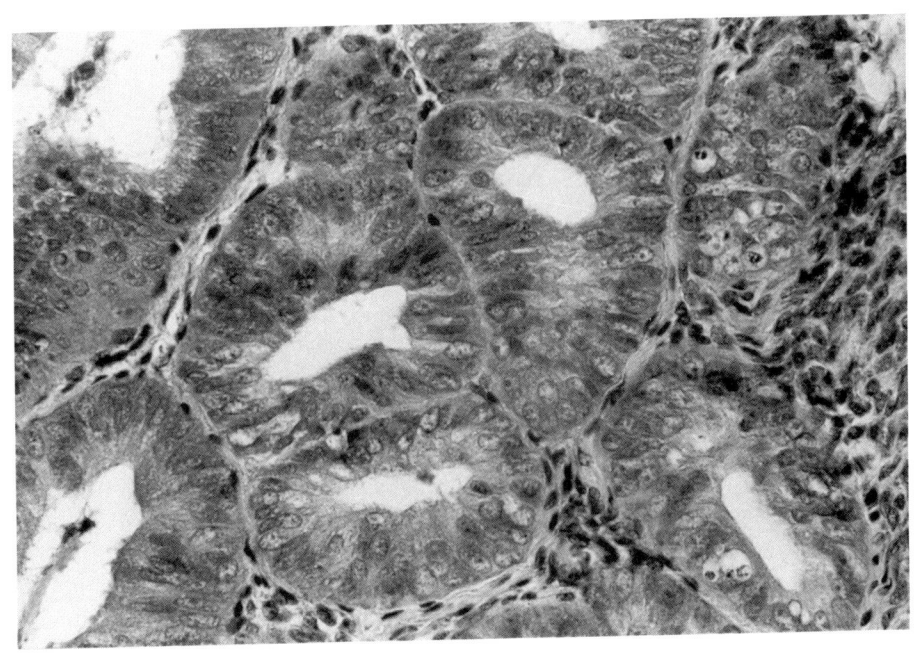

Figures 12-27, 12-28. Endometrial curettings of patient discussed in Figs. 12-25 and 12-26 showing atypical hyperplasia, r/o adenocarcinoma. (10×, 40×).

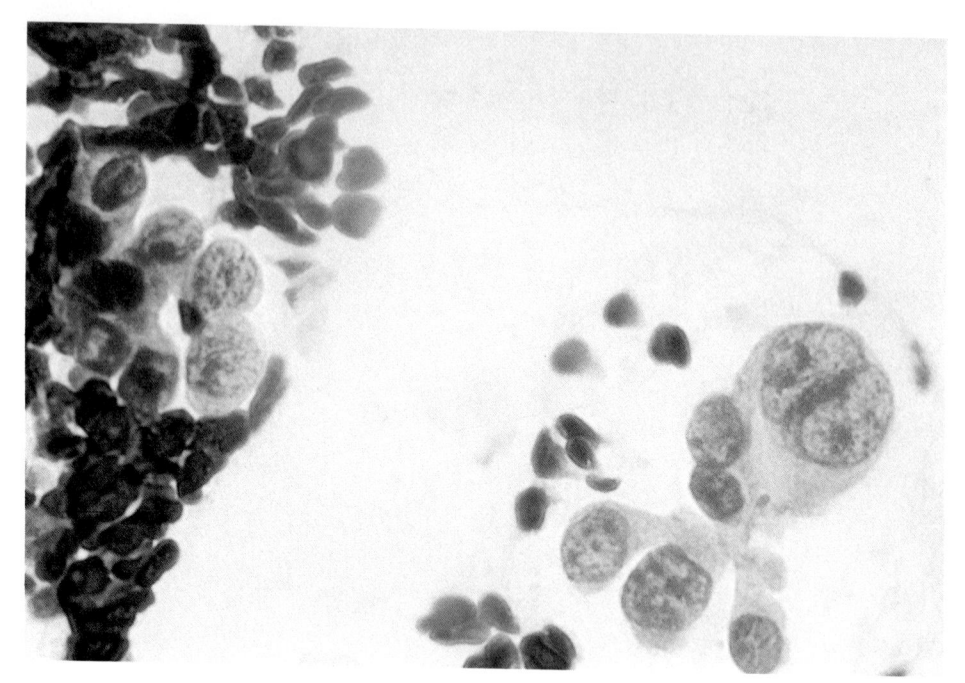

Figure 12-29. Endometrial adenocarcinoma cells. Note how closely the cells resemble their benign counterparts in size and amount of cytoplasm. The nuclei are enlarged and slightly polarized. A coarse chromatin pattern is present. (40×).

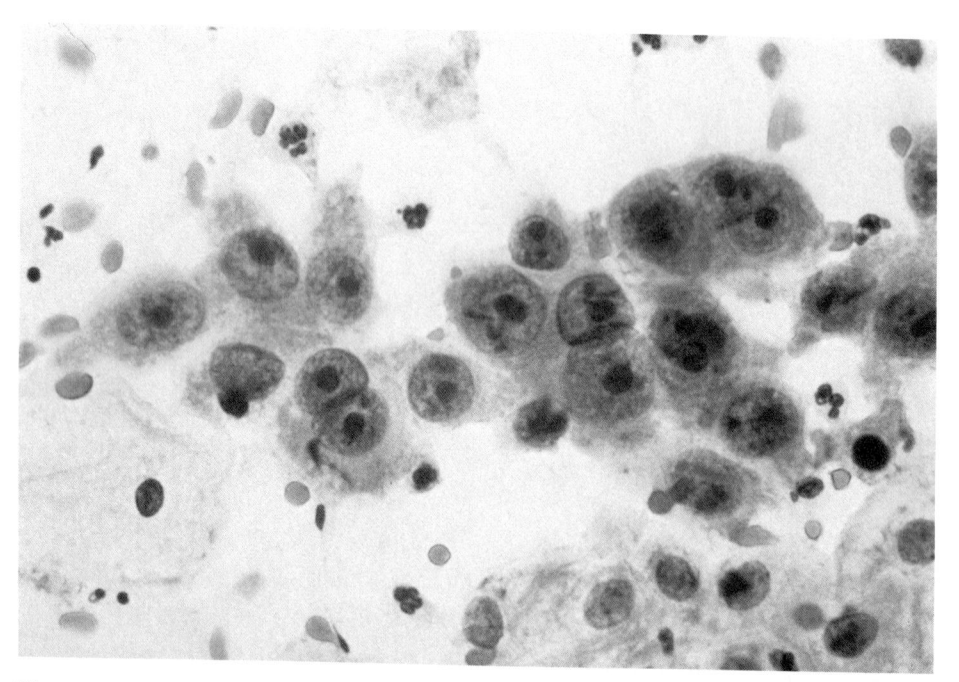

Figure 12-30. Endometrial adenocarcinoma cells. Note the finely vacuolated cytoplasm. Here we see single prominent eosinophilic nucleoli, which are not seen in benign glandular cells (refer to Fig. 12-1 for comparison). (40×).

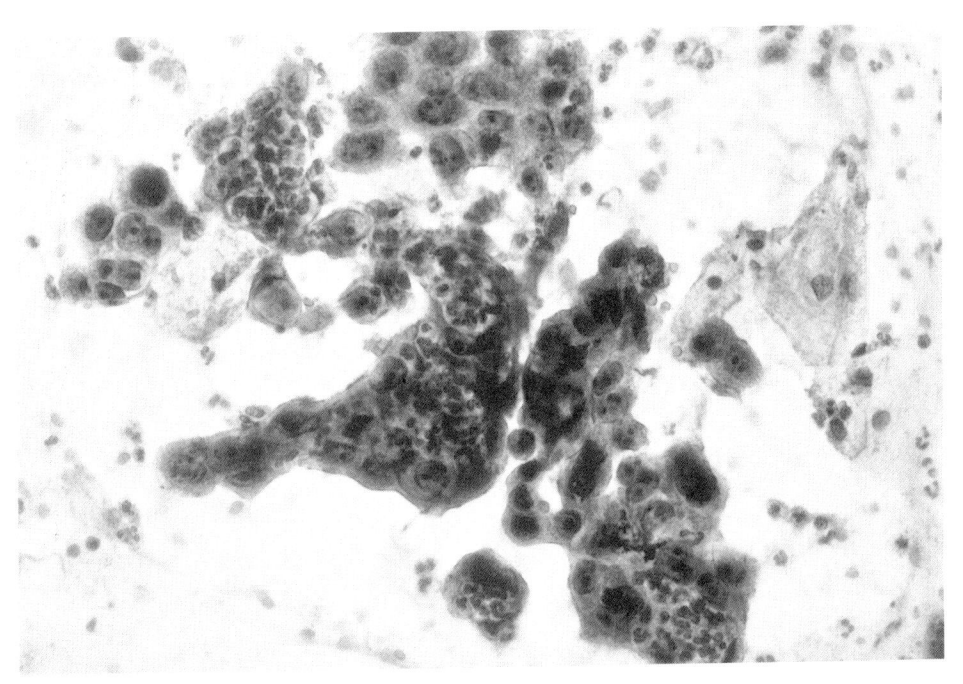

Figure 12-31. Clusters of endometrial adenocarcinoma. Intense cytoplasmic neutrophilic infiltration is present in this case. (20×).

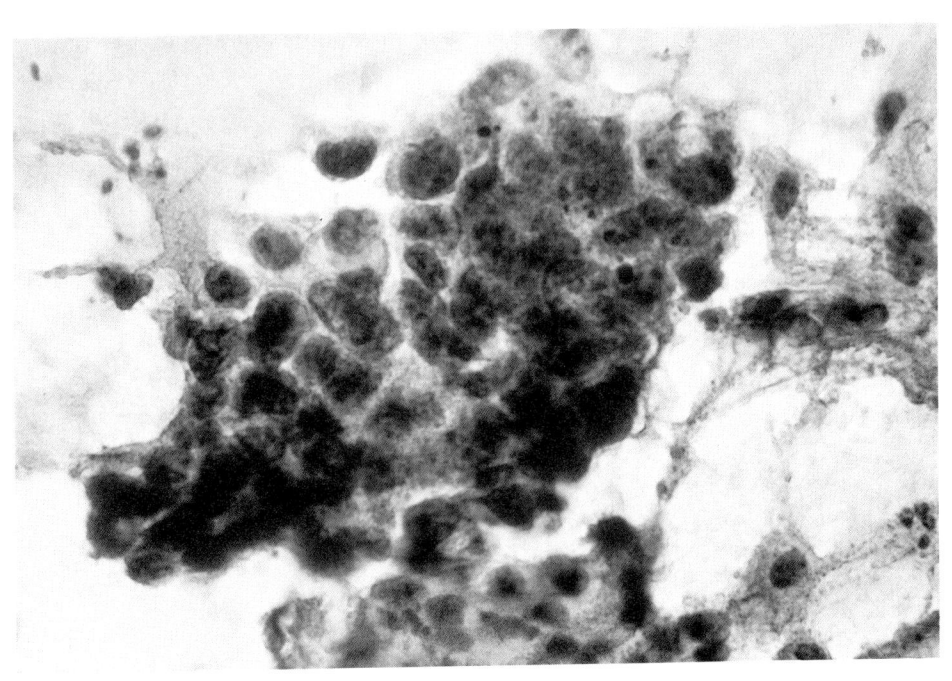

Figure 12-32. Cluster of endometrial adenocarcinoma. Note the indistinct cell borders, nuclear overlap, and loss of polarity seen here. These cells exfoliated from a poorly differentiated adenocarcinoma of the endometrium. The more disorganized and atypical the cytology, the less differentiated is the tumor. (40×).

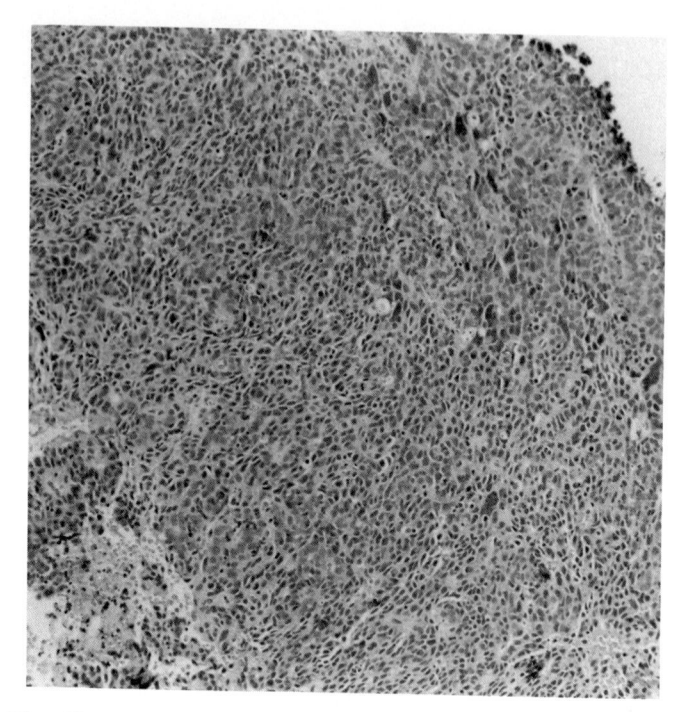

Figure 12-33. Endometrial curettings on the patient described in Fig. 12-32 showing poorly differentiated adenocarcinoma. There is a suggestion of gland formations, but well-formed lumina are not seen. (4×).

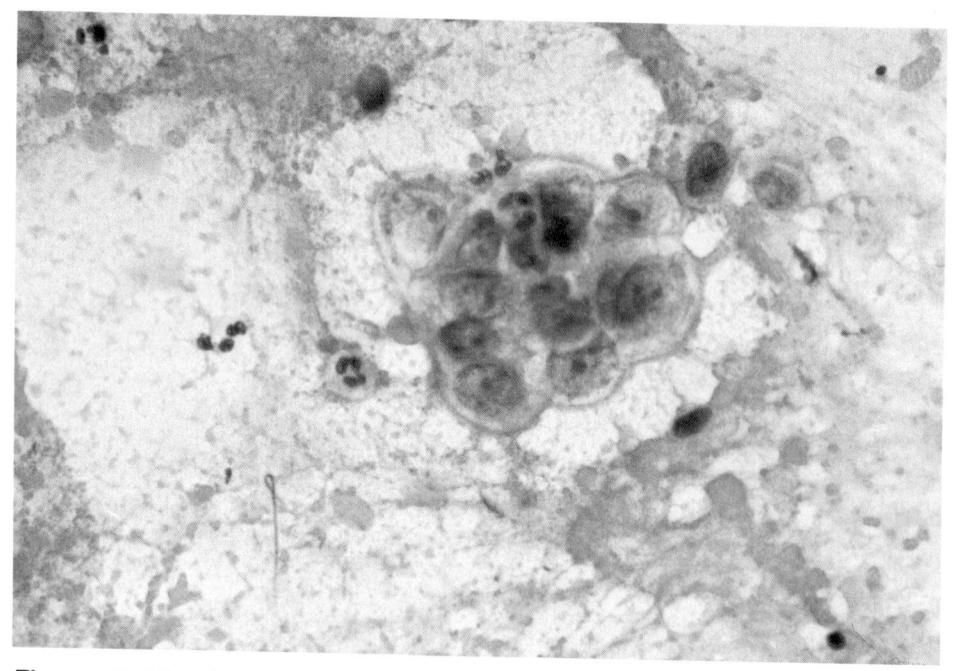

Figure 12-34. Cluster of endometrial adenocarcinoma. Peripheral nuclear protrusions impart a knobby surface to the cluster. Note the fresh and lysed blood in the background. (40×).

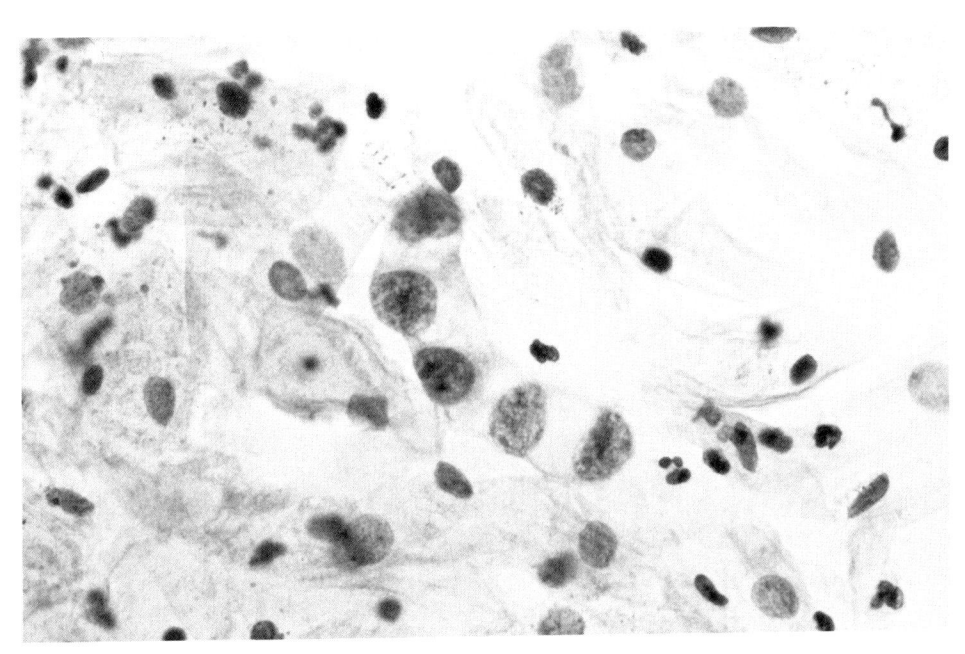

Figure 12-35. File or linear arrangement of endometrial adenocarcinoma cells from a patient noted to have a pelvic mass. The differential diagnosis here would be a breast primary that can also form linear arrays ("Indian files"). (40×).

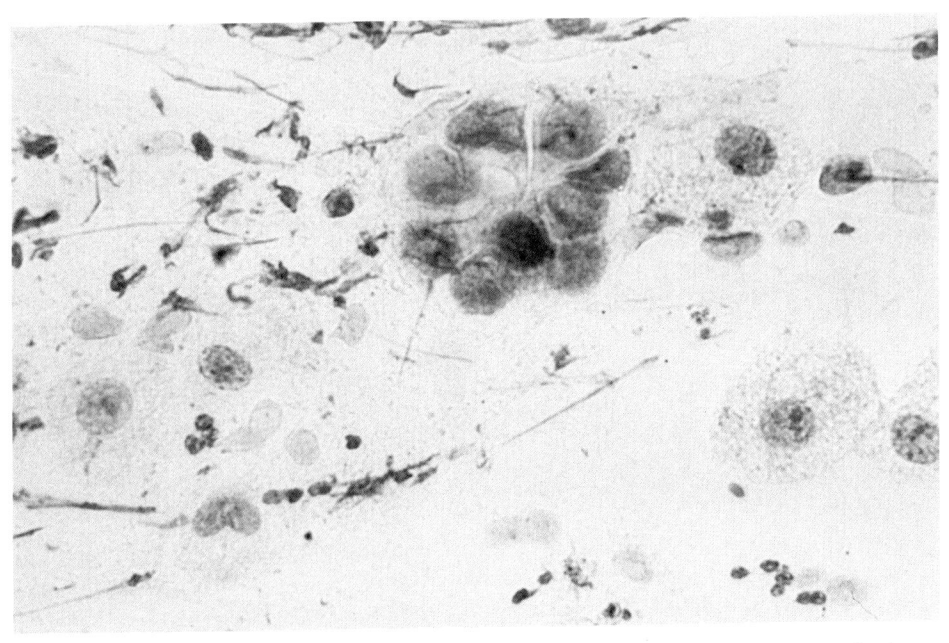

Figure 12-36. Rosette formation of endometrial adenocarcinoma cells in a 58-year-old postmenopausal patient noted to have bleeding. Note the slight nuclear eccentricity and scant cytoplasm. The background contains numerous histiocytes that can be recognized by their oval to reniform-shaped nuclei and finely vacuolated cytoplasm. (40×).

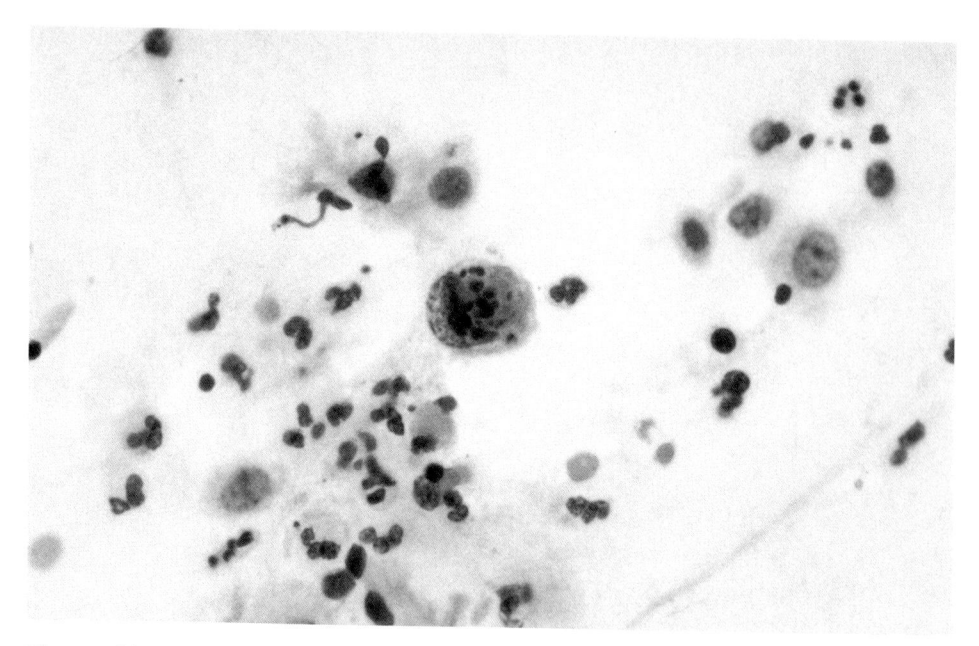

Figure 12-37. Signet ring endometrial adenocarcinoma cell. Note the crescentic configuration to the nucleus, which is displaced eccentrically. Coarse chromatin and sharp nuclear corners are malignant features. Signet ring cells are also seen in lobular carcinoma of the breast and gastric adenocarcinomas. (40×).

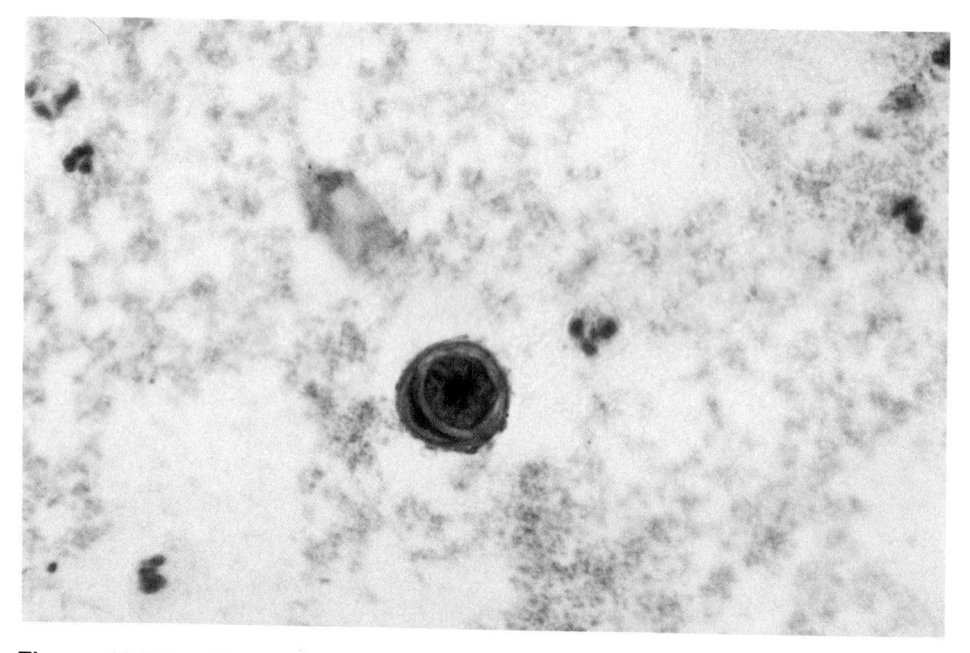

Figure 12-38. Signet ring endometrial adenocarcinoma cell. In addition to the features observed in Fig. 12-37, the cell-in-cell phenomenon is seen here. This is when a cell engulfs another cell; in this case both are malignant. Cell-in-cell is a feature that often helps suggest the glandular nature of a neoplasm. (40×).

tumor is, the more cohesive the cells are, and the more the cells and clusters resemble the native cells.

The importance of the smear background has been discussed in the literature. The background may be clean and unremarkable, or it may contain tumor diathesis (hemolyzed blood and necrotic debris). An elevated estrogenic effect (i.e., high squamous cell maturation) or numerous histiocytes, if present in a vaginal specimen, are considered significant by some.[1,3,13,14,17,18] Zucker et al,[3] in a retrospective study of 102 peri- and postmenopausal women with abnormal endometrial cytology by cervical Pap smear, reviewed the following six background criteria: (1) mononucleated histiocytes, (2) multinucleated histiocytes, (3) nonspecific inflammatory changes, (4) blood, (5) elevated squamous maturation, and (6) abnormal endometrial cytology. They found that only criterion 6, the degree of atypical endometrial cytology, had any statistical predictive value. It must be emphasized that the study was on cervical Paps, not vaginal Paps, and the study group was small.

OTHER MALIGNANCIES AND VARIANTS

Serous Papillary Carcinoma

This may be recognized by the presence of malignant papillary fronds or clusters. Psammoma bodies may also be seen. Differential diagnosis includes fallopian tube primary and ovarian primary.

Clear Cell Carcinoma (Uncommon)

This has a loosely cohesive pattern with many single cells present. The cytoplasm is often wispy and clear due to glycogen content.

Mucinous Carcinoma (Rare)

This exhibits a palisading picket-fence arrangement of cells that resemble goblet cells. Mucin pools may be present in the background. Metastases from ovary and colon must be considered.

Adenosquamous Carcinoma (Adenocarcinoma with Squamous Differentiation)

This is a mixed tumor composed of both malignant glandular cells (see description of adenocarcinoma above) and malignant keratinized or nonkeratinized squamous cells (cannot be differentiated from those derived from cervix, vagina, etc.) (Figs. 12-39 through 12-41).

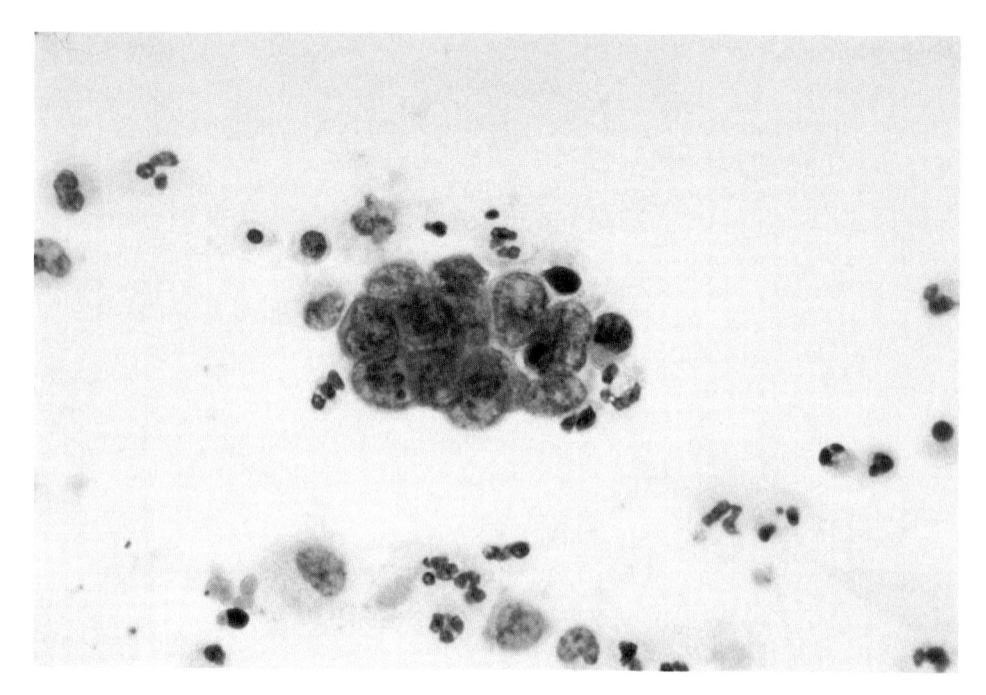

Figure 12-39. Adenosquamous carcinoma. Here we see the malignant glandular component which appears as a typical cluster of endometrial adenocarcinoma. Again note the scant cytoplasm and small cell size. (40×).

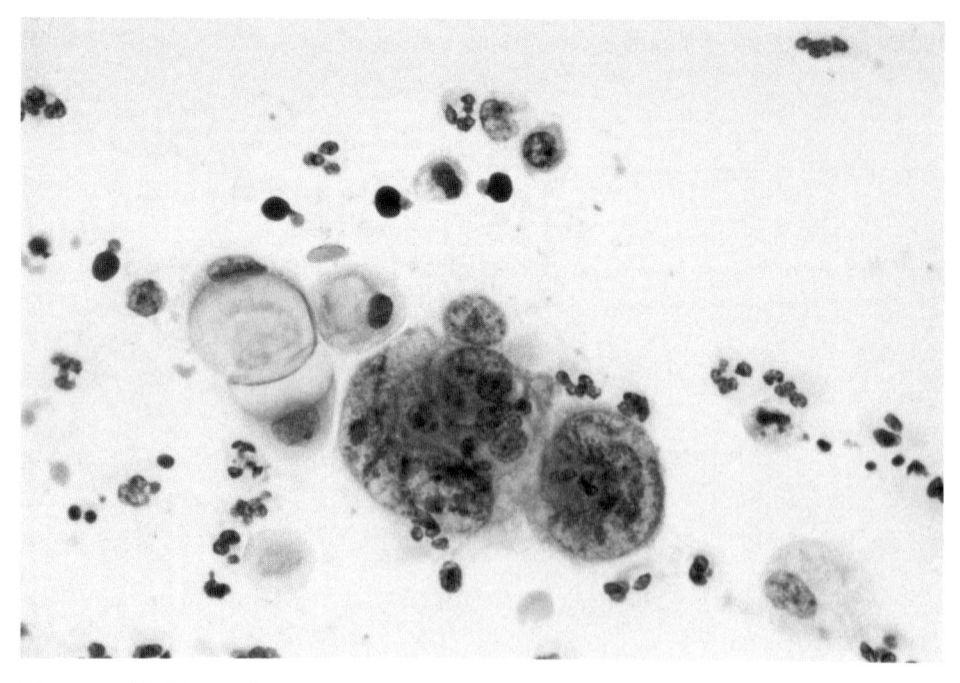

Figures 12-40. Adenosquamous carcinoma (same case as in Fig. 12-39). Other clusters of adenocarcinoma cells with more atypical features, prominent nucleoli, cell enlargement, nuclear overlap, and neutrophilic infiltration. (40×).

Other Malignancies and Variants

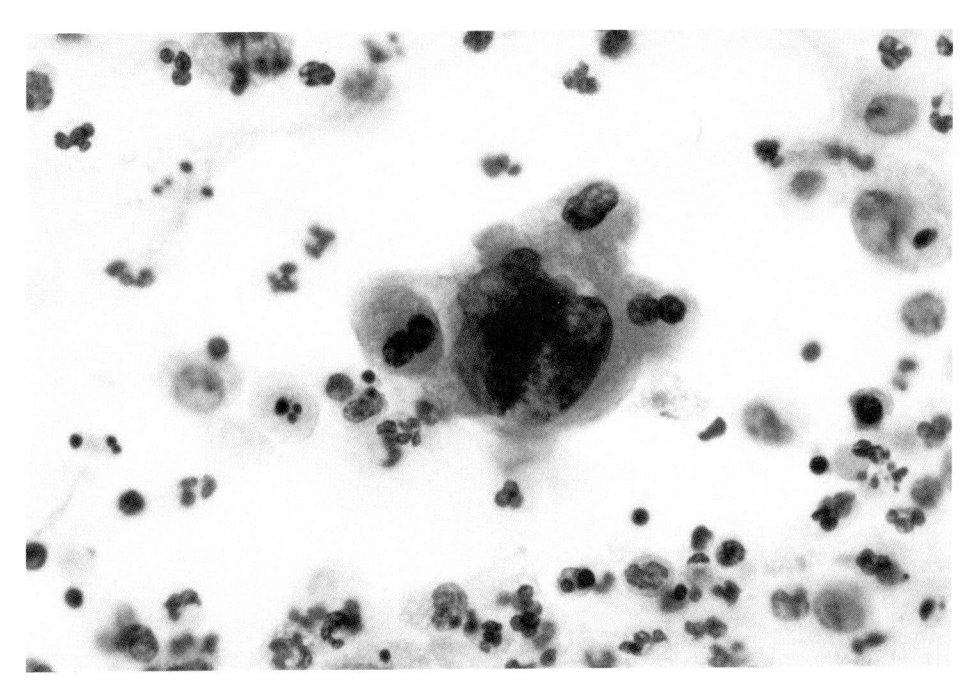

Figure 12-41. Adenosquamous carcinoma (same case as Figs. 12-39 and 12-40). Malignant squamous component. The cytoplasm is dense, and the nucleus is hyperchromatic and more centrally located. (40×).

Sarcomas (Rare)

Leiomyosarcomas and endometrial stromal sarcomas occur in the uterus. In these tumors the cells may vary from small, rounded, and wispy to elongated, spindly, and tapered.

Malignant Mixed Müllerian Tumor

This tumor contains both malignant epithelial (glandular and/or squamous) elements and malignant mesenchymal (stromal) element(s) (Figs. 12-42 through 12-44).

Choriocarcinoma (Rare)

This is characterized by syncytia of malignant syncytiotrophoblast cells.

Lymphoproliferative Disorders

In this group many atypical lymphocytes, histiocytes, or plasma cells are found in a single-cell distribution (Fig. 12-45).

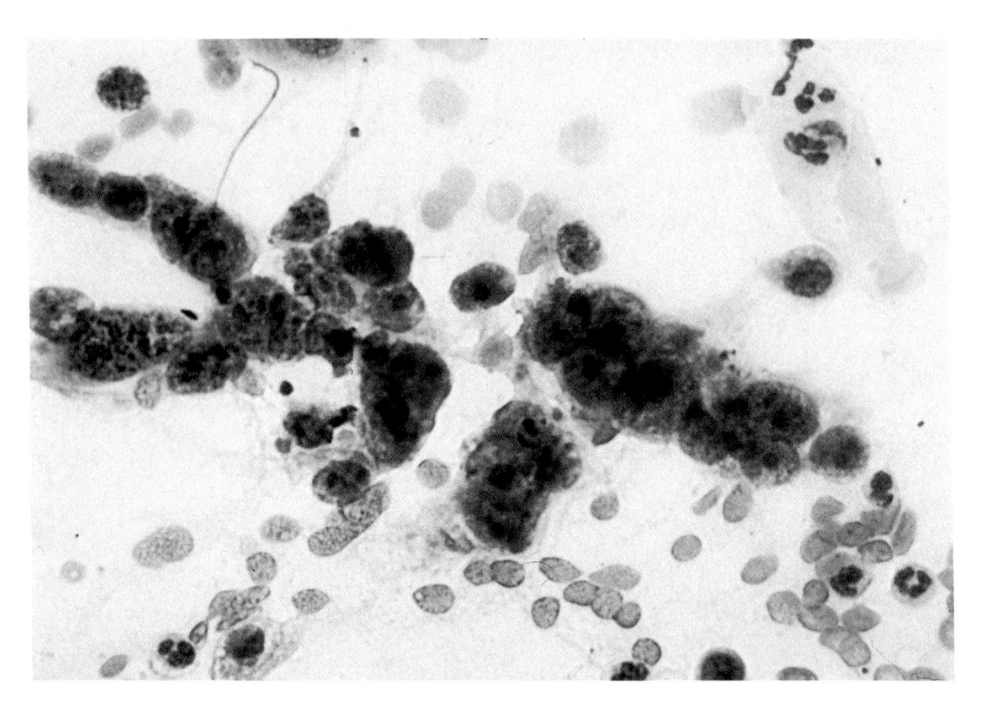

Figure 12-42. Malignant mixed Müllerian tumor. Malignant glandular component is seen here. Features of endometrial adenocarcinoma previously described can be recognized. (40×).

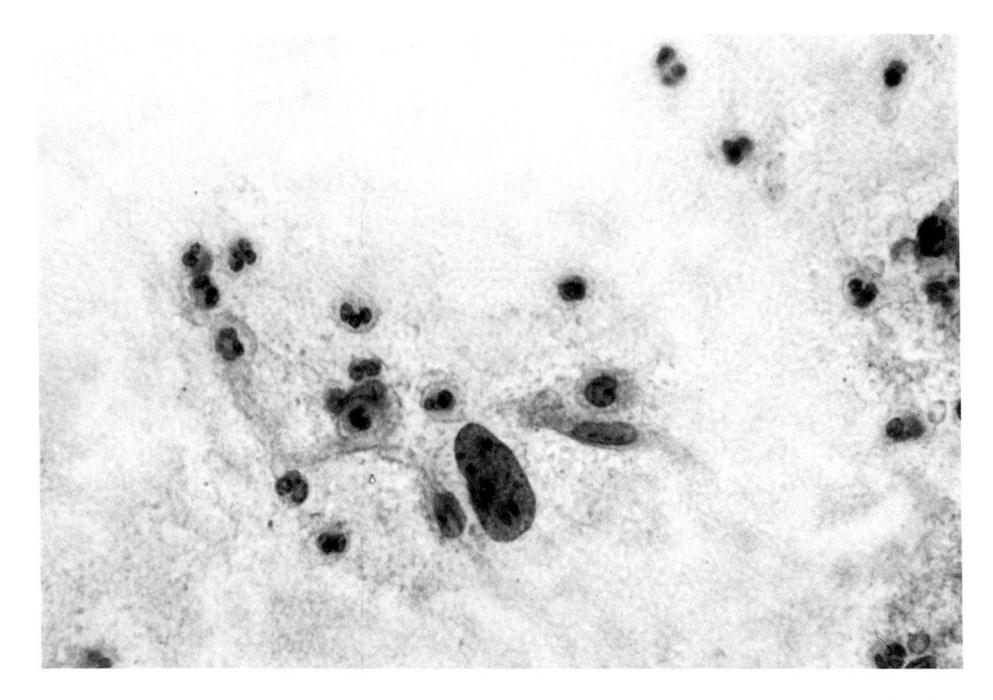

Figure 12-43. Malignant mixed Müllerian tumor (same patient as in Fig. 12-42). Here we see the malignant stromal component. Note the bizarre spindle cells; the large one is stripped of its cytoplasm. (40×).

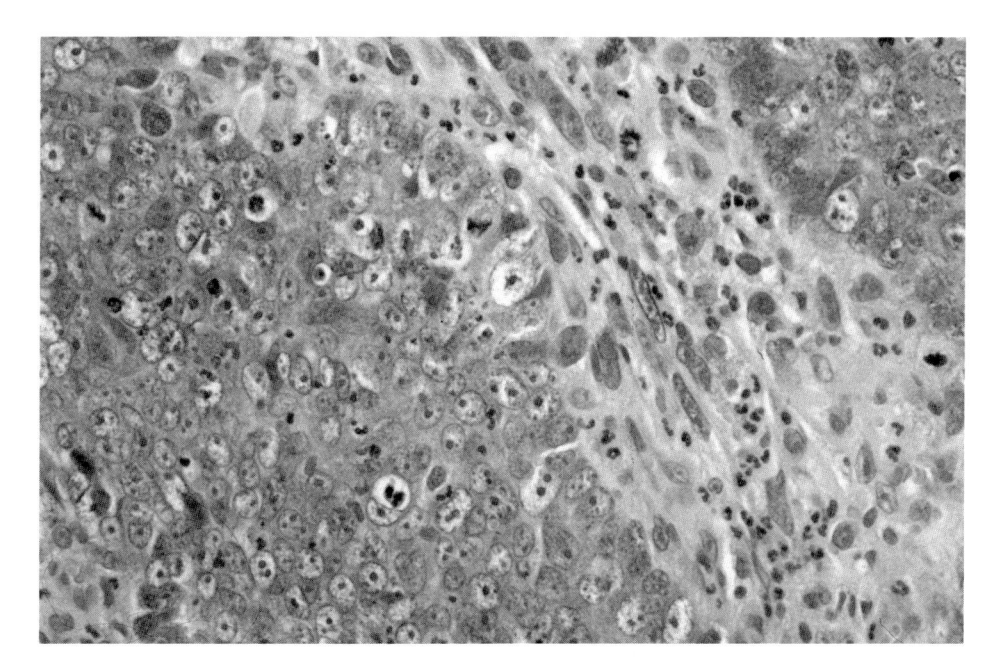

Figure 12-44. Malignant mixed Müllerian tumor (same patient as in Figs. 12-42 and 12-43). Endometrial biopsy shows the glandular epithelial elements on the left and far right. Note the open chromatin and prominent nucleoli. The malignant stromal (mesenchymal) elements are seen here in the center of the picture. The same nuclei as seen in Fig. 12-43 are in the stroma. (20×).

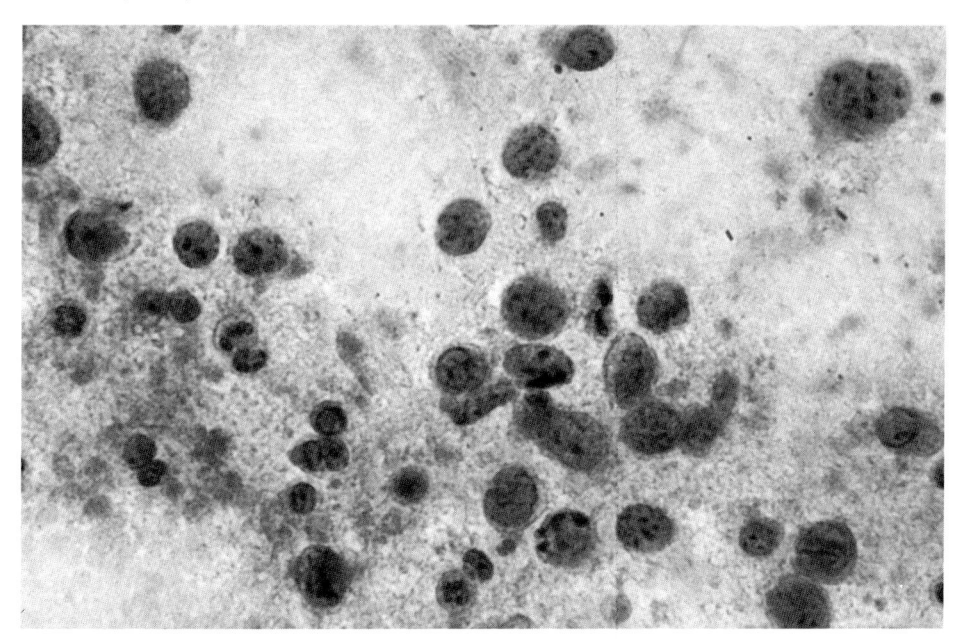

Figure 12-45. Highly atypical lymphoid cells seen on a Pap smear. Smear is suspicious for lymphoma. Note the chromocenters, nuclear indentations, and protrusions. Single cell distribution and karyorrhexis (nuclear fragmentation) are important features. Immunoperoxidase studies would be helpful in this case. (40×).

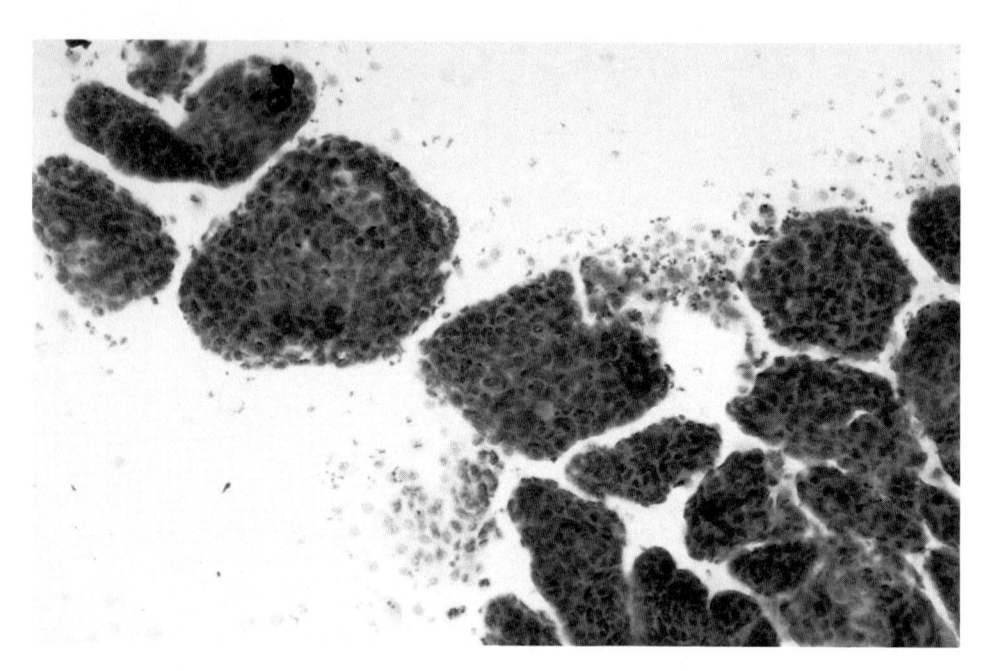

Figure 12-46. Metastatic papillary adenocarcinoma from ovary. Low-power view shows the distinctive papillary pattern in this case. Note the clean background, which often is the tipoff to the metastatic nature of the lesion. (10×).

METASTATIC TUMORS

Endometrial adenocarcinoma can usually be recognized by the characteristic small cell size. Metastatic disease may be considered when the cells are considerably larger, if the background is clean,[1,4,18] and if the patient is young. The most frequent sites of origin are ovary, GI tract, and breast.[1] Ovarian carcinoma should be considered when psammoma bodies and malignant papillary clusters are observed (Figs. 12-46, 12-47). If signet ring cells predominate, the GI tract or lobular carcinoma of the breast may be the primary site. An "Indian file" cell pattern may also be seen in the latter. A palisading arrangement of columnar cells and extracellular mucin deposits can be seen in colonic malignancies (Fig. 12-48).

Adenocarcinoma of the endocervix is usually more cellular than endometrial adenocarcinoma since the cells are more accessible to the cytobrush. Endocervical origin may also be suggested if the cells are more columnar in configuration and if a gradient of atypia is seen on the slide.

CONCLUSION

Although the cervical Pap smear has greatly contributed to the decline of cervical carcinoma, the same unfortunately cannot be said for endometrial

Conclusion

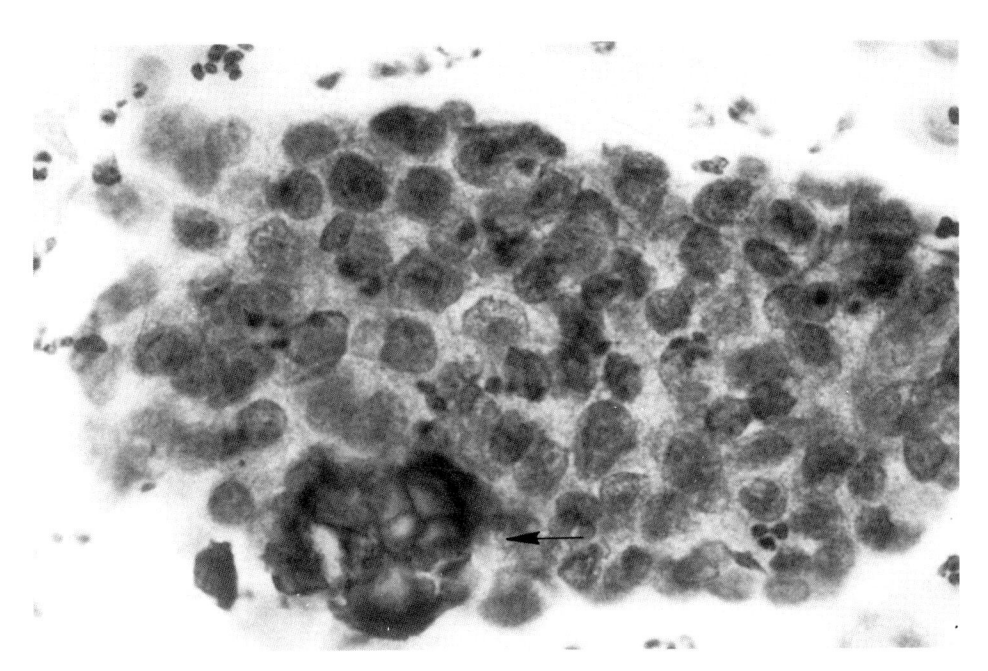

Figure 12-47. Metastatic papillary adenocarcinoma from ovary. Note the characteristic psammoma body (arrow), which is often seen in these ovarian lesions. (40×).

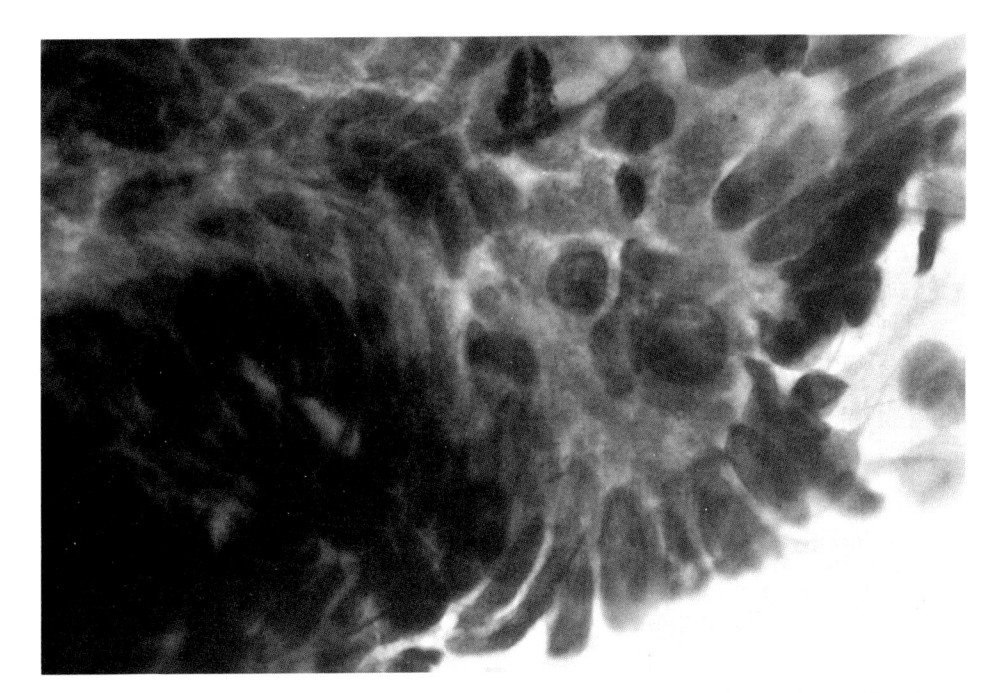

Figure 12-48. Metastatic adenocarcinoma from colon. Note the palisading or picket-fence arrangement of the tall columnar cells that are forming a gland.

carcinoma. The Pap smear has a limited role in detecting endometrial pathology. The following rules of thumb are used in regard to endometrial cells and the Pap smear:

A negative Pap smear in a symptomatic patient still requires further investigation. Benign endometrial cells found out of cycle still require an explanation (IUD, recent biopsy, etc.). Endometrial cells present in a smear from a postmenopausal patient regardless of whether they appear benign or atypical still necessitate further investigation until the underlying lesion is discovered.

REFERENCES

1. Nieberg RK: Cytology of the endometrium. In Astarita RW (ed): *Practical cytopathology.* Churchill Livingstone, New York, 1990.
2. Chambers, JT, Chambers SK: Endometrial sampling: When? Where? Why? With what? *Clin Obstet Gynecol* 35:28–39, 1992.
3. Zucker P, Kasdon EJ, Feldstein ML: The validity of Pap smear parameters as predictors of endometrial pathology in menopausal women. *Cancer* 56:2256–2263, 1985.
4. Shu Y, Ikle FA: *Cytopathology of the endometrium correlation with histopathology.* McGraw-Hill, New York, 1992.
5. Burk JR, Lehman HF, Wolf FS: Inadequacy of Papanicolaou smears in the detection of endometrial cancer. *NEJM* 291:191–192, 1974.
6. Koss LG, Schreiber K, Moussouris H, et al: Endometrial carcinoma and its precursors: detection and screening. *Clin Obstet Gynecol* 25:49–61, 1982.
7. Palermo VG: Interpretation of endometrium obtained by the EndoPap sample and a clinical study of its use. *Diagn Cytopathol* 1:5–12, 1985.
8. LaPolla JP, Nicosia S, McCurdy C, et al: Experience with the EndoPap device for the cytologic detection of uterine cancer and its precursors: a comparison of the EndoPap with fractional curettage or hysterectomy. *Am J Obstet Gynecol* 163:1055–1059, 1990.
9. Palermo VG, Blythe JG, Kaufman RH: Cytologic diagnosis of endometrial adenocarcinoma using the EndoPap sample. *Obstet Gynecol* 65:271–275, 1985.
10. Pritchard KI: Screening for endometrial cancer: is it effective? *Ann Intern Med* 110:177–179, 1989.
11. Meisels A, Jolicoeur C: Criteria for the cytologic assessment of hyperplasias in endometrial samples obtained by the EndoPap endometrial sampler. *Acta Cytol* 29:297–302, 1985.
12. Koss LG, Schreiber K, Oberlander SG, et al: Screening of asymptomatic women for endometrial cancer. *Obstet Gynecol* 57:681–690, 1981.
13. Koss LG: Diagnosis of early endometrial cancer and precancerous states. *Ann Clin Lab Sci.* 9:189–194, 1979.
14. Yancey M, Magelssen D, Demaurez A, et al: Classification of endometrial cells on cervical cytology. *Obstet Gynecol* 76:1000–1005, 1990.
15. Gondos B, King EB: Significance of endometrial cells in cervicovaginal smears. *Ann Clin Lab Sci* 7:486–490, 1977.
16. Ng ABP, Reagan J, Hawliczek S, et al: Significance of endometrial cells in the detection of endometrial carcinoma and the precursors. *Acta Cytol* 18:356–361, 1974.

17. Koss LG, Durfee GR: Cytologic diagnosis of endometrial carcinoma—result of ten years of experience. *Acta Cytol* 6:519–531, 1962.
18. Koss LG: *Diagnostic cytology and its histopathologic bases*, Vol. 1. Lippincott, Philadelphia, 1979.
19. Cherkis RC, Patten SF Jr, Dickinson JC, et al: Significance of atypical endometrial cells detected by cervical cytology. *Obstet Gynecol* 69:786–789, 1987.

Index

A
Actinomyces, 96–97
Acute endometritis, 92–93
Adenocarcinoma
 ciliated cell, 147
 clear cell, 148–152
 endocervical, endometrial adenocarcinoma, distinguishing, 154
 endometrial hyperplasia
  atypical, distinguished, criteria, 128–134
  distinguished, 114–136
   carcinoma in situ, 128
   clinical features, 115
   epidemiology, 115
   gross findings, 116
   microscopic findings, 116–126
    atypical hyperplasia, 124–126
    complex hyperplasia, 118–124
    simple hyperplasia, 116–121
   progression to endometrial carcinoma, risk of, 126–127
   therapy, 134–135
 mucinous, 148
Adenocarcinoma, with squamous differentiation, 209–210
Adenofibroma, and adenosarcoma, 160–162
Adenomatoid tumor, 101
Adenomyosis, 98
 endometrial carcinoma in, 154–155
Adenosarcoma, and adenofibroma, 160–162
Asherman's syndrome, 98
 hysteroscopy, 31, 36–37
 secretory phase of cycle, 31, 37
Atrophic endometrium, dysfunctional uterine bleeding, 78–79
Atypical hyperplasia, 124–126

B
Basalis, endometrial sampling, 47–48
Benign endometrial disorder, ultrasound, 15

Benign organic lesion, 91–102
 abnormal uterine bleeding, 91–92
 adenomatoid tumor, 101
 adenomyosis, 98
 Asherman's syndrome, 98
 endometriosis, 98
 endometritis, 91–96
  actinomyces, 96–97
  acute, 92–93
  chronic, 92–95
  granulomatous endometritis, 95
  tuberculous endometritis, 95–96
 leiomyomas, 96, 98
 polyp, endometrial, 98–101
  atypical polypoid adenomyoma, 98–101
  typical, 98–100
Biopsy
 Asherman's syndrome, secretory phase of cycle, 31, 37
 endometrial carcinoma and hyperplasia, 36
Bleeding, uterine
 abnormal, benign organic lesion, 91–92
 causes of, 3–4
 dysfunctional, 76–90
  atrophic endometrium, 78–79
  disordered proliferative endometrium, 78–79
  dyssynchronous secretory endometrium, 79–81
  endometrial patterns, 78
  hormone, effect of, 76–81
  irregular ripening, 79–81
  irregular shedding, 79–81
  nonsecretory patterns, 78–79
  out-of-phase secretory endometrium, 79–81
  progestational therapy, 82–85
  proliferative endometrium, 78–79
  secretory patterns, 79–81
  weakly proliferative endometrium, 78–79
  weakly secretory endometrium, 79–81
 polyp, hysteroscopy, 31
 second-trimester, 173
 third-trimester, 173
Bone fragments, fetal, hysteroscopy, 31, 33

C

Carbon dioxide insufflator, hysteroscopy, 28
Carcinoma
  in adenomyosis, 154–155
  association, 112
  classification, 139
  clear cell, 209
  diagnosis, 138–141
  endometrial, 137–141
  grading, 140
  hyperplasia, atypical, distinguished from, 137–138
  histological types, 141–154
    carcinoma metastatic to endometrium, 153–154
    ciliated cell adenocarcinoma, 147
    clear cell adenocarcinoma, 148–152
    endometrial adenocarcinoma, with squamous differentiation, 144, 146
    endometrioid adenocarcinoma, 141–144
    mixed-cell-type carcinoma, 153
    mucinous adenocarcinoma, 148
    secretory carcinoma, 146–147
    squamous cell carcinoma, 152
    undifferentiated carcinoma, 151–152
    uterine papillary serous carcinoma, 149, 151
  in situ, 128
  metastatic to endometrium, 153–154
  mixed-cell-type, 153
  mucinous, 209
  progression of endometrial hyperplasia to, risk, 126–127
  radiation effect on, 155–156
  papillary serous, on smear, 209
  squamous cell, 152
  staging, 140–141
  undifferentiated, 151–152
  uterine papillary serous, 149, 151
Cervical tissue, endometrial sampling, 48
Choriocarcinoma, 211
Chorionic gonadotropin, human, 166
Chronic endometritis, 92–95
Ciliated cell adenocarcinoma, 147
Ciliated cell metaplasia, 106
Clear cell adenocarcinoma, 148–152, 209
Clear cell metaplasia, 109
Complex hyperplasia, endometrium, 118–124
Conception, retained products of, ultrasound, 10–14
Cytology on cervicovaginal smear, 185–217
  adenosquamous carcinoma, 209–210
  atypical endometrial cells on Pap smear, 193–198
  benign endometrial cell on Pap smear, 186–193
  choriocarcinoma, 211
  clear cell carcinoma, 209
  endometrial hyperplasia, 197–198
  endometrial polyp, 195
  inflammation-related conditions, 191–195
  IUD, 195, 197
  lymphoproliferative disorder, 211, 213
  malignant criteria on, 198–209
  metastatic tumor, 214–215
  mixed Müllerian tumor, 211–213
  mucinous carcinoma, 209
  papillary serous carcinoma, 209
  regenerative endometrium, 197
  sarcoma, 211

D

Dalkon shield, fractured, 31, 34
Dating, of endometrium, 57, 71–72
Decidual changes, ultrasound, 10–14
Diethylstilbestrol (DES) exposure, 149
Disordered proliferative endometrium, dysfunctional uterine bleeding, 78–79
Dysfunctional uterine bleeding, see Bleeding, uterine, dysfunctional
Dyssynchronous secretory endometrium, 79–81

E

Ectopic pregnancy, 173, 175
Endocervical adenocarcinoma, endometrial adenocarcinoma, distinguishing, 154
Endocrine causes of uterine bleeding, 4
Endogenous hormonal therapy, effects of, 81–88
  endometriosis, 83, 85
  hormonal replacement therapy, 81–83
  oral contraceptive therapy, 81–82
  ovulation induction therapy, 86–88
  progestational therapy in dysfunctional uterine bleeding, 82–85
  tamoxifen therapy, 86, 88
Endometrial adenocarcinoma
  endocervical adenocarcinoma, distinguishing, 154
  with squamous differentiation, 144, 146
Endometrial artifacts, endometrial sampling, 53–54
Endometrial carcinoma, 137–141
  in adenomyosis, 154–155
  classification, 139
  diagnosis, 138–141
  grading, 140
  histological types, 141–154
    carcinoma metastatic to endometrium, 153–154
    ciliated cell adenocarcinoma, 147
    clear cell adenocarcinoma, 148–152
    endometrial adenocarcinoma, with squamous differentiation, 144, 146
    endometrioid adenocarcinoma, 141–144
    mixed-cell-type carcinoma, 153
    mucinous adenocarcinoma, 148
    secretory carcinoma, 146–147
    squamous cell carcinoma, 152
    undifferentiated carcinoma, 151–152
    uterine papillary serous carcinoma, 149, 151
  and hyperplasia, 36

Index

hyperplasia, atypical, distinguished from, 137–138
radiation effect on, 155–156
staging, 140–141
Endometrial hyperplasia
  adenocarcinoma, distinguishing, 114–136
    carcinoma *in situ,* 128
    clinical features, 115
    epidemiology, 115
    gross findings, 116
    microscopic findings, 116–126
      atypical hyperplasia, 124–126
      complex hyperplasia, 118–124
      simple hyperplasia, 116–121
    progression to endometrial carcinoma, risk of, 126–127
    therapy, 134–135
  atypical, distinguished from adenocarcinoma, 128–134
  cytology on smear, 197–198
  natural history of, 127
Endometrial malignancy, *see* Malignancy, endometrial
Endometrial metaplasia, 103–113
  carcinoma, association, 112
  epithelial, 103–109
    ciliated cell metaplasia, 106
    clear cell metaplasia, 109
    eosinophilic metaplasia, 106
    hobnail metaplasia, 109
    mucinous metaplasia, 109–110
    papillary syncytial metaplasia, 106
    squamous metaplasia, 103–105
    tubal metaplasia, 106
  stromal, 109–112
    malignant mixed mesodermal tumor, distinguishing, 109
    stromal foam cell, 111–112
Endometrial polyp, cytology on smear, 195
Endometrial sampling, 3–8, 43–44
  diagnostic pitfalls, 47–55
    basalis, 47–48
    cervical tissue, 48
    endometrial artifacts, 53–54
    foreign elements, 51, 53
    lower uterine segment, 47
    smooth muscle, 48, 51
  gynecologist, role of, 46
  limitations of, 44–47
  pathologist, role of, 47
  tissue limitations, 44–46
Endometrial stromal sarcoma, 157–160
Endometrioid adenocarcinoma, 141–144
Endometriosis, 98
  hormonal therapy, effect of, 8, 83
Endometritis, 91–96
  acute, 92–93
  chronic, 92–95
  granulomatous, 95
  tuberculous, 95–96
Endometrium, normal, *see* Normal endometrium
Eosinophilic metaplasia, 106–108

Epithelial metaplasia, endometrium
  ciliated cell metaplasia, 106
  clear cell metaplasia, 109
  eosinophilic metaplasia, 106–108
  hobnail metaplasia, 109
  mucinous metaplasia, 109–110
  papillary syncytial metaplasia, 106–108
  squamous metaplasia, 103–105
  tubal metaplasia, 106
Equipment, hysteroscopy, 28–29
Exaggerated implantation site, pregnancy, 172

F
FIGO (International Federation of Gynecologists and Obstetricians, staging of endometrial carcinoma, 140–141
Fetal bone fragments, hysteroscopy, 31, 33
First-trimester-pregnancy loss, 170–172
Flexible hysteroscope, 26–27
Foreign elements, endometrial sampling, 51, 53
Fractured Dalkon shield, 31, 34

G
Gestation, early, ultrasound, 10–14
Gestational trophoblastic disease, 178–184
  choriocarcinoma, 180, 182
  hydatidiform mole, 178–180
  invasive mole, 180
  placental site trophoblastic tumor, 182–184
Gonadotropin, chorionic, human, 166
Granulomatous endometritis, 95
Gynecologist, endometrial sampling, role of, 46

H
Hemorrhage, postpartum, 173–178
  placenta accreta, 176–177
  retained placenta, 176–177
  subinvolution of uterus, 176
Hobnail metaplasia, 109
Hormonal effect
  bleeding, uterine, dysfunctional, 76–81
  on endometrium, 76–90
Hormonal replacement therapy, effect of, 19–21, 81–83
Hormonal therapy, endogenous, effects of, 81–88
  endometriosis, 83, 85
  hormonal replacement therapy, 81–83
  oral contraceptive therapy, 81–82
  ovulation induction therapy, 86–88
  progestational therapy in dysfunctional uterine bleeding, 82–85
  tamoxifen therapy, 86, 88
Human chorionic gonadotropin, 166
Hydatidiform mole, 178–180
  pregnancy, 178–180

Hyperplasia, endometrial, see Endometrial hyperplasia
Hysteroscope, 27–29
Hysteroscopy
  Asherman's syndrome, 31, 36–37
  biopsy forceps, 26–27
  bleeding endometrial polyp, 31
  cancer
    with submucosal extension to endocervix, 31, 35–36
    with uterine isthmus involvement, 31, 35
  carbon dioxide insufflator, 28
  Dalkon shield, fractured, 31, 34
  endometrium evaluation, 26–40
  equipment used, 28–29
  fetal bone fragments, 31, 33
  hysteroscope, 27–29
  Lippes loop, 31, 34
  menorrhagia, 31–32
  menstrual endometrium, 40
  myoma
    pedunculated, 31–32
    submucous, 31–33
  normal cavity view, 30
  in office, 28, 30
  premenstrual endometrium, 40
  proliferative phase, early, 38
  resectoscopic morcellation, of myoma, 31, 33
  secretory phase
    early, 38–39
    late, 38–39
  technique, 26, 28

I
Immunohistochemistry, role of, in gestational trophoblastic disease, 184
Implantation site, exaggerated, pregnancy, 172
Induction, of ovulation, ultrasound, 21–22
Infertility, luteal phase defect, 89
Inflammation-related conditions, cervicovaginal smear, 191–195
Invasive mole, pregnancy, 180
Irregular ripening, dysfunctional uterine bleeding, 79–81
Irregular shedding, dysfunctional uterine bleeding, 79–81
IUD, cytology on smear, 195, 197
In-vitro fertilization, ultrasound, 21–22

L
Lactogen, placental, human, 166
Leiomyomas, 96, 98
Lippes loop, hysteroscopy, 31, 34
Loss of pregnancy, first-trimester, 170–172
Lower uterine segment, endometrial sampling, 47
Luteal phase defect, infertility, 89
Lymphoproliferative disorder, 211, 213

M
Malignancy, endometrial, 137–165
  endometrial adenocarcinoma, endocervical adenocarcinoma, distinguishing, 154
  endometrial carcinoma
    in adenomyosis, 154–155
    classification, 139
    diagnosis, 138–141
    grading, 140
    histological types, 141–154
      carcinoma metastatic to endometrium, 153–154
      ciliated cell adenocarcinoma, 147
      clear cell adenocarcinoma, 148–152
      endometrial adenocarcinoma, with squamous differentiation, 144, 146
      endometrioid adenocarcinoma, 141–144
      mixed-cell-type carcinoma, 153
      mucinous adenocarcinoma, 148
      secretory carcinoma, 146–147
      squamous cell carcinoma, 152
      undifferentiated carcinoma, 151–152
      uterine papillary serous carcinoma, 149, 151
    hyperplasia, atypical, distinguished from, 137–138
    radiation effect on, 155–156
    staging, 140–141
  mesenchymal neoplasm
    involving endometrium, 157
    pure
      heterologous, 158, 160
      homologous, 157–160
        endometrial stromal lesions, 157–160
        smooth muscle neoplasm involving endometrium, 158
  mixed epithelial-mesenchymal tumor, 160–163
    adenofibroma, and adenosarcoma, 160–162
    mixed Müllerian tumor, 162–163
  mixed Müllerian tumor, stromal metaplasia, distinguishing, 109
  pyometra, 155
  ultrasound, 15–19
Menarche
  during, normal endometrium, 72–73
  prior to, normal endometrium, 72
Menopause, normal endometrium, 73–75
Menorrhagia, hysteroscopy, 31–32
Menstrual cycle, normal endometrium, 59–72
Mesenchymal neoplasm
  involving endometrium, 157
  pure
    heterologous, 158, 160
    homologous, 157–160
      endometrial stromal lesions, 157–160
      smooth muscle neoplasm involving endometrium, 158
Metaplasia, endometrial, see Endometrial metaplasia

Metastatic tumor, 214–215
Mixed-cell-type carcinoma, 153
Mixed epithelial-mesenchymal tumor, 160–163
  adenofibroma, and adenosarcoma, 160–162
Mole
  hydatidiform, 178–180
  invasive, 180
Morcellation, resectoscopic, of myoma, 31, 33
Mucinous adenocarcinoma, 148, 209
Mucinous metaplasia, 109–110
Müllerian tumor, malignant mixed, 162–163, 211–213
Müllerian tumor, malignant mixed, stromal metaplasia, distinguished, 109
Myoma
  pedunculated, 31–32
  resectoscopic morcellation, 31, 33
  submucous, 31–33

N

Natural history of endometrial hyperplasia, 127
Neoplastic causes of uterine bleeding, 4
Nodule, placental site, pregnancy, 173–174
Nonsecretory patterns, dysfunctional uterine bleeding, 78–79
Normal endometrium, 56–75
  components of, 56–59
  dating of, 57, 71–72
  menarche
    during, 72–73
    prior to, 72
  menopause, 73–75
  menstrual cycle, 59–72
  proliferative, 60–63
  secretory, 61, 63–69

O

Oral contraceptive therapy, hormonal effect, 81–82
Out-of-phase secretory endometrium, 79–81
Ovulation induction
  therapy, hormonal effect, 86–88
  ultrasound, 21–22

P

Pap smear
  atypical endometrial cells on, 193–198
  benign endometrial cell on, 186–193
  malignant criteria on, 198–209
Papillary serous carcinoma, manico-vaginal smear, 209
Papillary syncytial metaplasia, 106–108
Pathologist, endometrial sampling, role of, 47
Patterns, dysfunctional uterine bleeding, 78
Perimenopausal uterine bleeding, causes of, 4
Placenta, retained, 176–177

Placenta accreta, 176–177
Placental lactogen, human, 166
Placental site plaque, 173–174
Placental site nodule, 173–174
Placental site trophoblastic tumor, 182–184
  pregnancy, 172
Plaque, placental site, 173–174
Polyp
  bleeding, hysteroscopy, 31
  endometrial, 98–101
    atypical polypoid adenomyoma, 98–101
    typical, 98–100
Postmenopausal endometrium
  hormone replacement, 19–21
  ultrasound, 19–21
Postmenopausal uterine bleeding, causes of, 4
Postpartum hemorrhage, 173–178
  placenta accreta, 176–177
  retained placenta, 176–177
  subinvolution of uterus, 176
Pregnancy, 166–184
  ectopic, 173, 175
  exaggerated implantation site, 172
  first-trimester-pregnancy loss, 170–172
  gestational trophoblastic disease, 178–184
    choriocarcinoma, 180, 182
    hydatidiform mole, 178–180
    invasive mole, 180
    placental site trophoblastic tumor, 182–184
  human chorionic gonadotropin, 166
  human placental lactogen, 166
  immunohistochemistry, role of, 184
  nodule, placental site, 173–174
  normal intrauterine, 166–169
  placental site trophoblastic tumor, 172
  plaque, placental site, 173–174
  postpartum hemorrhage, 173–178
    placenta accreta, 176–177
    retained placenta, 176–177
    subinvolution of uterus, 176
  second-trimester bleeding, 173
  third-trimester bleeding, 173
  ultrasound, 10–14
  uterine bleeding, causes of, 4
Premalignant endometrial disorder, ultrasound, 15–19
Premenopausal uterine bleeding, causes of, 4
Premenstrual endometrium, hysteroscopy, 40
Progestational therapy in dysfunctional uterine bleeding, hormonal effect, 82–85
Proliferative endometrium, 60–63
  dysfunctional uterine bleeding, 78–79
Proliferative phase, early, hysteroscopy, 38
Puberty, uterine bleeding, causes of, 4
Pyometra, 155

R

Radiation effect, on endometrial carcinoma, 155–156

Regenerative endometrium, cytology on smear, 197
Resectoscopic morcellation, of myoma, 31, 33
Retained placenta, 176–177
Retained products of conception, ultrasound, 10–14

S
Sampling, of endometrium, uterine bleeding workup, 5
Sarcoma, 211
Scarring, endometrial, Asherman's syndrome, 31, 36–37
Second-trimester bleeding, 173
Secretory carcinoma, 146–147
Secretory endometrium, 61, 63–69
Secretory patterns, dysfunctional uterine bleeding, 79–81
Secretory phase
  early, hysteroscopy, 38–39
  late, hysteroscopy, 38–39
Papillary serous carcinoma, on cervicovaginal smear, 209
Shield, Dalkon, fractured, 31, 34
Simple hyperplasia, endometrium, 116–121
Smear, cervicovaginal, 185–217
  adenosquamous carcinoma, 209–210
  atypical endometrial cells on Pap smear, 193–198
  benign endometrial cell on Pap smear, 186–193
  choriocarcinoma, 211
  clear cell carcinoma, 209
  endometrial hyperplasia, 197–198
  endometrial polyp, 195
  inflammation-related conditions, 191–195
  IUD, 195, 197
  lymphoproliferative disorder, 211, 213
  malignant criteria on, 198–209
  metastatic tumor, 214–215
  mixed Müllerian tumor, 211–213
  mucinous carcinoma, 209
  papillary serous carcinoma, 209
  regenerative endometrium, 197
  sarcoma, 211
Smooth muscle
  endometrial sampling, 48, 51
  neoplasm, involving endometrium, 158
Squamous cell carcinoma, 152
Squamous metaplasia, 103–105
Stromal foam cells, 111–112
Stromal lesion, endometrial, 157–160
Stromal metaplasia, 109–112
  malignant mixed Müllerian tumor, distinguished, 109
  stromal foam cell, 111–112
Subinvolution of uterus, 176

T
Tamoxifen therapy, hormonal effect, 86, 88
Third-trimester bleeding, 173
Tissue limitations, endometrial sampling, 44–46
Trophoblastic disease, gestational, 178–184
  choriocarcinoma, 180, 182
  hydatidiform mole, 178–180
  invasive mole, 180
  placental site trophoblastic tumor, 182–184
Trophoblastic tumor, placental site, 172
Tubal metaplasia, 106
Tuberculous endometritis, 95–96

U
Ultrasound, 9–25
  benign endometrial disorder, 15
  decidual changes, 10–14
  Doppler effect, 22–23
  gestation, early, 10–14
  In-vitro fertilization, 21–22
  malignant endometrial disorder, 15–19
  menstrual cycle changes, endometrium, 9–10
  normal endometrium, menstrual cycle changes, 9–10
  ovulation induction, 21–22
  postmenopausal endometrium, 19–21
  pregnancy evaluation, 10–14
  premalignant endometrial disorder, 15–19
  retained products of conception, 10–14
  technique, 9–10
Undifferentiated carcinoma, 151–152
Uterine bleeding
  causes of, 3–4
  endometrial sampling, 5
Uterine isthmus, cancer, 31, 35
Uterine papillary serous carcinoma (UPSC), 149, 151
Uterine pregnancy, normal, 166–169
Uterus, subinvolution, 176

W
Weakly proliferative endometrium, dysfunctional uterine bleeding, 78–79
Weakly secretory endometrium, dysfunctional uterine bleeding, 79–81